WOMEN AND
MENTAL HEALTH
POLICY

Volume 9
Sage Yearbooks in WOMEN'S POLICY STUDIES

WOMEN AND MENTAL HEALTH POLICY

Edited by

LENORE E. WALKER

WITHDRAWN

 SAGE PUBLICATIONS Beverly Hills London New Delhi

For information address:

SAGE Publications, Inc.
275 South Beverly Drive
Beverly Hills, California 90212

SAGE Publications India Pvt. Ltd.
C-236 Defence Colony
New Delhi 110 024, India

SAGE Publications Ltd
28 Banner Street
London EC1Y 8QE, England

Printed in the United States of America

Library of Congress Cataloging in Publication Data

Main entry under title:
Women and mental health policy.

(Sage yearbooks in women's policy studies ; v. 9)
Bibliography: p.
1. Women—Mental health. 2. Women—Mental health services—United States. 3. Mental health policy—United States. I. Walker, Lenore E. II. Series.
RC451.4.W6W646 1984   362.2'088042   84-9899
ISBN 0-8039-2257-4
ISBN 0-8039-2258-2 (pbk.)

FIRST PRINTING

CONTENTS

INTRODUCTION

Lenore E. Walker

Interest in women's mental health has existed for as long as we have records. References to women's emotional state exist in written mythology as well as oral tales passed down through the ages. Those behaving in deviant ways were labeled, ostracized, killed, or warehoused in jails or early versions of mental institutions. Mental health policy, if it existed at all, was formulated by male leaders, usually to force women to conform by punishing those who did not. Janet, Charcot, and other early pioneers in humanizing the mental institutions rarely commented on the societal implications of the disproportionate numbers of women who were in these mental institutions. Nor did Freud or any of the other nineteenth- or twentieth-century leaders in the mental health movement attempt to link women's high use of the mental health system to the negative effects of sexism until Phyllis Chesler's exposé, *Women and Madness*, published in the early 1970s. This volume reviews the major issues for women in mental health and links them to policy decisions in our country. In some areas such policy implications leap out at us, while in others a more careful weighing of the pros and cons seems more judicious. Many of these can be changes incrementally implemented if a long-term policy is adopted.

HISTORICAL OVERVIEW

The United States of America has one of the most extensive mental health system in the world. Not only do we have hospitals and institutions for our most seriously disturbed people, we also have a system of out-patient mental health services that ostensibly can be utilized by anyone, regardless of their personal financial condition. Government-supported mental health centers, school counselors, religious advisers, prepaid health maintenance organizations, employee assistance plans and benefits through medical insurance, and independent practitioners are among the cadres of mental health professionals trained to assist people whose mental health is in question. The economics of the health service industry indicates that it is big business. Despite the gathering of utilization statistics, analysis of patterns of use of this system by women is inadequate. (Russo & Sobel, 1981).

The mental health component of U.S. policy had its first growth spurt during World War II when the need arose for trained specialists to treat soldiers experiencing what was then defined as "combat shock" and today classified as "post traumatic stress disorder." Government funding poured into the universities, and numerous clinical psychology graduate departments sprang up to train doctoral-level psychologists. Many of these psychologists were better able to treat the soldiers than were the medically trained pyschiatrists who had most of their previous experience in hospitals with the more chronically mentally ill. It was less expensive and took less time to train a psychologist who could diagnose and treat emotionally disturbed people on outpatient basis. And so, in the late 1940s and early 1950s with government support, outpatient facilities began to appear, often utilizing the services of those trained during the war effort. This time, however, men were not the primary patients; rather, women and children sought services.

Another important development in the 1950s was the discovery and increased use of major tranquilizers, allowing for shorter hospitalization periods for the mentally ill. Outpatient clinics could dispense the medication and provide brief psychotherapy in a more cost-efficient manner. Women were given pills and counseled to adjust to what we now know were intolerable situations. Interdisciplinary teams, with representatives from psychiatry, psychology, social work, and psychiatric nursing, were thought to provide the best services. Mental health treatment moved away from the original goal of restoring a person's ability to function in society and instead began to focus first on adjustment, and then on personal growth. The goals changed as did the popularity of treatment philosophies.

In the early nineteenth century, the goal of humanizing the asylums was started by defining absence of mental health as another kind of illness. Once people's abberant behavior was understood as a medical illness, the fear of witchcraft or possession by the devil was reduced and the stigma of difference less powerfully called for isolation. Freud and his early colleagues' ability to treat patients without removing them from the community paved the way for the least-restrictive treatment mandate in place today. Lost in the usual historical analysis of the mental health movement is the differential impact on women and men.

Some researchers believe that Freud was given leeway by the medical community in Vienna because the development of psychoanalysis paralleled the rise of the women's movement. His theories demanded that women go back to their kitchens and children rather than continue joining in that first wave of feminist ideology. In the late 1800s, many women were involved in demanding the vote in this country and other reforms toward equality in Europe. That many of Freud's early female patients participated in such efforts has been forgotten or played down by the male-dominated psychoanalytic profession. It took another fifty or so years for women to get their right to vote in America, and almost one hundred years later, women still do not have their rights protected by the Constitution. The ERA might well be the most important preventive mental health strategy for women available. Its passage would give women's value legitimacy by recognizing our equality through the law—one of the most powerful ways of institutionalizing societal values.

Until the recent controversy over Freud's letters raised by Jeffery Masson (1984), a former projects director of the Sigmund Freud Archives, the exact impact of collegial pressure on Freud's thinking was not known. Masson presents compelling evidence that Freud's original theory that all neurosis comes from adult male's forceful sexual seduction of young female children was changed because he could not bear the pressure of ostracism by his colleagues and their invalidation of this theory by pretending they did not hear what he said. For example, his speech on "The Aetiology of Hysteria" in 1896 to the Society for Psychiatry and Neurology in Vienna appeared in the weekly medical journal without the customary summary or discussion of what was said. Masson reveals edited portions of previously published letters that were purposely removed so as not to confuse psychoanalysts with the earlier seduction theory; they instead focus on the unconscious wish fullfillment of what was later labeled children's sexual fantasies. He suggests Freud changed his theory, in part, to protect his friend Fliess—a good example of protecting collegial maleness at the expense of women. Today, of course, we are reevaluating Freud's original seduction theory as more accurate than the substituted fantasy theory in light of the large numbers of women still seeking therapy for the same kind of damages that occurred a century earlier when society would not tolerate acknowledgment of them. It remains to be seen whether or not present-day society will revise its policy to deal with such injustices done to women by more powerful men.

OVERVIEW OF THE BOOK

Many of the chapters in this book deal directly with these issues. The topics are not always popular with the larger male-dominated social structure or its mental health subsystem. The difficulty in getting research funded, not to mention disseminated, when it is not in keeping with the status quo is addressed by all of the authors, most of whom are women. Some of the contributors, such as Jessie Bernard, Del Martin and Phyllis Lyon, and Carol Nadelson and Malkah Notman, have been involved in this debate for several decades. Others such as Deborah Belle, Laura Brown, Maureen Hendricks, Sandy Kaplan and Janet Surrey, are researchers, academicians, and clinicians who chronicle the past with an eye to a new vision of the future. Those in policymaking positions, like Nancy Russo, Jacqueline Bouhoutsos, Nick Cummings, and Donna Stringer and Nancy Welton, share a hope for a more sex-fair future. Lorna Cammaert, Lynne Rosewater, and I attempt to apply these new ideas to the practice of psychology. Each chapter provides the data necessary to support the relevant policy changes recommended. If the issues were popular or the policy changes in the country's leaders' best interests, these data would be sufficient to get the process moving. But that has not happened. We must examine the issues carefully, within the economic and political structures of our country, to learn why day-care centers are not funded, reproductive freedom is not granted to individuals in what purports to be an individualistic society, and myths about women's high rate of depression when children leave home flourish despite evidence to the contrary.

The threat of women's sexuality is one of the book's major themes. Martin and Lyon discuss the role homophobia — the fear of loving same-sex persons — plays in policy legislation. They see current policy, which forces many to keep such relationships a secret, as detrimental to the mental health of at least ten percent of the population, and they are critical of the mental health profession for its role in maintaining the status quo. Secrets about sexual behavior between male professionals and female clients are also detrimental, as discussed in Bouhoutsos's chapter on sexual exploitation of psychotherapy clients. She speculates that the attitudes that deny that such behavior is harmful are learned in graduate schools where most universities have refused to interfere in professors' (usually male) sexual behaviors with students (usually females); these attitudes are then reinforced by a society that does not punish offenders (usually male) for their physical, sexual, and psychological violence against women (as is examined in my chapter).

Attitudes toward women's sexuality have traditionally been defined by men and when dysfunctional, treated by men. Cammaert's chapter on new sex therapies for women documents how women have made an impact and perhaps turned that process around. Education, she feels, will help women get the treatment they need while also redefining sexual pleasure for women as broader than genital intercourse, an understanding that may obviate many dysfunctions in the future. Such policies will have an impact on the medical profession as they devise new ways to protect women's mental health while treating serious illnesses in the reproductive system. Psychiatrists Nadelson and Notman acknowledge the dangers of male gynecologists creating policy decisions for women patients suffering from what used to be secretly whispered about as "women's troubles." The average person believed that any reproductive function disorders would have a negative impact on women's moods and, thus, enforced the conspiracy of silence. Even normal women were said to be victims of their raging hormones at least once a month as the age old taboo about menstruating women was perpetuated. The recent controversy over the impact of premenstrual syndrome (PMS) on women's mental health continues this debate. Some feminists decry PMS as the same old argument to keep women out of the executive boardrooms while others suggest that noxious environmental chemicals and food allergies do cause biochemical reactions that affect the hypothalamus, where the reproductive center regulating hormones is located. Such biochemical sensitivity can cause the behavior reactions associated with PMS. Some victims' symptoms disappear with progesterone treatment — a compelling argument to use it cautiously, despite its political implications.

In political and economic societies where labor has been divided between men and women into sex-assigned jobs, regulation of women's sexuality and reproductive functions becomes the interest of a broad group of policymakers. In agrarian societies, where labor is divided by sending both men and women into the fields, and assigning home chores like cooking and child care to women and care of the livestock to men, there are fewer reports of mental health problems other than the occasional deviate who could not or would not do his or her share. Such a community usually cared for its own mentally ill without assistance from the larger society. Jessie Bernard traces the sociological development of how such divided roles produces differences in the expectations of men and women regarding marriage and family roles.

Any discussion of women's mental health must include the critical impact of children. Although Russo documents the weakening of the "motherhood mandate," most women were socialized to believe their sense of self develops from how well they raise their children. Guilt is induced by not wanting children, not being able to bear children, or voluntarily electing abortion and use of contraceptives to prevent bearing children. Yet, Russo, Sales and Frieze, Belle, and Bernard, all provide data indicating the profound negative impact child bearing and childraising have on women's mental health. Walker reports that violence in families is commonly experienced by women and children. Only Kaplan and Surrey suggest children have any positive influence on the development of women's relational self.

If our society puts a high premium on families, why are these data ignored by policymakers? Perhaps it is due to the economic interests, which use women's inability to control their reproductive functions to justify keeping them in lower status jobs. They are not impressed with the cost this policy has on the very fabric of family life they wish to preserve. The image of the male executive going out to work while his wife works at taking care of his children and home so that he is unburdened by the daily details of organizing these other parts of his life is still attractive to many men and some women. The articles in this book cannot be interpreted in any other way but to demonstrate exactly how detrimental that role is for women. Men may be incapable of designing new women-oriented policies, as it eliminates a model that they see as good for them. This point is elaborated in Stringer and Welton's chapter. They suggest that male policymakers rarely can understand a woman's experience, no matter how sensitive they may be, and therefore are usually incapable of designing policies that genuinely address women's needs. Further, some men are not interested in policies that address women while others are openly hostile to such policies. Stringer and Welton believe it is critical for women to become policymakers. The recommendations of the President's Commission on Mental Health's Subpanel on Women that discuss ways to design and implement new policies and procedures to reverse such patterns are discussed by Russo.

In labor-intensive societies, such as modern-day China, past discrimination of women has been addressed by the communist government by deemphasizing male and female differences and encouraging unisex standards in dress, jobs, and educational opportunity. While such denial of any gender differences by policy has had a major effect on reversing sex discrimination, there is no indication that it has had a concommitant effect on women's (or men's) mental health. In fact, mental illness was also ruled to be anti-country, and the mental health profession was dismantled during the Cultural Revolution. Education toward the correct way was deemed more appropriate by communist cadre leaders. Recent trips to China by myself as well as other psychologists indicate that the reeducation approach to mental health is only partially successful. The Chinese government is eager to learn modern American psychology techniques so as to motivate and treat the growing numbers of emotionally disturbed people. Women's groups have expressed concern over the social policy of allowing only one child per family, and persistent reports about amniocentisis to discover the sex of the fetus and subsequent abortion should the fetus be female continue to surface despite official denials by the People's Republic of China's government.

Many attribute the same concerns for women's mental health in our own capitalistic and democratic society. In our economic structure, women are at the lower end of the job hierarchy, still earning about 59¢ to every dollar earned by a man, even though large numbers have reached middle management levels in the past decade. Childraising decisions figure prominently into women's career motivation as do the other mental health issues described by Sales and Frieze. Yet, unless the male economic power structure is ready to allow women and men equal access to all levels in the job market, women are going to be stopped from fair competition in any way available to policymakers. It is no accident that corporate America with its vested interest in retaining the male-dominated power structure eagerly supports limitations to women's own control of their reproductive functions and sexuality. Pressure on government policymakers against freedom of choice to abortions, so called "squeal rules," to inform parents about teenagers' requests for birth control, lack of funded day-care, and programs that give more incentive for mothers to remain on Aid to Dependent Children grants rather than to get adequate job training all must be viewed in light of business interests (including those of organized religion, as discussed by Hendricks). Minority and low income women are disproportionately affected by these policies, as is discussed by both Belle and Russo. Even when mental health services are available to this group of women, it is most often by service providers who have a personal interest in maintaining the economic status quo so that they can maintain their own standard of living.

There are some who suggest that workers receive mental health benefits from their companies precisely because psychotherapy encourages adjustment and not radical action. Anger is channelled into safer directions instead of toward revolt and demands for equality or better working conditions. This may have been true in the 1950s and early 1960s, but in the last two decades issues about women's mental health have figured prominently in radicalizing the women's movement. The heavy tranquilization of women by drugs prescribed by male doctors was exposed by feminist women's groups. Rosewater describes the rise of feminist therapy as a response to women's needs to separate the crazy-making aspects of living in a world where to be a woman invites discrimination of all kinds from the actual internal mental health problems of an individual. Johnson and Auerbach raise the controversial issue of who decides what is good psychotherapy and, even more important, how therapy is paid for. At present, guild-and-turf issues prevent resolution of this controversy, but economics may ultimately dictate compromises.

Johnson and Auerbach note that research on women and psychotherapy has decreased markedly following a lot of activity during the 1970s. They recommend that attention to the effects of gender be made a part of all subsequent psychotherapy research. They discuss existing efforts to educate therapists, clients, and students about gender effects but concede that such efforts cannot be mandated. There is growing pressure on the community of psychologists and psychotherapy researchers to demonstrate the effectiveness of psychotherapy. In considering policy implications, they find it useful to divide policy into efforts at education and at legislation. They cite recent examples to demonstrate that efforts at legislation are fraught with difficulties. On important issues of therapy practice, there are likely to be differences of opinion within the therapeutic professions as to which changes should be made. The vagaries of governmental action constitute another obstacle in the way of correcting gender inequities.

The impact of the environment, and especially social interactions upon a person's mental health, seems to be even more critical for women than for men. Laura Brown describes the growth of the media psychologist and its potential to get relevant mental health education to women. Some feminists have, for a time, believed that acknowledging any differences could be used to strengthen the arguments by those who wish to retain sex-typed role division. Thus, it became politically important to present a unified view of the correct feminist philosophy. Clearly, communication and dissemination of the new knowledge base about the psychology of women and a sense of having many women's issues validated has relaxed the demand for political correctness. Many women who might not otherwise have self-identified as feminists have found a freedom in the elimination of a party line, and the original goal of feminism — to promote equality through acceptance of diversity of life choices — has been reaffirmed. Responsible reporting of the issues by the media can be of tremendous assistance, in continuing to affirm these values, as Brown discusses.

Kaplan and Surrey present an exciting new understanding of women's personality development that accounts for women's need for social relationships. In their work, they have found that women's self-esteem develops from a relational self rather than the autonomous self proposed by previous personality theorists who were male. Women's ability to feel and express deeper emotions more easily than can men may well come from childraising patterns that encourage development of their relational self. It may also explain women's more humanistic morality, as discussed by Gilligan (1982), and why so many women continue to function even while experiencing extreme emotional distress.

It is possible that women experience emotions in a different way than do men, which can allow for women to be more intense and perhaps even seem to become lost or enmeshed in their feelings without losing their sense of self (as is suggested in earlier literature). Many women diagnosed as borderline may actually be functioning in a normal way for a woman, even though their behavior may make male-identified therapists anxious. The diagnostic labeling of women's emotional experience into categories proposed by the male-dominated psychiatric structure has been challenged by Kaplan (1983) in an article in *American Psychologist*. She suggests that categorizing women's emotional responses may be a way of reifying the sex role stereotypes into pejorative groupings rather than providing meaningful assessment and treatment planning. In fact, all of the authors suggest that past discrimination against women has permeated the mental health profession as well as the mental health of women in insidious as well as directly observed ways.

Women's spirituality has also suffered through oppression by organized religions. Hendricks discusses how the major patriarchal religious systems influence women's mental health. She suggests that if women do not reclaim their spirituality, mental health policy appropriate for holistic care cannot be achieved. Hendricks argues that mental health professionals' refusals to acknowledge religion's positive as well as negative influence on people's attitudes and belief systems merely continues the patriarchal oppression of women. It is striking that the more affluent and businesslike religions, especially those espousing the newer fundamentalism, are the most involved in keeping women in subordinate roles, no matter what the cost to women's mental health. Even in this country, where separation between church and state has been an idealistic cornerstone, we must question whether or not religions sell women's souls to protect state's interest.

Johnson and Auerbach's review of the research on psychotherapy with women helps to account for the potential success of new policy implications, which all are recommending. Their review of the data on efficacy of psychotherapy is consistent with what we already know: The more experience a therapist has and the closer together therapist and client goals are, then the more successful is the outcome of therapy. Those therapists least likely to have successful outcomes with women clients are young, recently trained male therapists. Yet, graduate programs persist in admitting and training male students without any attempts at remediating the difficulties caused by their gender, much less even seriously offering formal coursework on the psychology of women. Efforts to get information about the psychology of women into the curriculum of every course in every mental health training program in the country have not been successful. Women psychologists and professionals in various training programs around the country often speak to the loneliness and ostracism they face, should they attempt to organize other women for support. Attempts to withhold accreditation for inadequate curriculum or supervision are met with responses by those finding the whole issue trivial as compared to the more basic elements of training. However, considering that over 70 percent of all psychotherapy users are women, updated information about their psychology surely ought to be considered basic. Psychologists taking the standard licensure examination will soon be facing specific questions on pertinent women's issues. It is hoped that other professions will follow this alternative way to force its professionals to learn about the psychology of women.

Not being taken seriously is a frequent complaint made by women. Many feel that no one really understands them. This is especially true for women who use the mental health system, whether they are the ethnic minorities or low income women as Belle discusses, lesbians as Martin and Lyon discuss, sexually exploited women as discussed by Bouhoutsos, victims of violence as my own chapter discusses, or those bound by religious traditions, as discussed by Hendricks. Rosewater's description of a therapy in which women perceive they are understood offers some hope for the future. Although the knowledge is slowly being introduced into training programs, a more rapid dissemination can be expected as more students find they cannot pass licensing examinations and as the general public becomes more sophisticated and knowledgeable than the old guard in academia. Brown's description of giving psychology away via the media, Stringer and Welton's description of women psychologists in policymaking positions, and Russo's discussion of disseminating data to government sources through the Presidential Commission on the Status of Mental Health's report indicate that the general public may become better informed than many experienced male-identified mental health practitioners who do not keep up with the expanding literature. Women consumers do not have to tolerate not being understood in the competitive mental health profession. Most women therapists, especially those with credentials practicing feminist therapy, report successful independent private practices. Economics rather than ethics may force some less knowledgeable to seek reeducation.

New policy guidelines for nonsexist research being developed by a task force in the American Psychology Association Division on the Psychology of Women should be an important guideline from which to evaluate current and proposed research as well as reexamine the limits of generalizability of past studies' findings. Studies that only include male subjects, those which measure hypotheses constructed from outdated sexist beliefs, and entire personality theories fashioned from male-dominated thinking do not inform us about women's feelings, thinking, and behavior. Researchers must familiarize themselves with the new guidelines and knowledge base at the same time as the new literature becomes published. Walker describes some difficulties in applying psychology to the legal arena where scientific bias is not recognized or is even deliberately misrepresented by those who have a vested interest in denying women their rights.

Nicholas Cummings describes the policy changes of his presidential administration of the American Psychological Association during the late 1970s when strong efforts were being made to eliminate such discrimination in the psychological profession. The fact that the policymaking body of the American Psychological Association in 1984 has a proportional number of women representatives elected to council and appointed to boards and committees indicate that the policy changes discussed by Cummings have been successful even if many people's attitudes toward women remain unchanged. The success within the psychology governance structure, however, has not sufficiently penetrated the scientific or professional training communities. But, it is hoped that such changes will be forthcoming now that female policymakers are in position.

There are those who question the ability of the mental health industry to effect social change. Such political thinking would suggest that any big business will have established political allies and stances that are too intertwined with other interest groups to make necessary changes. Certainly this seems true if fundamental changes that call for the elimination of that business are needed. Some radical feminist women's groups feel this is true and are therefore disassociating themselves with the mental health movement. Such groups feel that the values of feminism have been diluted by their appeal to so many people. They believe that the original feminist goal to create equality for women and men needs to take place in a classless society and thus cannot occur in a capitalistic political and economic system. Patriarchy is seen as supporting all forms of discrimination; changing the existing institutions in order to accommodate sex-fair equality is viewed as an impossible task.

The articles in this book will not answer the questions raised by those who hold such ideology. Hendricks suggests the patriarchally organized religions might be flexible enough to accommodate women as equals. Russo's data suggest the mental health industry might have the potential to do the same. None of the authors propose destructive approaches, but rather evidence hope that our economic and political system is elastic enough to accommodate the tremendous social change advocated.

Policy changes that will make women's lives more meaningful and satisfying have to come from all levels. The education of women is seen as a critical element, whether it be formal schoolroom learning or informal knowledge gained from daily living. Women's roles are changing, bringing along the changes in our social structure. The average marriage lasts six years, according to the 1980 census data. Serial relationships with children relating to several sets of stepfamilies may be the family structure of the future. I am struck by the resemblance such non-blood family networks have to the kinship patterns in traditional tribal cultures. As others begin to share the family responsibilities previously fulfilled by women, perhaps the rate of women's mental illness will decrease. However, this can only occur if women learn to measure their self-worth through a variety of successful experiences and not just by the way they keep their homes or mother their children.

It is clear that the current federal administration policy that supports the maintenance of the nuclear family has not supported a kinship family network development. Such changes come inadvertantly from the impact other policy decisions have had on grassroots people. It can be expected that many of the policies eliminated, weakened, or not implemented will result in keeping women in an inferior place. Mental health professionals are both morally and ethically responsible for recognizing and addressing the current dangers. As women become stronger and more organized, the articles in this book suggest they will be less likely to need mental health services. Only time will tell if a backlash will arise, strong enough to keep women in an inferior place. I doubt that the struggle will fail this time.

REFERENCES

Chesler, Phyllis. (1973). *Women and madness.* New York: Avon Books.

Freud, Sigmund. (1896). Aetiology of hysteria. In *Sigmund Freud: Collected papers, vol. 1* (E. Jones, trans.). New York: Basic Books.

Gilligan, Carol. (1982). *In a different voice: Psychological theory and women's development.* Cambridge, MA: Harvard University Press.

Kaplan, Marcie. (1983). A woman's view of the DSM-III. *American Psychologist, 38*(7), 786-792.

Masson, Jeffrey. (1984). Freud and the seduction theory. *The Atlantic Monthly,* (February), 23-60.

Russo, N. F. & Sobel, S. B. (1981). Sex differences in the utilization of mental health facilities. *Professional Psychologist, 12*(1). 7 19.

1

WOMEN IN THE MENTAL HEALTH DELIVERY SYSTEM: IMPLICATIONS FOR RESEARCH AND PUBLIC POLICY

Nancy Felipe Russo

Participation in the development of public policy is not a new role for mental health professionals. With the rise of the professional class in the United States, experts from many fields began to play a variety of roles in shaping the policies of our public institutions. If we look at those contributions from a feminist perspective, the experts do not receive high marks as advocates of equality for women. The long-standing sexism found in societal institutions required justification, and psychologists and psychiatrists played an influential role in perpetuating the status quo (Ehrenreich & English, 1978; Shields, 1975).

THE EMERGENCE OF A FEMINIST PERSPECTIVE IN MENTAL HEALTH RESEARCH AND PUBLIC POLICY

The decade of the 1970s brought a transformation in beliefs and expectations about women's roles and feminine identity. A feminist scholarship emerged and began to document the complex ways that sex bias, sex role stereotyping, and devaluation of women affect the nature, diagnosis, and treatment of mental health problems (Zuckerman, 1979).

Women's health did not emerge as a policy issue on the Washington agenda until 1976, when the formation of the Women and Health Roundtable and the organization of the National Women's Health Network (which opened its offices in Washington in the spring of

Author's Note: *I would like to thank Arnold Kahn for his comments on earlier drafts of the manuscript.*

1977) gave a national focus to those concerns. Mental health issues received only minor attention by those groups. However, their ability to lobby on behalf of women's health issues became an important foundation for the activities of advocates on behalf of women's mental health. (See Lear, 1983, for a history of the policy activities of women's health advocates during the 1970s.)

The President's Commission on Mental Health (PCMH) was established by President Carter on February 17, 1977, to review the mental health needs of the nation and to make recommendations to the president as to how this country might best meet those needs. The commission received the assistance of special fact-finding panels, including a Task Panel on Special Populations: Minorities, Women, and Physically Handicapped. That task panel was divided into seven subpanels, one of which was the Subpanel on the Mental Health of Women. The report of the subpanel, which will be discussed in more detail, remains a blueprint for the development of mental health policy responsive to women's needs and has become an organizing platform for women's mental health policy advocates.

From the beginning, the PCMH was concerned with underserved groups. Children, adolescents, minorities, and the elderly were identified as priority populations. Given that women were overrepresented in the mental health delivery system, subpanel members were concerned that women's needs would not receive adequate commission attention. Further, as the subpanel pointed out, consideration of women's needs requires a recognition of the impact of the social context on mental health, a position that challenges traditional intrapsychic, biomedical approaches to mental illness. The subpanel thus focused on issues of access to appropriate services, documenting how sex bias and sex role stereotyping detracted from the provision of appropriate care.

The subpanel's report detailed the social, economic, and psychological effects of inequality, recommending modifications in the areas of mental health training, service, and research, as well as strategies for prevention considered necessary for a mental health delivery system appropriately and positively responsive to the needs of women (Subpanel on the Mental Health of Women, 1978).

In this context, subpanel members considered the commission report (PCMH, 1978) a significant advance in mental health policy when it began with the recognition that

> Because of their age, sex, race, cultural background, or the nature of their disability, far too many Americans do not have access to personnel trained to respond to their special needs. (p.2)

The commission also affirmed that "changes in public attitudes have led to an awareness of the lack of appropriate services for many women" (p. 4).

Sex bias has long detracted from the quality of mental health research and service delivery. However, the detrimental effects of sex bias have become exacerbated as the stereotypes about women's roles and family structure increasingly diverge from the reality of women's family and work responsibilities. This discrepancy between stereotypes and reality presents a special challenge to mental health professionals and policymakers who are responsible for the design and delivery of mental health services. The commission recognized this challenge, as follows:

> The rapidly changing role of women has left many traditionally trained mental health practitioners ill-prepared to deal with the new problems that women face as a result. We know that women have expressed realistic concerns about the quality of their lives and their place in society. Many report that the response of the mental health services systems is often "treatment" aimed at encouraging them to accept the status quo and their "natural" position in life. We are concerned by the failure of mental health practitioners to recognize, understand, and empathize with the feelings of powerlessness, alienation, and frustration expressed by many women. (p.7)

The remainder of this article highlights some of the changes that have exacerbated the discrepancy between the stereotypes and the realities of women's lives—changes that underlie the feelings of powerlessness, alienation, and frustration of women, and that have special implications for mental health policies. It profiles women's utilization of mental health services, pointing out findings with special implications for research, training, and public policy, concluding with the subpanel's recommendations for change.

WOMEN'S CHANGING ROLES

Changes in women's work and family roles have been dramatic. In less than a generation, the size of the female workforce has doubled. The most recent statistics from the Women's Bureau of the U.S. Department of Labor (1983) reveal that from 1971 to 1981 alone, the number of women in the work force increased by more than 15 million. The 47 million women workers in 1981 accounted for more than 43 percent of all workers.

That year 62 percent of women 18 to 64 years of age were workers, compared with 91 percent of men. Labor force participation was highest among women aged 20 to 24, at 70 percent. The more education, the higher probability a woman will be in the labor force. Among women with four or more years of college, about 58 percent worked. Labor force participation rates for women are similar across racial/ethnic groups: 53 percent for black women (5.4 million); 52 percent for white women (40.2 million); and 48 percent for Hispanic women (2.2 million). Black women made up nearly half of the black labor force (49 percent); white women, 42 percent of white workers; Hispanic women, 39 percent of workers of Spanish origin.

Women represented 63 percent of all persons below the poverty level who were over 15 years old in 1981. It is clear that the majority of women work because of economic need. In March 1982, more than one in five woman workers had husbands whose 1981 earnings were less than $15,000. An additional 45 percent were either single (25 percent), widowed (5 percent), divorced (11 percent), or separated (4 percent).

Compared to men, women are still more likely to be concentrated in low status, low paying occupations and to experience salary discrimination. In 1981 they were 80 percent of clerical workers, 62 percent of service workers, and 63 percent of retail sales workers. In contrast, they constituted 45 percent of professional and technical workers, 28 percent of nonfarm managers and administrators, and 6 percent of craft workers.

Women workers with four or more years of college education had slightly less income than men who had only one to three years of high school—$11,085 and $11,936, respectively, in 1981. When employed full time, women high school graduates with no college had about the same average income as fully employed men who had not completed elementary school—$12,332 and $12,866, respectively.

Among full-time year-round workers the average woman still earns only about 59 percent of the average man's earnings. This global figure masks racial differences. In 1981, median salary figures by sex and race were white men, $20,160; black men, $15,119; white women, $12,287; black women, $11,312. The proportional impact of sex versus race on salary can be seen in the fact that black men make 72¢ for every dollar white men make, while the comparable figure for white women is 58¢. Black women make 93¢ for every dollar white women make. Belle (1984) explores the mental health implications of poverty and discrimination in further detail. (See Chapter 7 in this book.)

Nonetheless, the nature of women's work is also changing, with increasing numbers of women assuming jobs with higher status and responsibility, and entering traditionally male-dominated fields. The movement of 21 million women into jobs that were 80 percent male in the early 1960s is a major factor underlying the 95 percent increase of women in the labor force in the past 20 years. The comparable increase for males, starting from a larger base, was 31 percent (Ehrenhalt, 1983). Sales and Frieze (this volume) provide a fuller discussion of the mental health implications of the changing nature of women's work and the relationships among mental health and work and family roles.

The relationship between work and family roles has changed dramatically. While the number of working women has more than tripled since 1940, the number of working mothers has increased more than ten times. In March 1982, 59 percent of all mothers with children under 18 years of age (18.7 million mothers) were in the labor force; for mothers with preschool children (7.4 million mothers) the figure was 50 percent. About 55 percent of all children under age 18 (32 million) have working mothers that year; for children under age 6 (8.5 million) the figure was 46 percent.

Except for age of child, few studies have examined the relationship between the characteristics of children and whether or not their mothers work. Breslau, Salkever, and Starnch (1982) report that caring for a disabled child in the home exerts a negative impact on the labor force behavior of married mothers. Child disability interacts with race and income, however, having a greater negative effect on labor force participation in black, compared with white, mothers. The reduction of labor force participation is correlated with severity of disability. More research on the relationship of maternal and child health and women's work and family roles is needed if effective mental health policies are to be designed in this area.

The discrepancy between the stereotype of the two-parent family and the reality of the single-headed household family life has increased. In 1982, about 16 percent of families were maintained by a woman, up from 12 percent in 1972. More than 7 out of 10 of such families are maintained by white women (71 percent); 27 percent are maintained by black women; 8 percent by Hispanic women. Blacks are disproportionally represented in such households. Of black families 41 percent are maintained by women, compared to 23 percent of Hispanic families and 13 percent of white families. The proportion of poor families headed by women increased from 40 percent in 1971 to 47 percent in 1981. In 1981, 70 percent of poor black families, which included

3.1 million related children under 18 years of age, were maintained by women. Similarly, 50 percent of poor Hispanic families, which included 909,000 related children, and 39 percent of poor white families, which included 3.1 million related children, were headed by women.

Today women have smaller families. Surveys of birth expectations report that married women 18-44 years of age expect an average of 2.2 lifetime births; the comparable figure in 1967 was 3.1. After a decline from 1960 to 1976, birth rates in the United States have been increasing, partly because of postponed births. For 1980, the birth rate was 69 births per 1,000 women 15-44 years of age. First births to women over 30 years of age have increased (National Center for Health Statistics, 1982).

Childbearing takes place in the context of a social structure, and the implications of parenthood for mental health policy will change depending on that social structure. Historically, childbearing has taken place in the context of what I have described as a "motherhood mandate"—a sex role proscription that women must have at least two children and raise them "well" (Russo, 1976, 1979). In the last decade access to birth control and the increasing legitimization of voluntary childlessness has weakened the motherhood mandate and profoundly changed the motherhood context. Consider: In the 1960s, 1 in 5 marital births was unwanted by one or both parents at the time of conception. A decade later, in 1976, the figure was 1 in 12. The development of reproductive technology that permits surrogate motherhood and selection of sex of offspring has further altered the social context for childbearing and child rearing in unknown ways.

The importance of understanding the relationship between motherhood and mental health is underscored by the work of researchers Veroff, Douvan, and Kulka (1981). Their major survey of mental health in the United States reaffirmed earlier findings that women experience more symptoms of mental stress than do men: Women report more worries; more often say they have felt they were going to have a nervous breakdown; say that bad things happen to them more frequently; more frequently feel overwhelmed by bad events when they do happen; experience greater feelings of inadequacy as parents; and turn to professional help for personal problems more often. More women than men also report slightly more psychological anxiety and endorse slightly lower self-evaluation and personal efficacy statements (p. 374).

Veroff et al. suggest that the consistency of their findings reflect the worries and feelings of helplessness induced by the societal demand that women assume responsibility for children. Furthermore, sex differences do not completely disappear when parental status is controlled. Thus, even women without children appear affected by a cultural context that defines a women's identity in terms of her childbearing and child rearing roles. The motherhood mandate can exact a price in women's mental health whether or not it is fulfilled. Mental health policies can determine the nature and extent of that price.

These changes in women's lives are occurring in the context of significant increases in life expectancy for females compared with males. In 1982, life expectancy at birth reached 78.2 years for females and 70.8 years for males. Thus women live an increasing number of years after their children have left home and can expect to be widowed for a longer period of time (Gordon, 1979). Care for aged parents, which often falls to women, should become an increasingly important issue for both feminists and policy makers. During 1979-1980, an estimated 4.7 million adults in the civilian noninstitutionalized population needed assistance in personal care or home management activities; more than half of this group was age 65 or older. Nearly one in five of persons 85 and older require such assistance (National Center for Health Statistics, 1984).

While social change can be a source of stress, the point of this discussion is not that stress is associated with changing sex roles. The point is the urgent need for mental health professionals and policymakers to shed their stereotypes and to develop an appreciation of the nature of women's changing roles and circumstances. But even if women's roles were not changing, stereotypes would detract from delivery of services. As will be discussed later, even women who choose traditional roles are harmed by stereotyping on the part of mental health professionals (Russo & VandenBos, 1981).

WOMEN'S UTILIZATION OF MENTAL HEALTH SERVICES

Sex differences in use of mental health facilities vary with type of disorder and situational factors that affect men and women differently in different populations, such as minorities, youth, and the aged. A model that considers occurrence of symptoms, identification of the symptom, the definition of the symptom as a problem, the decision to seek help, actually seeking help, the diagnosis that is received, and the treatment model applied is needed if a full understanding of the differences is to be achieved.

Women are more likely to use mental health services than men, particularly outpatient services. In 1977, an estimated 5.6 percent of females compared with 3.5 percent of males visited ambulatory health care services (in either the specialty mental health care or general medical health care sectors) in conjunction with a mental health-related problem (Horgan, 1982).

A look at the utilization patterns in Table 1 (taken from Russo & Sobel, 1980) reveals dramatic differences by age, sex, and race/ethnicity across type of facility. Although males account for 51 percent of admissions overall, more females than males receive services from private mental health centers (57 percent), community mental health centers (52 percent), general hospital inpatient units (63 percent), and

TABLE 1

Utilization of Selected Psychiatric Facilities,
Number of Patients, and Percentage Female
by Age and Race (United States, 1975)

Patient Population	State and County Mental Hospitals[a]	Public General Hospital Psychiatric Inpatient Units[b]	Nonpublic General Hospital Psychiatric Inpatient Units[b]	Private Mental Hospitals	Outpatient Psychiatric Facilities[c]	Community Mental Health Centers[d]
All patients	385,237	139,352	376,185	129,832	1,406,065	919,037
percentage female	35	49	63	57	55	52
Adults—white	290,488	105,042	311,423	105,503	890,695	643,763
percentage female	36	50	63	58	60	55
Adults—other races	86,245	23,243	33,139	8,903	157,309	128,683
percentage female	35	49	64	54	66	53
Younger persons—white	17,548	7,599	26,928	13,853	280,501	118,085
percentage female	37	35	57	51	37	38
Younger persons—other races	7,704	3,468	4,695	1,573	77,560	28,506
percentage female	33	52	65	46	34	40
Age 18-64—white	261,220	98,234	281,272	93,146	846,284	558,144
percentage female	35	49	63	57	60	55
Age 18-64—other races	78,306	22,794	32,407	8,343	148,633	111,379
percentage female	34	49	64	54	64	53
Elderly—white	17,383	6,808	30,151	12,357	44,411	30,757
percentage female	38	63	64	65	76	57
Elderly—other races	3,176	449	732	560	8,676	6,150
percentage female	48	—[e]	—[e]	53	88	56

SOURCE: The data in this table were assembled from tabulations contained in Rosenstein and Milazzo-Sayre, (Tables 1a-1f). Reprinted from Russo and Sobel 1981, pp. 7-19.

a. Admissions.

b. Discharges.

c. Admissions, excluding federally funded community mental health centers, Veterans Administration psychiatric services, and private mental health practitioners.

d. Additions.

e. Five or fewer sample cases. Estimate not shown because it does not meet standards of realiability.

outpatient psychiatric facilities (55 percent). The situation reverses in state and county mental hospitals and public mental hospitals. Note that women are 1 percent of patients in Veterans Administration hospitals.

The obvious interaction effects of age, race/ethnicity, and type of facility with sex as seen in Table 1 suggest that mental health statistics derived from patient studies have limited usefulness to policymakers unless the sex, race/ethnicity, and age of patients as well as type of facility, are known. Further, any discussion of differences between females and males should be appropriately qualified unless the data are specifically age-adjusted, or the data on the subpopulations of younger persons, adults, and the elderly are specifically reported. The use of the terms "men" and "women" should be confined to describing populations at least 14 years of age and over.

Sex differences in the use of mental health services also differ depending upon whether or not one is considering the specialty mental health or the general medical sectors. In 1977, of the 5 percent of the U.S. population who had at least one ambulatory visit in conjunction with a mental health problem, three-fifths received their care in the general medical sector (i.e., physician and nonphysician health care providers exclusive of psychiatrists, psychologists, psychiatric social workers and mental health counselors). Knowledge about women's patterns of use in this sector are lacking. Data from the National Medical Care Expenditure Survey (NMCES) do suggest that women are even more likely to have visits in the general medical sector.

Of females using ambulatory mental health care services, 66.3 percent had the majority of their visits in the general medical sector; for males, the figure was 51.1 percent. Of persons with the majority of their visits in the specialty mental health sector, 53.8 percent were female; for the general medical sector, the comparable figure was 68.7 percent. These differences may reflect an age by sex interaction. Over 60 percent of users aged 18 years or younger (more likely to be male) had their visits in the specialty mental health sector. Over 88 percent of users aged 65 and over (more likely to be female) had the majority of their visits in the general medical sector (Horgan, 1982). Belief in the medical model to explain mental illness has been shown to detract from the appropriate treatment of patients (Farina & Fisher, 1982). Given that physicians in the general medical sector are trained in the medical model of illness, its detrimental effects would have a disproportionate impact on women, particularly older women.

While a larger percentage of persons had mental health-related visits in the general medical sector, users of the specialty sector had a higher average number of visits (9.6 versus 2.9). Males and females did not appear to differ in mean number of visits. Unfortunately the data are not broken out by age and sex, so whether or not women and men have similar numbers of visits is unknown.

The PCMH specifically identified the need for more precise demographic and socioeconomic data if we are to understand and meet the different needs that exist in our society, recommending

- Immediate efforts to gather reliable data on the incidence of mental health problems and the utilization of mental health services. Particular attention should be paid to population groups within our society known to have special needs, such as children, adolescents, the aging, women, and racial and ethnic minorities.

- Increased research efforts designed to produce greater understanding of the needs and problems of people who are underserved or inappropriately served or who are at high risk for mental disorders.

- Expanded research on the ways mental health services are delivered and the policies affecting these services (PCMH, 1978, p. 49).

While gathering of data is important, appropriate analysis of the data is critical if we are to comprehend fully women's service needs. There are considerable epidemiological data collected on the use of mental health services. Current knowledge is limited by the failure to analyze adequately the data now collected. Reports are developed to assist policymakers and planners in making decisions on the design and delivery of mental health services (e.g., the *ADAMHA National Data Book,* Vischi et al., 1980), but they are devoted to global data summaries that mask interaction effects with important policy implications in misleading and potentially harmful ways. An expanded discussion of the inadequacies of the epidemiological picture can be found in Russo and Sobel (1981).

Although age, race/ethnicity, and marital status affect utilization patterns, there are few analyses of the simultaneous interaction effects of age, sex, race/ethnicity, and martial status on service utilization (Rosenstein & Milazzo-Sayre, 1982; Rosenstein, 1980). Only some interaction effects have been explored (Russo & Sobel, 1981; Russo & Olmedo, 1983). Interaction effects vary by type of disorder, but little has been done to examine the basis of this variance. Further, the reports are not intended to place the data in a theoretical context, and the implications of the interaction effects for research, service, and policy are not discussed. To meet the long-term goal of designing and delivering appropriate and cost-effective mental health services to subpopulations in need, psychologists and epidemiologists must work together to ensure the relevant variables in the social context are included in the collection and analyses of the data.

It is inappropriate to draw conclusions about differences in prevalence of mental disorders across subgroups based on utilization statistics. The use of mental health facilities by subgroups of the population varies for complex reasons. Utilization data can, however, be used to draw conclusions about the types of knowledge needed to design mental health policies that will be responsive to the special service needs of women.

THE NEED TO INCREASE THE KNOWLEDGE BASE

The PCMH defined the task of mental health professionals and policymakers as

> to begin to understand that the causes of mental health problems are as varied as their manifestations. Some are physical. Some are emotional. Some are rooted in social and environmental conditions. Most are a complex combination of these and other factors, some of which are unknown. (p. 57)

In considering the importance of expanding the knowledge base regarding mental disorder, the PCMH concluded that "research must also begin to address a wide variety of issues relating to women" (p. 75). If access to appropriate mental health services is to be obtained, we must increase our knowledge about the processes involved in the development, diagnosis, and treatment of mental disorders in special populations. Although there has been considerable interest in stereotyping by mental health professionals, until recently the literature has been predominantly atheoretical (Sherman, 1980). Inconsistency of definitions and conceptualizations has often resulted in a divergence of opinion regarding the conclusions to be drawn from the research as to whether and how stereotypes affect therapeutic judgments (e.g., Sherman, 1980, in contrast to Davidson & Abramowitz, 1980; and Whitley, 1979). Recent theory and research on stereotyping, however, provide useful theoretical perspectives (Wallston & O'Leary, 1981).

There is a substantial literature on the causes and effects of sex typing and the consequences to individuals who violate sex role norms (Wallston & O'Leary, 1981). Such research has shown that the effects of stereotyping differ with age, sex, race, ethnicity, marital status, education, and geography (Crovitz & Steinmann, 1980; D'Arcy & Schmitz, 1979; Del Boca & Ashmore, 1981; Gatz, Pearson, & Fuentes, 1984). These effects have important implications for mental health research, training of mental health providers, and the design of mental health services. The failure of research to explore differences within ethnic and gender groups means that the literature on minority women in particular is overwhelmingly anecdotal in nature, perpetuating stereotypes devoid of empirical foundations (Espin & Lovelace, 1981; Olmedo & Parron, 1981; Senour, 1977; Staples, 1971). Knowledge of how the interactions of these characteristics relate to diagnosis and treatment is necessary for development of solid mental health policy.

Interaction effects of age, sex, and race on the most frequently diagnosed types of disorders reflect the paradoxical effects of sex role stereotyping. For disorders that are congruent with the societal feminine stereotype, such as depression, females show higher rates of service utilization than males (see Figure 1). In contrast, for disorders that are incongruent with society's view of idealized femininity and the proper role of "good" women (such as alcoholism) women's needs are neglected (Carmen, Russo, & Miller, 1981; Russo & Sobel, 1981; Russo & Vanden-Bos, 1981). Further, once patients receive a diagnostic label, they are subject to the beliefs and stereotypes attached to that label (Farina & Fisher, 1982; Rosenfeld, 1982; Wolinsky, 1981).

Beliefs about mental disorder can be placed in the larger context of attribution theory. People deduce their own intentions and dispositions by what they do and the effects of their actions. They seek counseling and therapy when their attributional conclusions lead them to define their behavior as ineffective or maladaptive, and themselves as responsible or ill.

Policies that assume belief in a medical model of mental disorder may contribute to the differential use of mental health facilities for men and women. We are beginning to understand about how beliefs about the nature of mental disorders affect the behavior of mental health service providers toward clients. For example, Cohen & Struening (1962) assessed attitudes of mental health workers toward mental health disorders. They found that the length of time patients spend in the community during the first year could be predicted from the responses of the staff members. In hospitals where the staff members believed that mental illness was specific type of illness, former patients spent fewer days in the community, compared to former patients from hospitals with a social learning view. These researchers showed that results could not be attributed to differences across hospitals in the degree of emotional disturbance of the patients.

Facility by Race	Number	Percent Distribution

Percent Distribution
☐ % Female ▓ % Male
10 20 30 40 50 60 70 80 90 100

Alcohol Disorders White

State & County	82,610	14%
Private	10,070	25%
Outpatient	42,109	24%

Other Races

State & County	24,005	29%
Private	757	28%
Outpatient	11,016	23%

Drug Disorders White

State & County	11,770	24%
Private	2,717	41%
Outpatient	13,049	47%

Other Races

State & County	2,665	17%
Private	360	33%
Outpatient	9,045	23%

Depressive Disorders White

State & County	41,165	53%
Private	51,957	66%
Outpatient	154,761	69%

Other Races

State & County	3,800	36%
Private	3,111	63%
Outpatient	25,974	89%

Schizophrenia White

State & County	90,631	45%
Private	24,865	58%
Outpatient	115,118	51%

Other Races

State & County	38,794	40%
Private	3,450	51%
Outpatient	33,115	64%

SOURCE: This figure was developed from statistics contained in Rosenstein and Milazzo-Sayre (in press), reprinted from Russo and Sobel, 1981, pp. 7-19.
NOTE: Statistics on outpatient facilities exclude federally funded community mental health centers, Veterans Administration psychiatric services, and private mental health practitioners.

Figure 1: Admissions to State and County Mental Hospitals, Private Mental Hospitals, and Outpatient Facilities for Selected Disorders by Sex and Race, 1975

Whitman and Duffey (1961) found newly admitted patients treated exclusively with drugs significantly shifted their beliefs toward viewing their condition as having a physical origin. They concluded that chemotherapy can result in strong denial of interpersonal difficulties and functional reasons for hospitalization, suggesting a vicious circle of inability to cope, seeking help, receiving drugs, having belief change, coping less satisfactorily, increasing dependence, continuing as patients, receiving more drugs. We know that women are more likely than men to use prescription drugs, particularly psychotropic drugs (Cafferata, Kasper, & Bernstein, 1983). In 1975, females received 87 percent of amphetamines, 67 percent of tranquilizers, and 60 percent of the barbiturates/sedatives prescribed (Subpanel on the Mental Health of Women, 1978). Research has shown that women have a higher median length of stay in inpatient service facilities. How drug-prescribing practices affect women's duration in treatment definitely needs to be studied.

Farina (1982) suggests that belief in a medical model influences mental health attributions in another way. He points out that a central tenet of the medical model is "the earlier the diagnosis and treatment, the better." This becomes translated into advice to monitor oneself for signs of problems and to seek help quickly. Most people will have trouble sleeping, have anxiety, or be depressed at some time or another. Belief in a medical model may increase the likelihood that normal conditions become defined as "illness" and result in help-seeking behavior.

We know that women report more emotional problems than do men. In addition, women seek psychiatric help at a higher rate than do men with comparable emotional problems. Evidence suggests that this difference is largely due to the fact that women more readily translate nonspecific feelings of distress into conscious recognition that they have an emotional problem. An estimated 10-28 percent of the difference in male-female morbidity is due to this sex difference in problem recognition (Kessler, Brown, & Broman, 1981). The tendency for women to have a "biology is destiny" principle applied to their behavior, to make self-attributions for their problems, and to be prescribed drugs as a treatment for their problems may all combine to affect women's use of mental health facilities.

A larger number of studies have examined various aspects of sex roles to explain sex differences in occurrence, diagnosis, and treatment of mental disorders (for a sampling of the literature, see Aneshensel, Frerichs, & Clark, 1981; Gove, 1972, 1979; Gove & Geerken, 1977; Goves, Hughes, & Style, 1983; Lewine, 1981; Rosenfeld, 1982; Veroff, Douvan, & Kulka, 1981; Weissman & Klerman, 1977). Most of the work reporting interaction effects has focused on how a limited number of variables relate to the occurrence and diagnosis of depressive and affective disorders in an attempt to explain the higher proportion of women experiencing them (cf. Radloff, 1975). But even work that has focused on sex differences in diagnosis and treatment of disorders with lower proportions of women (e.g., schizophrenia [Lewine, 1981; Test & Berlin, 1981], and alcoholism [Gomberg, 1981; Sandmaier, 1980]) has suggested the presence of interactions. The sex by age interaction effect on diagnosis and treatment is so powerful for schizophrenia that it has been suggested that separate norms for each sex be developed (Klorman, Strauss, & Kokes, 1977).

A number of findings in stereotyping literature have implications for the labeling of symptom severity for disorders associated with one sex. For example, Costrich, Feinstein, Kidder, Marecek, and Pascale (1975) found that an aggressive woman was rated as even more dominant than an aggressive man with an identical script. Coie, Pennington, and Buckley (1974) found that persons who acted in a manner incongruent with their sex role were seen as more maladjusted than those who acted in a sex role congruent manner. The consequences for sex role deviance appear to be more severe for females compared with males in some, although not all, contexts (Feinmen, 1981; O'Leary, Kahn, & Weber-Kollman, 1980; Shaffer & Johnson, 1980).

Rosenfeld (1982) directly examined the relationship of stereotype violation and treatment decisions in a psychiatric emergency room. She found that for disorders in which females predominate (neuroses and depression), males were significantly more likely to be hospitalized than females. For disorders in which males predominate (personality disorders and substance abuse), females were more likely than males to be hospitalized. This study focused on a limited population and did not explore the interaction of patient characteristics (race, ethnicity, marital status, education) with decision to hospitalize. More sensitive measures of intensity of treatment, such as number of hours of therapy, were not included. Nonetheless, the findings provide a powerful case for the importance of exploring the relationship between sex role stereotypes and treatment decisions.

TOWARD AFFECTING MENTAL HEALTH POLICY

Women have the power to influence mental health policy priorities, but we have yet to exert fully that power on our own behalf. If we are to have appropriate policy development, whether at federal, state, or local levels, women must participate in all levels of the decisionmaking process. It is crucial to understand, however, that policy development alone is insufficient. Policies must be implemented. Translation of statutes into gains for women requires enforcement. To be most effective, executive, legislative, and judicial strategies should be developed and evaluated in conjunction with each other (Sobel & Russo, 1981). It should also be understood that as long as the nation's economic crisis continues, women's mental health will not be high on the domestic policy agenda unless women themselves play an active part in developing that agenda.

As mentioned earlier, the recommendations of the subpanel provide a blueprint for developing mental health policies responsive to women's needs. Space limitations prohibit a full discussion of them, but I have reproduced them below in their entirety in the hopes that their wider dissemination will serve as catalyst for action.

Recommendations of the subpanel to the PCMH were as follows:

1. Set the eradication of sex and race bias in the mental health training, research, and service delivery as a priority.

2. Ensure that women—as policymakers, administrators, providers, researchers, and consumers—are active participants at all levels of the decisionmaking process in the mental health delivery system.

3. Establish administrative positions with the responsibility for reviewing policies, regulations, and programmatic decisions for their impact on the lives of women.

4. Staff such positions with individuals who have demonstrated knowledge of, sensitivity to, and empathy with women's issues.

5. Priority should be given to:
   (a) the examination and development of curriculum materials devoted to the new psychology of women.
   (b) the development of programs for training a variety of new and established mental health care providers in the psychology of women.
   (c) training programs for lay caregivers to develop appropriate listening and referral skills as an important preventative strategy in the delivery of mental health services.

6. Stop the funding of programs that perpetuate sex bias on the part of mental health care providers that results in inappropriate diagnosis and treatment of women.

7. Ensure that all programs receiving Federal funds, especially training funds, have demonstrated an active affirmative action commitment.

8. Develop alternative, nonmedical models such as crisis shelters as part of a comprehensive approach to the delivery of mental health services.

9. Ensure that agencies that fund such alternative models give priority to community-initiated self-help groups that have demonstrated expertise in the delivery of services designed for the special needs of women.

10. Evaluate reimbursement mechanisms such as National Health Insurance, Medicare, and Medicaid for their possible discriminatory impact on women, both as providers and consumers.

11. Promote the concept of consumer "freedom of choice" of medical and nonmedical mental health professionals.

12. Ensure that the data collection activities of the Federal Government are relevant to women's experiences.

    (a) Review the data gathering activities of the various agencies and reorganize them to maximize their potential policy impact.

    (b) Coordinate the fragmented and incompatible data gathering efforts of the various Federal agencies and make the data accessible to research and policymaking as well as public interest groups.

    (c) Provide Federal, State, and other jurisdictions with comparable planning and monitoring information regarding the appropriateness and equity of allocated health and social services funds.

13. Give priority to research that expands the knowledge base regarding the special mental health needs of women.

14. Ensure that all new research be designed, conducted, and staffed with an awareness of potential sex and race bias in existing theory, methodology, instrumentation, and interpretation.

15. Evaluate all ongoing programs for:

    (a) the criteria for determining their target population.

    (b) the reality of the assumptions that are made about women's lives.

    (c) the degree to which program objectives are related to women's needs.

    (d) the degree to which the special needs of women are met in the delivery of the services.

Any carefully conceived strategy for the prevention of mental illness and the promotion of mental health must have as one of its basic goals eradication of sexism and racism in the larger society. The Subpanel recommends that the President's Commission:

16. Articulate the damaging effects that the inability to control reproduction has on mental health.

17. Support the concept of reproductive freedom for women—i.e., ensure that women have access to the means to control their reproduction, without coercion.

18. Recommend to the president reconsideration of his position on Federal funding for abortion services and to work with the Congress to ensure that all restrictions on Federal funding for abortion be eliminated.

19. Endorse the Equal Rights Amendment as a strategy for primary prevention and call on the president as well as mental health professionals to work actively for its passage.

20. To endorse the International Women's Year National Plan of Action and request that the president set implementation of its recommendations as a priority for the Administration.

IN SUMMARY

Complex processes of sex bias and sex role stereotyping detract from the quality of mental health services to both sexes, but particularly to women because of their disadvantaged status. Understanding how such processes can at the same time create barriers to service access and create inappropriate service delivery will require an expansion of our knowledge base, but is essential to ensure quality mental health services. Ameliorating the problems of women in the mental health delivery system will require policymakers who have a sophisticated understanding of the nature of those problems and a firm commitment to seek creative solutions to them.

REFERENCES

Aneshensel, C. S., Frerichs, R. R. & Clark, V. A. (1981). Family roles and sex differences in depression. *Journal of Health and Social Behavior, 22,* 379-393.

Breslau, N., Salkever, D., & Starnch, K. S. (1982) Women's labor force activity responsibilities for disabled dependents: A study of families with disabled children. *Journal of Health and Social Behavior, 23*(2), 169-182.

Brodsky, A. M., (1982). *Sex, race, and class issues in psychology (master lecture Series).* Washington, DC: American Psychological Association.

Cafferata, G. L., Kasper, J. & Bernstein, A. (1983). Family roles, structure, and stressors in relation to sex differences in obtaining psychotropic drugs. *Journal of Health and Social Behavior, 24*(2), 132-143.

Carmen, E., Russo, N. F. & Miller, J. B. (1981). Inequality and women's mental health: An overview. *American Journal of Psychiatry, 138*(10), 1319-1330.

Cohen, J. & Struening, E. L. (1962). Opinions about mental illness in the personnel of two large mental hospitals. *Journal of Abnormal and Social Psychology, 64,* 349-360.

Coie, J. D., Pennington, B. R. & Buckley, H. H. (1974). Effects of situational stress and roles on the attribution of psychological disorder. *Journal of Clinical and Consulting Psychology, 42,* 559-568.

Costrich, N., Feinstein, J., Kiddler, L., Marecek, J. & Pascale, L. (1975) When stereotypes hurt: Studies of penalties for role reversals. *Journal of Experimental Social Psychology, 11,* 520-530.

Crovitz, E. & Steinmann, A. (1980). A decade later: Black-white attitudes toward women's familial role. *Psychology of Women Quarterly, 5,* 170-176.

D'Arcy, C. & Schmitz, J. A. (1979). Sex differences in the utilization of health services for psychiatric problems in Saskatchewan. *Canadian Journal of Psychiatry, 24*(1), 19-28.

Davidson, C. V. & Abramowitz, S. I. (1980). Sex bias in clinical judgment: Later empirical returns. *Psychology of Women Quarterly, 4,* 377-395.

Del Boca, F. K. & Ashmore, R. (1981). Sex stereotypes through the life cycle. In L. Wheeler (Ed.), *Review of Personality and Social Psychology* (Vol. 2). Beverly Hills, CA: Sage.

Ehrenhalt, S. M. (1983). Cited in *Women Today,* Women moving into many male-dominated professions. p. 120.

Ehrenreich, B. & English, D. (1978). *For her own good: 150 years of the experts' advice to women.* Garden City, NY: Doubleday.

Espin, O. M. & Lovelace, V. (1981). A brief annotated bibliography on third world minority women: Resources for mental health practitioners (1955-1980). *JSAS Catalog of Selected Documents in Psychology, 11,* 70.

Farina, A. (1982). The stigma of mental disorders. In A. G. Miller (Ed.). *In the eye of the beholder.* New York: Praeger.

Farina, A. & Fisher, J. D. (1982). Beliefs about mental disorders: Findings and implications. In G. Weary and H. F. Mirels (Eds.), *Integrations of clinical and social psychology.* New York: Oxford University Press.

Feinmen, S. (1981).. Why is cross-sex-role behavior more approved for girls than for boys? A status characteristics approach. *Sex Roles, 7,* 289-300.

Gatz, M., Pearson, C. & Fuentes, M. (1984). *Social and psychological problems of women: Prevention and crisis intervention.* Washington, DC: Hemisphere.

Gomberg, E.S.L. (1981). Women, sex roles and alcohol problems. *Professional Psychology, 12,* 146-155.

Gordon, N. M. (1979). Institutional response: The federal income tax system. In Smith (Ed.), *The subtle revolution: Women at work.* Washington, DC: Urban Institute.

Gove, W. R. (1972). The relationship between sex roles, marital status, and mental illness. *Social Forces, 51,* 34-44.

Gove, W. R. (1979). Sex differences in the epidemiology of mental disorder: Evidence and explanation. In E. S. Gomberg and V. Franks (Eds.), *Gender and disorder behavior.* New York: Brunner/Mazel.

Gove, W. R. & Geerken, M. R. (1977). The effect of children and employment on the mental health of married women and men. *Social Forces, 56,* 66-76.

Gove, W. R., Hughes, M. & Style, C. B. (1983). Does marriage have positive effects on the psychological well-being of the individual? *Journal of Health and Social Behavior, 24*(2), 122-131.

Horgan, C. M. (1982). *A comparison of utilization and expenditure patterns for ambulatory mental health services in the specialty mental health and the general medical sector.* Paper presented at the annual meetings of the American Public Health Association, Montreal, Canada, November.

Kessler, R. C., Brown, R. L. & Broman, C. L. (1981). Sex differences in psychiatric help-seeking: Evidence from four large-scale surveys. *Journal of Health and Social Behavior, 22*(1). 49-64.

Klorman, R., Strauss, J. & Kokes, R. (1977). The relationship of demographic and diagnostic factors to measures of premorbid adjustment in schizophrenia. *Schizophrenia Bulletin, 3,* 214-225.

Lear, J. G. (1983). Women's health and public policy: 1976-1982. In I. Tinker (Ed.), *Women in Washington: Advocates for public policy.* Beverly Hills, CA: Sage.

Lewine, R.R.J. (1981). Sex differences in schizophrenia: Timing or subtypes. *Psychological Bulletin, 90,* 432-444.

National Center for Health Statistics. (1982). *The nation's health: 1982.* DHHS Pub. No. (PHS) 83-1232. Public Health Service. Washington, DC: U.S. Government Printing Office.

National Center for Health Statistics. (1984). *Health—United States, and prevention profile.* DHHS Pub. No. PHS 84-1232. Washington, DC: U.S. Government Printing Office.

O'Leary, V. E., Kahn, A. & Wever-Kollman, R. (1980). *The price of sex-role deviance: It costs men less.* Paper presented at the Annual meetings of the American Psychological Association, Montreal, Quebec, Canada, September.

Olmedo, E. L. & Parron, D. L. (1981). Mental health of minority women: Some special issues. *Professional Psychology, 12,*103-111.

President's Commission on Mental Health. (1978). *Report to the President, Volume I.* Washington, DC: U.S. Government Printing Office.

Radloff, L. (1975). Sex differences in depression: The effects of occupation and marital status. *Sex Roles, 1*(3), 249-265.

Rosenfeld, S. (1980). Sex roles and societal reactions to mental illness. The labeling of "deviant" deviance. *Journal of Health and Social Behavior, 23,* 18-24.

Rosenstein, M. (1980). *Hispanic Americans and mental health services: A comparison of Hispanic, black, and white admissions to selected mental health facilities, 1975.* Series CN No. 3. DHHS Publication No. (ADM) 80-1006, Superintendent of Documents. Washington, DC: U.S. Government Printing Office.

Rosenstein, M. & Milazzo-Sayre, L. J. (1982). *Characteristics of admissions to selected mental facilities, 1975: An annotated book of charts and tables.* U.S. Public Health Service Publication. Washington, DC: U.S. Government Printing Office.

Russo, N. F. (1976). The motherhood mandate. *Journal of Social Issues, 32*(3), 143-154.

Russo, N. F. (1979). Overview: Sex roles, fertility, and the motherhood mandate. *Psychology of Women Quarterly, 4*(1), 7-14.

Russo, N. F. & Olmedo, E. L. (1983). Women's utilization of outpatient psychiatric services: Some emerging priorities for rehabilitation psychologists. *Rehabilitation Psychology, 28*(3), 141-155.

Russo, N. F. & Sobel, S. B. (1981). Sex differences in the utilization of mental health facilities. *Professional Psychology, 12,*;7-19.

Russo, N. F. & VandenBos, G. (1981). Women in the mental health delivery system. In Wade Silverman (Ed.), *A health sourcebook for board and professional action.* New York: Praeger.

Sandmaier, M. (1980). *The invisible alcoholics: Women and alcohol abuse in America.* New York: McGraw-Hill.

Senour, M. N. (1977). Psychology of the Chicana. In J. L. Martinez, Jr. (Ed.), *Chicano psychology.* New York: Academic Press.

Shaffer, D. R. & Johnson, R. D. (1980). Effects of occupational choice and sex-role preferences on the attractiveness of competent men and women. *Journal of Personality, 48,* 505-519.

Sherman, J. (1980). Therapist attitudes and sex-role stereotyping. In Annette Brodsky & Rachel T. Hare-Mustin (Eds.) *Women and psychotherapy.* New York: Guilford Press.

Shields, S. A. (1975). Functionalism, Darwinism, and the psychology of women. *American Psychologist, July,* 739-754.

Sobel, S. B. & Russo, N. F. (1981). Equality, public policy, and professional psychology. *Professional Psychology, 12*(1), 180-189.

Staples, R. (1971). The myth of the black matriarchy. In R. Staples (Ed.), *The black family: Essays and studies.* Belmont, CA: Wadsworth.

Subpanel on the Mental Health of Women, President's Commission on Mental Health. (1979). *Task Panel Report, Vol. III, Appendix 1022-1116.* Washington, DC: U.S. Government Printing Office.

Test, M. A. & Berlin, S. B. (1981). Issues of special concern to chronically mentally ill women. *Professional Psychology, 12,* 134-144.

Veroff, J. Kulka, R. A. & Douvan, E. (1981). *The inner American: Self-portrait from 1957-1976.* New York: Basic Books.

Vischi, T. R., Jones, K. R., Shank, E. L. & Lima, L. H. (1980). *The alcohol, drug abuse, and mental health national data book.* DHEW Publication No. ADM 80-938. Washington, DC: U.S. Government Printing Office.

Wallston, B. S. & O'Leary, V. E. (1981). Sex makes a difference: The differential perceptions of women and men. In L. Wheeler (Ed.), *Review of Personality and Social Psychology* (Vol. 2, pp. 9-41). Beverly Hills, CA: Sage.

Weissman, M. M. & Klerman, G. L. (1977). Sex differences in the epidemiology of depression. *Archives of General Psychiatry, 34,* 98-111.

Whitley, B. E. (1979). Sex roles and psychotherapy: A current appraisal. *Psychological Bulletin, 86,* 1309-1321.

Whitman, J. R. & Duffy, R. F.(1961). The relationship between type of therapy received and a patient's perception of his illness. *Journal of nervous and mental disorders, 133,* 288-292.

Wolinsky, F. D. & Wolinsky, S. R. (1981). Expecting sick-role legitimation and getting it. *Journal of Health and Social Behavior, 22,* 229-242.

Women's Bureau, U. S. Department of Labor. (1983). *Twenty facts about women workers.* Washington, DC: U.S. Government Printing Office.

Zuckerman, E. (1979). *Changing directions in the treatment of women: A mental health bibliography.* DHEW Publication N. ADM 79-749. Washington, DC: ADAMHA.

2

FEMALE PSYCHOLOGISTS IN POLICYMAKING POSITIONS

Donna M. Stringer
Nancy R. Welton

This chapter discusses the importance of women as policymakers, including risks involved and necessary qualifications for policymakers, special contributions that women trained in psychology can bring to policymaking, and how women in different roles can work together to effect policy. Our definition of policymaking includes participation in three separate activities: the development of a *policy* (a statement of what is to be done); the development of *regulations* (a statement of how the policy will be enacted); and the development of *legislation* (establishing the legal power to implement and fund policies).

This chapter addresses itself specifically to women, regardless of ethnicity, age, class, sexual preference, or other inherent or elected differences. The tenets we discuss related to female policymakers who focus on issues affecting women also apply to other traditionally excluded groups (ethnic minorities, lesbians and gays, physically challenged, and older or younger persons). We will discuss female policymakers as if they were specifically committed to working on issues affecting women although this is not always the case. Female policymakers are needed to affect *all* types of policies, not just those defined as "women's issues."

We will also discuss policymaking in a generic way. We do not refer exclusively to a narrow definition of "mental health policy" because it is our belief that any public policy that touches women's lives (e.g., housing, energy, criminal justice, health) has an effect on women's mental health. While a discussion of licensing mental health professionals clearly has a direct impact on women's lives whether they are clients or practitioners, other public policy is equally important. Stress placed on women, from unemployment, lack of housing, lack of child care, lack of access to shelters for victims of violence, or the presence of nuclear plants in one's backyard, all affect women's mental health.

WHY POLICYMAKING ROLES ARE IMPORTANT FOR WOMEN

Policy systems must include a wide range of representation in order to develop policies that include all subgroups within a society. Since women and other subgroups are not adequately represented in policymaking systems, they are often not considered in terms of policy impact. When only white males develop policy, they frequently do not think about potential impact on women; when they do express concern about women they may have difficulty understanding what the impact will be. It is important, therefore, to include women as policymakers if women's needs are to be addressed. Feminist psychologists are ideally prepared to bring understanding of the full range of women's social, economic, and psychological needs to bear on policy systems (Sobel & Russo, 1981).

It would appear that the mere presence of a woman, regardless of her sensitivity to women's concerns, has an impact on the way policy is developed. This impact occurs for two reasons: First, the physical presence of a woman may cause men to think more readily about how a policy will affect women. Second, the female policymaker is likely to have a different perspective from men simply because of differential world experiences resulting from gender. Perhaps the most publicly visible example of this impact is Supreme Court Justice Sandra Day O'Connor whose experiences include parenting, relocating for a spouse's career, and blatant sex discrimination in employment. While these experiences have not necessarily meant she always favors feminist positions on issues, Justice O'Connor's history clearly indicates a different perspective on issues affecting women than has historically been represented in the Supreme Court. Schafran (1981) states,

> Whatever her judicial philosophy, Sandra Day O'Connor will bring to the Supreme Court a solidly grounded understanding of the real lives of women in contemporary society—she will bring to the Court's deliberations on these issues the touchstone of reality that has been so glaringly absent.

Second, it is important for female psychologists to be in policymaking roles in order to look below the surface of what appears to be equal *treatment* but which, in fact, may be discriminatory in its actual *impact*. While policies that treat the sexes equally are usually to be advocated, there are instances where past discrimination, sex role socialization, or actual physical differences, may necessitate policies that treat the sexes differently in order to achieve equal impact. Historically, both differential treatment and equal treatment have been used in policy to discriminate against women in their impact.

An example of *differential treatment* used to discriminate against women is labor laws. Originally designed to "protect" women, laws that limited the hours a woman could work and the weight she could be required to lift resulted in women being denied lucrative overtime hours and jobs that required physical strength and lifting. Through alliances with unions, these laws were revised to protect men and women equally from the abusive use of long hours or unreasonable physical demands of employers (Peterson, 1983; Rawalt, 1983).

On the other hand, a current example from the criminal justice system demonstrates *equal treatment* that results in disparate impact. Most criminal systems assume that inmates who are parents leave an intact family and return to the intact family upon release—therefore, no family living arrangements are considered. Women prisoners, however, reflecting the larger society, are more likely than men to be single heads of household. Therefore, children of women prisoners are more likely to be separated from their siblings and placed with different extended family members and/or foster homes. When the mother leaves prison she must collect her children and reestablish a nuclear family. A man, on the other hand, is more likely to have an intact family waiting for him when he is released. Returning to an intact family requires substantially different skills than recreating a nuclear family, and yet most prison systems treat male and female prisoners the same way on release. Unfortunately, the treatment is usually to give little or no preparation for reentering any kind of family setting. The impact of these gender-related differences, however, can be profound for children of women prisoners who experience both the stigma of an incarcerated parent as well as family disruptions and sibling separation (Hunter, 1983).

Differential policies should be developed only when they are necessary to achieve equal impact. Differential treatment should be used only until historical or social inequities are remedied. Affirmative action policies are an obvious example. If women and ethnic minorities achieve employment equity with majority males, affirmative action programs can be discarded and we can move to an equal treatment policy.

One advantage to women psychologists as policymakers is specifically related to the issues of treatment versus impact. Psychologists are trained to examine and understand the impact of treatment at both a societal and an individual level; therefore, a psychologist as policymaker can use the data of social science to demonstrate whether equal or disparate policies should be written. Further, if the policymaker recommends disparate policy to undo the effects of social history, she can also make some recommendation about when and how to review the policy to see if it is time to change it to an equal treatment policy because historical effects have been eradicated.

Using the examples of labor laws and prison policies can demonstrate the role of psychologists in policymaking. Psychologists are likely to understand how protective laws can be used to develop learned helplessness in women, thus restricting their career goals. Psychologists could also use available data to demonstrate the developmental needs of children for familial stability in order to draft policies that consider individual parental situations and best meet the needs of children and parents, including exploration of nuclear family prison settings. These policies could be revised if social science data told us that parenting and family traditions had changed in such a way that mothers entering prison were leaving children with a male parent in an intact family.

A third major reason it is important for women to be included in policymaking roles is to complete the connection between direct services, advocacy, research, and policy. Women have historically been involved in provision of direct services such as teaching, nursing, and counseling. More recently women have become involved in advocacy through the development of community organizations specifically aimed at meeting needs that have gone unnoticed and unserved by the larger society, such as crisis counseling for rape victims and shelters for battered women. Also during the past two decades women have begun to conduct research and publish work that challenges traditional methodology, content that ignores women, and the assumption of males as the "norm" (Roberts, 1981; Stanley & Wise, 1983). Examples of this recent research include the areas of psychological androgyny, achievement motivation, and menopause. To complete the cycle, women have most recently become involved in policymaking via elected and appointed positions.

To meet women's needs fully, it is critical to understand the link between the four roles of direct service, advocacy, research, and policy. For example, if a female policymaker is advocating for a mental health policy within a city, she must rely on the researcher to provide her with data about women's mental health needs[1]; she must rely on the direct service provider to give her information about the specific unmet needs of women within that city; and she must rely on the community advocate to provide "outside" community pressure on city government while the female policymaker is advocating "inside" city government. Barriers between people in these four roles will make policies less effective in meeting the needs of women. Some potential barriers include lack of information and understanding about the nature and limitations of each role, lack of open communication, personal or professional territoriality or jealousy, and mistrust of the motives of people in other roles. An understanding and appreciation of each others' roles can reduce the traditional barriers that arise between such seemingly disparate groups. This is important to decrease hostilities that can make it appear (both to women and to those who would like to sabotage women's efforts) that women are not working together toward the same goals. Those "inside" and those "outside" policymaking spheres can learn to complement each other's roles, resulting in maximum effectiveness in reaching long-term goals.

It is particularly important to find ways to communicate the nature and limitations of each role because of the natural tendency to reduce the unknown to stereotypes (Frieze et al., 1978). For example, researchers have been stereotyped as elitist and isolated from the real world. Direct service providers are labeled as being "touchy-feely" but out of touch with the "facts." Legislators are seen as uncaring powermongers, and policymakers are viewed as coopted bureaucrats whose only concern is self-aggrandizement. Each person has some responsibility for not allowing these stereotypes to interfere with her working relationships. The sensitive nature of each of these roles, of course, requires that some information be kept confidential, and yet sharing secrets is often a way groups establish trust and overcome stereotypes. Other forms of establishing group trust need to be developed, therefore, including the following: establishing basic principles of agreement, developing a shared vision; developing short- and long-term goals; developing a strategy for achieving goals together; disclosing all information that can be shared as well as clarity about information that cannot be shared; developing genuine friendships in which trust allows each person to limit information disclosure without being suspect. Effective mentoring also has an important place here. The less experienced a woman is in these roles, the more she will need assistance understanding the distinct responsibilities to ensure that she does not become ineffective or destructive through stereotyping her potential colleagues and allies.

The fourth and final reason policymaking roles are important is the issue of empowerment. Women who are in policymaking positions are professionally empowered by the system to make changes. Through role modeling for other women and men, the female policymaker helps personally empower those who see themselves as equally capable of being policymakers. The female policymaker also encourages collective empowerment for women insofar as she creates public policy that recognizes women's needs as legitimate. More battered women are now asking for legitimate assistance as a result of the collective work of advocates, researchers, service providers, and policymakers who have changed laws and regulations to respond to needs of battering victims. Finally, female policymakers help empower women by forcing power brokers to recognize the community's advocates and direct service providers.

RISKS FACED BY WOMEN IN POLICYMAKING ROLES

One risk faced by women entering a policymaking role is the expectation that she will make a difference quickly. It has been said that a "camel is a horse designed by a committee." Perhaps nowhere does progress move more slowly than in the area of public policy. Most public policy requires considerable negotiation among affected interest groups and often across governmental bodies. In order to develop, implement, or revise public policy it is usually necessary to involve citizens, professions in the area affected by the proposed public policy, and myriad public policymakers. Examinations of legislative history find policy changes occurring incrementally. Ideal changes may take several policy revisions over years to reach the ultimate goal. Rape legislation is a prime example: Almost two decades after women began changing rape laws we finally see a sprinkling of states outlawing marital rape — a change that could not have been won without years of incremental shifts, public education, and data gathering. This can be particularly frustrating if the advocacy, research, and direct service people are leaning on the policymaker to move quickly. It is important for a female policymaker to recognize the time constraints under which she is operating and to communicate those time constraints honestly to women working in other roles. It is equally important that she not attempt to prove her "credentials" by promising to move something quickly. Such promises are rarely kept and can lead to the female policymaker losing credibility with a constituency. The policymaker must keep her own ultimate goals in mind; occasionally she may need simply to put an issue on hold temporarily rather than compromising it beyond recognition. If the policymaker decides that a delay is strategically helpful, she should communicate this to the women's community so they do not see the delay as abandonment.

A second risk female policymakers face is that of becoming so integrated into the system that their original commitment to women is forgotten. This is sometimes called "cooptation," or "being bought off." This is a very touchy issue. A female policymaker must be enough of a chameleon to be able to work within the system. Thus, when a policymaker compromises it may mean that she is simply recognizing the constraints of the system within which she is operating, not that she has lost commitment.

A third risk of being a policymaker is that of losing contact with women who have been disenfranchised from the policymaking system. To work inside any system is to risk insulation from the rest of the world. One way to guard against insulation is by consistently communicating with the community.

A fourth risk is the desire, and occasional attempt, to draft policy that can meet all women's needs equitably and simultaneously. Women's diverse needs make such an attempt impossible. Policymakers must be willing to seek information from a diversity of women and write policy that is complex enough to address different needs. For example, domestic violence legislation needs ultimately to recognize diverse lifestyles by protecting nonmarried people (including lesbians) from violence by a primary partner rather than using only the traditional terminology of "spouse."

The final, and perhaps most personally destructive danger of being a female policymaker is the stress resulting from being in a male-dominated system, which can lead to a sense of isolation, misunderstanding, and alienation (Forisha & Goldman, 1981). The problem of isolation is, to some degree, inherent in the role of policymaker. The woman policymaker will never be part of the "male" system; there will always be some sense of distance between her and her male colleagues simply by virtue of her gender. Neither is she truly a part of the "women's community" (or the ethnic minority community if she is a woman of color); there will always be some sense of distance between her and other women by virtue of her role in the male system.

An effective policymaker, regardless of the issues about which one is concerned, must maintain enough separation to evaluate effectively all options and potential results of policies being considered. In order to do this, one cannot be so enmeshed in any single issue or community that a sense of encompassing vision is lost. A policymaker who is deeply involved in the "violence" community, for example, must not work on violence policies to the exclusion of issues like housing, employment, child care, taxes, and the like, or she may lose credibility with colleagues. In order to maintain a sense of balance, then, she cannot "belong" exclusively to any one group or issue.

Using Merton's (1938) model, if a female policymaker cannot maintain a balance between the cultural change goals of the women's community and the institutional methods for attaining such change, she is most likely to have one of two responses. She may withdraw from the women's community and become a "Queen Bee" or a hardened, play-it-by-the-book bureaucrat to avoid confronting criticism from the women's community. Or she can withdraw from her policymaking colleagues and become the "rebel" within the system, which almost always results in less effectiveness in achieving policy goals. For neither of these responses to occur, the female policymaker must develop a complex set of skills and support systems that include conformity to the rules of policymaking systems while retaining commitment to social change issues. Here again we see the value of psychology: The psychologist as policymaker should be well equipped to identify and correct dissonance, stress, and burnout if she experiences it; she should be skilled in communicating with everyone with whom she needs to work; and she will surely be able to use the tenets of both organization and learning theories to persuade her colleagues regarding necessary policy changes.

Since burnout results from an imbalance between job demands and the worker's resources, several courses of action may prevent the burnout that would otherwise result from the pressures of a policymaking role (Cherniss, 1980). One strategy involves reducing external job demands by setting priorities, setting limits based on established criteria, and carefully explaining these limitations to the community. A second strategy involves modifying one's own level of expectations, preferences, and/or goals so that unrealistic pressure is not placed on oneself. A third strategy is to expand resources for meeting job demands by sharing the work with others, increasing staff when possible, and making maximum use of outside resource people and materials. A fourth strategy is to seek contact and support from other female policymakers who understand the complexities and pressures involved. Several organizations have been established for the purposes of this type of support including Women in Municipal Government,

Washington Elected Women, and the Congressional Caucus for Women's Issues at the federal level. Personal support systems and the pursuit of balance between policy and nonpolicy work can also be helpful. Both trust and communication must be built into personal and community connections if the female policymaker is to be nurtured enough to stay in her role and remain effective.

REQUIRED QUALITIES FOR POLICYMAKERS: PSYCHOLOGY AS AN IDEAL TRAINING

The first set of requirements for policymakers includes categories of *education, training, and experience.* These might also be seen as cognitive or "left brain" types of training. Policymakers must understand research methodology and findings in order to conduct policy analyses, needs assessment, evaluations of policy and potential impacts; the policymaker may need to know who to ask for such analyses (e.g., Does she need a forensic psychologist, a demographer, or a child clinician to provide background data?). Psychology training programs generally include heavy emphasis on research methodology including analysis, assessment, and evaluation that are effectively translated into the public policy arena. Finally, in order to implement any policy as discussed above, policymakers must be able to work with a large number of groups and individuals. The understanding of individual behavior, group process, communication styles, and persuasion techniques are all part of most psychology training programs and are central to policy roles. To be able to identify and select the most effective option for policy without being able to implement the policy is useless. The understanding of people, group process, and communication makes psychology training a profoundly useful education background for policy roles.

A second major set of requirements for public policymakers falls under the label of *professional abilities.* These might also be called political or interpersonal skills, creativity, and/or "right brain" training. These include the following:

- creative analysis (finding sexism between the lines of policy language and/or implications);
- communication skills (talking about women's issues without making others defensive and hearing sexism without acting in a defensive or counterproductive manner);

- political skills (getting things done, intuitiveness about timing, process, developing allies inside/outside the organization);
- ability to develop credibility, including honesty and fairness, both inside and outside the organization;
- patience;
- ability to live with long-range goals;
- risk taking;
- independence.

This list is, of course, not exhaustive, but includes the more critical qualities required for an effective public policymaker. Many of these professional skills are addressed in psychology training programs.

A final set of qualities is generally not taught in formal training programs but results largely from life experiences. These are the category of *personal qualities* including a deep commitment to women, a willingness to establish diverse community contacts who will help identify policy needs, a personal independence and strength that will survive standing alone, and the ability to articulate women's needs without complete support from either "inside" or "outside" sources.

COMMUNITY RESPONSIBILITIES TO THE POLICYMAKER

In order for a policymaker to be effective, she can use assistance in three major ways. First, it is important that the policymaker receive community assistance in identifying needs. This means information about policies that are deficient or need revision if they are to meet women's needs. Key actors in this assistance are direct service providers who find policy ineffective in meeting the needs of their community or actually blocking the ability to provide services. A feedback system from citizens who attempt to get necessary services but cannot is important so the policymaker can evaluate how to connect services effectively to citizens. Also, researchers will often be needed to identify "hard" data about the need for a policy and/or the impact of various policy options.

Once a policy has been drafted the policymaker needs the support of the women's community in order to see the policy implemented. Specifically, the policymaker will need citizens to testify at public hearings regarding the need for a policy, direct service providers to provide both data and anecdotal information about the impact of the proposed policy, and researchers to provide necessary data. It is often very necessary for the feminist community to provide a show of public support for a policymaker when she comes under attack for advocating policy that addresses itself to the needs of women. Female policymakers are criticized for a number of things, some of which may be legitimate. Most critically, however, when a female policymaker proposes policy aimed at improving the lives of women, she will find herself under assault for being "too interested in women." It is important when this occurs for the feminist community to give the female policymaker both public and private support if she is to continue being an effective advocate for policies related to women's needs. This support may be demonstrated through a substantial number of women attending a public hearing and putting "outside" pressure on her to support a specific issue. This decreases the potential for her male colleagues to believe that the issue is her personal concern and not related to community needs.

Finally, the community has the responsibility not to expect "political purity" from female policymakers. It is the community's responsibility to understand the policymaker's role, including the need to negotiate and compromise in order to get any issue related to women addressed and to understand that political process (which is what public policy is all about) is always slow, often painful, and frequently results in less than "all we want." Feminists need to be more aware of the need to define their compromise positions and communicate them to the policymaker. If the feminist community expects a policymaker to move quickly and effectively toward "getting it all," they will be disappointed in her performance and consequently may make her ineffective within the political system, thus robbing women of an important "inside" ally.

The overall position we wish to communicate is that there is a mutual responsibility between female policymakers and women in the community. A very effective combination of two-way communication, mentoring, networking, and empowerment has been occurring in the feminist community during the past decade in the form of training workshops, lobbying alliances, and political action committees. An example is Washington Women United (WWU), a statewide organization within the State of Washington which was formed when the state women's commission was abolished by the governor during the 1970s. This organization is composed of both individual and organizational members who employ a single lobbyist to work on women's issues in the state legislature. Each year prior to the legislative session,

WWU presents legislative forums throughout the state to determine which issues will be targeted for action during that session. Female legislators and appointed policymakers attend these sessions for two purposes. First, they provide training regarding the legislative process and information about attitudes of individual legislators. Second, they listen to the women in attendance to gather information about what issues are important and why. This is a good example of the women's community and the policymakers working together to empower themselves and develop effective alliances and strategies for policy change. In one recent legislative session alone this strategy resulted in enacting almost two dozen bills covering a wide range of issues including comparable worth, marital rape, Aid for Dependent Children, pensions and insurance, abortion, child care, and women-owned businesses. It is generally the community's responsibility to set up such training sessions and lobbying efforts while it is the policymakers' responsibility to empower the community to use policy systems effectively.

POLICY MAKES A DIFFERENCE: EXAMPLES

There are three major areas in which policy makes a difference in women's lives: policy and procedures, funding, and legislation or law.

Policy. In 1983 a new Job Training Partnership Act (JTPA) was implemented by the United States Congress. This act is the replacement for what was previously called the Comprehensive Employment Training Act (CETA). In order to implement this new program each community obtaining JTPA funds was mandated to appoint a committee (Private Industry Council, or PIC) that would be responsible for determining target populations and occupations for training, developing the policy regarding which employment and training programs are funded, how much funding each receives, how trainees are selected, and how trainees are reimbursed. In Seattle, the PIC was appointed jointly by the mayor and the county executive. Because the Seattle Office for Women's Rights (OWR)[2] is part of the mayor's executive division and had developed considerable credibility in the area of advocating for women's employment equity, both the mayor and the county executive asked this Department to make recommendations for appointments to the policy committee. Virtually every woman and ethnic minority recommended by OWR was appointed to the committee. As a result of these appointments, the Seattle/King County PIC has established a high target percentage for women participants and has instituted the maximum allowable funds to provide child care as a support service for women enrolled in job training programs. This same level of targeting women and allowing child care funding has not occurred in other communities. Child care is a substantial barrier to women's full involvement in employment and has critical economic and psychological impact on women and their children (Children's Defense Fund, 1982; Congressional Caucus for Women's Issues, 1983). Involvement of women in policy (both in recommending committee members and in participating as committee members) has, therefore, had a significant impact on women in Seattle.

Funding. In most communities two major sources of funding are the Community Development Block Grant (CDBG) through city agencies and United Way as a private fundraising entity. In those communities where substantial numbers of women participate in the CDBG process and fund allocation, women's programs have received an equitable share of these public funds. In the same manner, United Way, which has women at the policymaking level, is beginning to fund some agencies that address the needs of women and girls (battered women's shelters, rape relief programs, girls clubs, etc.). This is not to say, of course, that either CDBG monies or United Way monies have yet attained an equitable funding for women's programs. Women have been ignored for a long time and have to face the reality that women's programs are the "new kid on the block." Having women at the policymaking level advocating for meeting the needs of women, however, has made a difference in providing more funding to women's programs (Griffin, 1981).

Legislation. Legislation that addresses itself to women's needs has been profoundly noticeable in the last two decades. Rape laws, laws related to battered women, incest victims, and sexual harassment are all notable examples. It was not until women were evident as advocates, lobbyists, and legislators that laws addressing these issues began to find their way into legal codes. Had Eleanor Norton Holmes not been the director of the Equal Employment Opportunity Commission (EEOC), could we expect to have federal legislation relative to sexual harassment in the workplace today? We think not. This is not to say, of course, that male legislators have not supported legislation affecting women's lives; without support from men such legislation would not be on the books today since most legislators are men. It has been critical, however, to have women legislators who have often been willing to sponsor or track a bill through to implementation. Further, as women legislators work in city, state, and federal offices, men begin to think about women's issues simply by virtue of working with women. It is easy to forget any group of people when they are not represented. It is far more difficult to forget women when they sit on committees, chair hearings, and work as colleagues.

The Congressional Caucus for Women's Issues is a notable example of an alliance that was created by congresswomen committed to women's issues and that has been effective for three major reasons: First, it has increased the visibility of female policymakers and women's issues; second, they have done an extraordinary amount of homework, always being fully informed and articulate regarding the issues; and third, it has established solid relationships with men willing to work on women's issues. While the motivation for men in joining this caucus has been questioned by some constituents, the fact is that the results obtained from such legislative alliances are unquestionably positive for women and are to be applauded.

As women continue to be more and more prevalent in policymaking positions, we will see both an increase in quantity and quality of policy-related issues that affect women's lives.

WORKING TOGETHER

In summary, policy is critical in serving the needs of women in a pluralistic society. We believe that as women become policymakers, women's needs will receive far more attention and resolution. Further, we believe that policymakers are a part of the team that includes researchers, advocates, and direct service providers. Communication and understanding among people in all four roles must occur if any of the four areas are to be fully effective for women. Psychology training provides an effective foundation for policymakers. As psychology programs address themselves more completely to women's issues, the training for policymakers will be even more effective. A sexist psychology training merely provides a sexist foundation for policymakers. It is equally important, then, that we affect the educational system if we are to affect the world of policy. As with everything else, this will require communication and cooperation among women at virtually all levels of society if we are to achieve equitable participation.

NOTES

1. Tangri and Strasburg (1979) outline several ways in which researchers can affect and assist policymakers, while Wallston (1981) argues that the policymaking implication of research should be considered as early as the hypothesis and methodology development stages. Further, Wallston points to both current and future policy as valuable sources of research questions.

2. The Seattle Office for Women's Rights is an executive-branch city department mandated by a city council ordinance to promote social and economic equity for women and sexual minorities (lesbians and gays). The department devotes the majority of its attention to policy work including monitoring and analyzing city, state and federal policies that may affect women and sexual minorities; advocating for changes where barriers are found; writing ordinances where needed; and educating the community and other policymakers regarding the roles they can play in achieving equitable policies.

REFERENCES

Cherniss, C. (1980). *Staff burnout: Job stress in the human services.* Beverly Hills, CA: Sage.

Children's Defense Fund. (1982). *A children's defense budget: An analysis of the president's budget and children.* Washington, DC: Children's Defense Fund.

Congressional Caucus for Women's Issues. (1983). *Update, 3,* 3, March 31.

Forisha, B. & Goldman, B. (1981). *Outsiders on the inside.* Englewood Cliffs, NJ: Prentice-Hall.

Frieze, I. H., Parsons, J. E., Johnson, P. B., Ruble, D. N. & Zellman, G. L. (1978). *Women and sex roles: A social psychological perspective.* New York: Norton.

Griffin, M. (1981). Funding for women's programs. *Responsive Philanthropy,* (Spring).

Hunter, S. Warden, Iowa Correctional institution for women. (1983). Personal communication.

Merton, R. K. (1938). Social structure and anomie. *American Sociological Review, 3,* 672-682.

Peterson, E. (1983). The Kennedy Commission. In I. Tinker (Ed.), *Women in Washington: Advocates for public policy* (pp. 21-34). Beverly Hills, CA: Sage.

Rawalt, M. (1983). The equal rights amendment. In I. Tinker, (Ed.), *Women in Washington: Advocates for public policy* (pp. 49-78). Beverly Hills, CA: Sage.

Roberts, H. (1981). *Doing feminist research.* London: Routledge & Kegan Paul.

Schafran, L. H. (1981). Sandra O'Connor and the supremes. *MS,* (October), 71-87.

Sobel, S. B. & Russo, N. F. (1981). Equality, public policy and professional psychology. *Professional Psychology, 17*(1), 180-189.

Stanley, L. & Wise, S. (1983). *Breaking out: Feminist consciousness and feminist research.* London: Routledge & Kegan Paul.

Tangri, S. S. & Strausberg, G. L. (1979). Can research on women be more effective in shaping policy? *Psychology of Women Quarterly, 3,* 321-343.

Tinker, I. (1983). *Women in Washington: Advocates for public policy.* Beverly Hills, CA: Sage.

Wallston, B. S. (1981). What are the questions in psychology of women? A feminist approach to research. *Psychology of Women Quarterly, 5,* 597-617.

3

WOMEN AND PSYCHOTHERAPY RESEARCH

Marilyn Johnson
Arthur H. Auerbach

The focus of this chapter is on psychotherapy research rather than psychotherapy itself. After providing an overview of the history of research on gender effects in psychotherapy, we discuss the current status of research and its implications for policy. Following this, we discuss briefly two issues that bring women to therapy (weight problems and chemical addiction) that seem particularly ripe for new approaches. We then outline the current policy debate that is dominating the field of psychotherapy research. The resolution of this debate will no doubt affect the psychotherapeutic experiences of women but, as we suggest, resolution lies somewhere in the future. We conclude with policy recommendations, including the proposal that we heed Miller's (1969) call to "give psychology away."

OVERVIEW OF THE RESEARCH LITERATURE

In Brodsky's (1981) comprehensive synopsis of the history of research in this area, she describes a 10-year cycle starting with a classical psychotherapy research tradition that rarely considered gender effects, followed by a "blitz" of publications and presentations that cited bias, followed by reports of replications showing no or only occasional bias, followed by critical attacks of the methodology, followed by calls for methodological changes to single case studies and clinical field studies. This cycle is a useful framework in which to review some of the influential literature of the past 10-15 years and to discuss some policy implications of the current status of the field.

The first stage in the cycle is exemplified by the presence of exactly two index entries under "sex differences" in the major overview of psychotherapy research in the early 1970s (Bergin & Garfield, 1971).

One book appearing in 1970 which reviewed some of the same literature *did* examine several studies for gender effects but reported that neither client nor therapist gender significantly affected process or outcome (Meltzoff & Kornreich, 1970). Attention to gender was more the exception than the rule.

Three publications in the early 1970s focused attention on the topic of women and psychotherapy—the Broverman et al. (1970) study of therapists' attitudes, Chesler's book on sexism in psychotherapy (1972), and Weisstein's (1971) critique of the educational foundation and philosophy of clinical psychology. These works began the "blitz" of studies, most of which examined therapists' attitudes for responses to hypothetical clients. Reports of these studies filled journal pages and convention programs until the late 1970s. By the mid-1970s, findings of bias began to disappear, probably due in part to the reaction of the therapist-subjects who had read the journals and attended the conventions and could report more socially approved attitudes. Then two major critiques of the research appeared, faulting the politics of the researchers as well as their methodologies (Smith, 1980; Stricker, 1977).

What now appears to be the watershed on this topic was a 1979 conference on women and psychotherapy, cosponsored by the National Institute of Mental Health and the American Psychological Association. Invited experts reviewed the status of the attitude, process, and outcome research as well as that of prevalent disorders and therapeutic approaches; the report of this conference concluded with a number of recommended research priorities (Brodsky & Hare-Mustin, 1980). This marked the final stage of the cycle, the recommendations of new methodologies.

The conference report that contained summaries of the literature appeared during a period when several other summaries of the literature were published (Abramowitz & Dokecki, 1977; Davidson & Abramowitz, 1980; Whitley, 1979; and Zeldow, 1978). The assembly of this group of reviews allowed Richardson and Johnson (in press) to summarize present knowledge by examining the basis of that knowledge, its empirical foundation. They selected 154 studies of psychotherapy with adults that were cited in at least one of the review articles appearing between 1977 and 1980 and they categorized them in terms of methodology (experimental or naturalistic), citation frequency, and time period of publication. On the basis of this analysis, they concluded that only 35 percent of the studies described actual therapy (naturalistic, archival, and interview studies); the other 65 percent comprised experimental (analogue and questionnaire) studies that frequently used college student subjects. They concluded that much of what we believe about gender effects in psychotherapy is based upon hypothetical examples of therapists' or students' reports.

In addition, Richardson and Johnson (in press) found that although only some of the research reports found gender effects, these were the reports most frequently cited, and they speculated that this has tended to promote the belief that such effects are common. Finally, they reported that the number of naturalistic studies remained steady (and small) over the past decade while experimental studies mushroomed. The conclusion of their analysis has been echoed by others (Brodsky & Hare-Mustin, 1980; Orlinsky & Howard, 1980): Examination of gender differences should be built into all psychotherapy research and not studied in experimental isolation.

So the current status of the field is rather uncertain. The prominent literature of the past five years has consisted of reviews (e.g., Brodsky & Hare-Mustin, 1980), methodological critiques (Smith, 1980; Stricker, 1977), and reports on the current status of the field (Davidson & Abramowitz, 1980; Brodsky, 1980, 1981). Relatively little empirical work has appeared. Although clinicians publish theoretical and clinical reports on the conduct of psychotherapy with women (Collier, 1982), research reports have been rare in this period. Several authors agree that widespread bias has not been proven empirically (Stearns et al., 1980); at the same time, a number of them also urge continuation of vigilance (Brodsky, 1981; Franks, 1977; Murray & Abramson, 1983). To paraphrase Parloff's statement about outcome research results, many therapists still believe that "there's a pony in there somewhere" (1979, p. 303).

Richardson and Johnson (in press) referred to a hiatus in research in gender effects in psychotherapy; it is equally possible that research efforts are essentially over. The zeitgeist of the 1970s that favored attention to the impact of gender on therapy has changed for several reasons. First, when it became apparent that naturalistic research was needed to advance the area beyond the use of experimental methods, researchers confronted many of the same problems that psychotherapy researchers had struggled with for years: access to clinical populations, therapist reluctance to participate, criterion measurement, and so on. This has resulted in attrition of effort. Second, many of the investigators who conducted research in this area have shifted their emphases to other fields of investigation, whether due to academic pressures or to a broadening of interest. They often retain a focus on sex roles in later research but move away from psychotherapy research. Third, there are new emphases in psychotherapy research including demonstrations of efficacy and cost effectiveness, the development of therapy manuals, and the like. Finally, government funding for "social research" has been reduced, making it unlikely that studies of gender effects in psychotherapy would be supported (APA, 1983).

These factors may strike the death knell for research on gender effects in psychotherapy as it has been conceptualized during the 1970s. Nevertheless, should our pessimism prove untrue, we have two recommendations for the conduct of future research. Neither is unique to us, but both bear repeating. First, the search for a main effect should be abandoned. Every study which looks only for differences between male and female therapists ignores Kiesler's (1966) examination of the uniformity myth (all male therapists are *not* alike). It is in interactions that revealing results may appear (Brodsky, 1981, Orlinsky & Howard, 1980).

The best examples of research focusing on interactions are those of Orlinsky and Howard (1976, 1980) in their reanalyses of old data. In both the process (1976) and outcome (1980) studies, they reported findings that may have real meaning for the practice of psychotherapy. For example, they found that young single women had better psychotherapy experiences with female therapists but that therapists gender was unrelated to process for other life-status groups of female clients. It may be that, if identical data were collected on a present-day sample, women from other life-status groups would also do better with female therapists. In their outcome study, the initial finding that the clients of female therapists had better outcomes than those of males was explained more precisely when therapist experience level was examined; it was the inexperienced males who accounted for nearly all of the poor outcomes. It is possible that current efforts to educate therapists in training about sex roles and their effects in treatment might reduce the likelihood of such a finding if this study were replicated today. We commend this research and regret that it has not stimulated others to pursue this line of investigation.

Our second recommendation has also been made by others. With Brodsky and Hare-Mustin (1980), Orlinsky and Howard (1980), and Richardson and Johnson (in press), we believe that examination of gender effects should become a routine part of all psychotherapy research. The widespread attention to gender effects in psychotherapy has led some but not all psychotherapy researchers to build in examination of gender (Waskow, 1983). Despite the potential importance of assessing gender effects, this can only be recommended—not mandated.

The following are two examples of current projects that would benefit from attention to gender effects. A national survey has recently been proposed that would survey numbers of clients and therapists concerning psychosocial and self-help practices. While sex roles are not a focus of the research, the detailed data that would result could provide an excellent opportunity for assessing their impact on both parties in the therapeutic encounter (Mellinger, 1983). Such information is necessary in order to evaluate systematically the current effect of gender on therapy. Another study that might provide interesting data, although it is not designed to study gender effects, is Hill's (1983) new work linking therapists' intentions to their interventions. In this research, therapists tape-record a therapy session and then, during a replay of the tape, define the purpose of each intervention. Given that therapist-subjects would respond honestly, their intention-intervention patterns may give some indication of how intentions colored by bias determine choice of intervention. The client's response is not a focus of Hill's design but it could be examined as well.

IMPLICATIONS FOR MENTAL HEALTH POLICY

Policy can be considered in two senses—one relatively restricted, and the other more broad. The restricted sense is an official course adopted and followed by a government or institution. The broader sense includes the practices and attitudes of the relevant groups whether or not they represent an official course.

EFFECTS ON POLICY IN THE BROADER SENSE

Despite the uncertain picture resulting from a decade of research, there have been practical effects flowing from the attention given gender effects. Most of these effects were recommendations directed at clinicians of assorted disciplines, many of which were supported by the American Psychological Association. The Task Force on Sex Bias and Sex Role Stereotyping in Psychotherapeutic Practice (1978), which conducted a survey of women psychologists in several APA divisions, developed a set of guidelines for practice, which was published in the *American Psychologist*. In addition, a set of 13 principles for counseling and therapy with women was developed by the (then) Ad Hoc Committee on Women of APA Division 17; the principles were endorsed by a number of APA divisions and were published in the *Counseling Psychologist* (Hill, Birk, Blimline, Leonard, Hoffman, & Tanney, 1979). While there is at present no way to enforce adherence to these guidelines and principles, the Division 17 Committee on Women has developed a document outlining methods of implementing the principles (American Psychological Association Division 17 Committee on Women, 1983). Their dissemination of this document will be of special help to psychotherapists who are unfamiliar with this topic. They are also developing sets of questions concerning the psychology of women for submission to state licensing boards for use in credentialing examinations.

The devotion of special journal issues to the topic of counseling women (Birk & Tanney, 1976; Fitzgerald & Harmon, 1973; Hill et al., 1979), the allocation of program time for symposia and workshops on the topic at national, regional, and local professional meetings, and the organization of the NIMH-APA conference on women and psychotherapy have all served to inform professionals and to shape policy. Although it is usually assumed that all of the information is directed by feminists toward biased practitioners, there has been a moderating effect on the theory and practice of psychotherapists who have examined their own inclinations to impose their feminist values on clients and supervisees (Brodsky, 1977; Kenworthy, 1979; Rogers, 1978). They have urged examination of therapists' countertransference feelings and consequent interventions, and greater understanding toward clients whose goals lie outside a feminist vision.

Many of the policy recommendations have been directed primarily at experienced practitioners, but some efforts have been focused specifically on graduate students. As an example, the Division 17 Committee on Women distributed to all counseling psychology graduate training programs a set of existing models for training counselors of women (American Psychological Association, 1981). These models can be applied in individual courses, in clinical supervision, in several-week institutes, and in special graduate tracks. No assessment has been made of the degree to which the models have been implemented in graduate programs; such an evaluation would be useful in determining the extent to which these efforts have actually affected education. The Division 17 Committee on Women has also begun the development of curriculum modules that provide for the addition of new content from the psychology of women to courses in counseling theory and career development theory.

Certain policy efforts have been directed to some degree toward female clients. The publication of a consumer's handbook on women and psychotherapy (Federation of Organizations for Professional Women, 1981) is a milestone in that it synthesizes the best and most current information for women to consider when contemplating psychotherapy. Its existence is not widely enough known; we would recommend its distribution to traditional mental health institutions, religious institutions, and educational institutions to ensure the greatest impact. The Division 35 Task Force on Clinical Training and Practice is devoting its efforts to increasing the availability of this excellent resource to all women, with particular emphasis on reaching those women least likely to be informed about psychotherapy.

It is not our charge to assess psychotherapy itself. However, two examples of problems brought to therapy where women's unique needs were previously ignored but are now being considered deserve comment. These are alcohol and drug abuse and the weight/body-image problem. The implications of these problems for physical health as well as for emotional health increase our interest and concern.

ALCOHOL AND DRUG ABUSE

One of the groups most ignored by service providers has been women with alcohol and other drug problems. Theoretical examinations of these problems have grown (Gomberg, 1977) but they have not had a sufficiently strong impact on clinical services. Gomberg (1977) and Stephenson and Walker (1981) have pointed to the need for clinical programs designed for women because models of female addiction are underdeveloped. One reason for this is that, until recently, the number of women seeking help for reducing alcohol and other drug use was relatively small. The cultural belief that a drunk woman is more offensive than a drunk man has no doubt made women's needs seem less worthy to themselves as well as others. Treatment programs are still designed primarily for men, so women often avoid or drop out of these programs because of the lack of child care facilities or because there is no allowance for pregnancy. Addicted lesbians have special difficulties in such programs because of sexism that encourages women to be "superfeminine."

In addition, many traditional treatment programs use a punishment model in which members are urged to participate in often destructive encounter group self-revelations; such emphasis also leads to attrition (Cushey, Berger, & Densen-Gerber, 1981). Women's dislike of aggression and confrontation in groups has been noted by Lieberman in a study of C-R groups (1979); in postgroup assessments, the members cited aggressive confrontation and advice giving as the most negative factors of the group. Service providers should consult such research in designing treatment programs.

In addition to psychotherapeutic services, it is essential that prevention be promoted through educational efforts. We consider the greatest risks of addiction to lie in women's relationships with what we call 'the three Ds'' (doctors, dealers, and darlings), the persons, primarily men, who often lead them into addiction. It requires a strong sense of identity, a lot of assertiveness and a knowledge of drug dangers to resist them; well-designed educational and clinical services would promote these strengths. The optimal programs would provide psychotherapy (individual, group, marital, and/or family), assertiveness training, career counseling, and health education; this broad spectrum approach would address individual and social system issues and would place the treatment component within a larger context.

WEIGHT/BODY-IMAGE PROBLEMS

Women have been the major sufferers of eating disorders (Garfinkel & Garner, 1982) as well as the predominant clients of weight-reduction programs (Fodor, 1982). Treatment of anorexia nervosa and bulimia has focused on psychodynamic (Bruch, 1983) and, to a lesser extent, family systems formulations (Minuchin, Rosman, & Baker, 1978). On the other hand, efforts to aid women in losing weight emphasized behavioral approaches like those pioneered by Stuart (1967) in the 1970s. However, this method has not lived up to the perhaps unrealistic hopes it inspired (Fodor, 1982; Wooley, 1980). This failure to help clients sustain weight loss has led to a feminist analysis that suggests that professionals have colluded with the society at large to promote the idea that slenderness is a desirable goal for all women. "The very existence of treatments participates in the cultural designation and definition of physical and emotional disorders, thereby shaping the way people feel about themselves and what they do" (Wooley & Wooley, 1980, p. 135).

New treatment alternatives allowing clients more control have had some measure of success (Boskind-Lodahl, 1976; Loro, Fisher, & Levenkron, 1979) and Orbach (1979). Orbach's method, which includes exploration of body image in a supportive group context, has not been assessed empirically, but we would recommend the development of such research because of the method's apparent clinical wisdom.

Fodor (1982) had developed a cognitive-behavior treatment that, like Orbach's, questions the value of a universal striving for slimness. One element of her treatment is to encourage women to accept and even love themselves when they consider themselves overweight. While this is an appealing idea, it creates a dilemma for therapists who, on the one hand, want to undermine society's pressure for all women to resemble Twiggy and, on the other hand, want to respond to the genuine pain of their clients. This is an area badly in need of reevaluation and renewed attention.

IMPLICATIONS FOR POLICY IN THE RESTRICTED SENSE

Policy in the restricted sense (i.e., the official doctrines of institutions or government entities) presents us with a different kind of problem. First, we feel obliged to have a very firm foundation for our recommendations. Since these recommendations might become hardened into doctrine it is not enough that they merely appear reasonable to us or satisfy our current sense of what is proper. We would prefer an empirical foundation for them, so that we may confidently argue for their adoption. Second, we have to concern ourselves with the actual likelihood of their translation into policy.

Regarding the empirical foundations, we have noted earlier that there are few solidly grounded research findings about the therapy of women that have held up over time. What then are we to do? We may want to consider making recommendations not specifically about the therapy of women but about therapy in general. Let us tentatively consider the possibility that what would benefit women the most are those policy recommendations that would benefit both sexes the most. If we thus broaden the scope of our interest, we have more research findings to draw upon. We also have before us certain examples of the fate of actual policy recommendations regarding psychotherapy that have been made. We believe that those who recommend policies should give some thought to the probable vicissitudes of their suggestions; otherwise, making recommendations becomes an empty exercise.

When we look at real-life instances of recommendations, we find more complications than we may have thought. Our original set of assumptions was probably something like this: A policy recommendation begins with the recognition of an inequity in therapeutic practice. Psychotherapists will generally agree on the existence of the inequity because they are professionals acting in good faith. Their professional knowledge plus commonsense will lead them to policy recommendations that will correct the inequity. There will be no significant opposition to these recommendations, either from the ranks of policymakers or from the interested sectors of the community.

Let us compare this scheme with two actual current situations involving policy recommendations for psychotherapy. For one situation, the locus of activities and interest is policymakers—chiefly, Congress and the administration. For the second, the locus of activities and interest is a few leading professionals in the mental health care field.

The first situation was described in a series of papers devoted to governmental efforts to set policy on the psychotherapy enterprise. DeLeon, VandenBos, and Cummings (1983) and Banta and Saxe (1983) describe how Congress, through its concern about which Medicare expenses to reimburse, developed an interest in the effectiveness of psychotherapy. The idea was that demonstrated effectiveness would serve as a basis for reimbursement. This reasonable ideal led to some constructive results: the report on psychotherapy effectiveness for the Office of Technology Assessment (Office of Technology Assessment, 1980), the institution by the National Center for Health Care Technology of a program for assessing the psychotherapies (Perry, 1983), and the introduction of a bill in the United States Senate that would have set up the machinery needed for rational decisions about psychotherapy reimbursement (Banta & Saxe, 1983). This program would have included research on therapy effectiveness. However, the bill did not become law (Banta & Saxe, 1983), and the National Center for Health Care Technology ceased operations when its funds were cut off (Perry, 1983). Thus, we must conclude that even when there are strong forces within the policymaking establishment favoring action that would benefit psychotherapy, there is no guarantee that that action will occur. Opposition forces may arise that will reverse the policy and cancel the steps already taken.

The second situation illustrates the strong differences of opinion on fundamental issues that can occur within the psychotherapy professions before the policymakers even get involved. Along with others, Gerald Klerman has for some time been dissatisfied with the lack of demonstrated efficacy and safety of the various kinds of psychotherapy practiced in this country. While he was director of the Alcohol, Drug Abuse and Mental Health Administration, he called for research that would demonstrate the efficacy and safety of the various psychotherapies. Recently he and Perry London have joined in advocating a far-reaching national program to improve the quality of psychotherapy and correct inequities in its reimbursement. Their position has been stated in journal articles (Klerman, 1983; London & Klerman, 1982) and in scientific meetings, notably in a debate held at the 1983 meeting of the American Psychiatric Association (Klerman, London, Michels, & Sharfstein, 1983).

In conformity with the scheme referred to above, the London/Klerman (1982) proposal began with an observed inequity. They noted that large amounts of public money were supporting psychotherapies whose safety and efficacy had not been demonstrated. (In the following we will use the word "effectiveness" to designate safety and efficacy). This expenditure of public funds occurred through payments for federal employees and their dependents. London and Klerman (1982) also noted that the number and variety of these therapies were increasing, and that the great majority of them showed no interest in adequately demonstrating their own effectiveness, although they asserted it confidently. Klerman (1983) stated that an excessive amount of public money went for the support of long-term psychotherapy of relatively minor emotional conditions. He referred to such therapies as "growth enhancement" or "happiness enhancement." Since the amount of money for reimbursement is limited, and is likely to become more scarce relative to need, London and Klerman called for a more rational reimbursement policy for the distribution of public funds. It should be guided by the principle of "humane priorities," according to which reimbursement decisions would represent a balancing of considerations of general equity, the urgency of the condition to be treated, and the effectiveness of the proposed treatment. They advocated a long-term policy consisting of a public statement of commitment to the principle of humane priorities, the creation of a public body to assess treatments, the support of research to provide data of effectiveness, and a means of linking research findings to reimbursement decisions.

We think most impartial observers would acknowledge that this proposal is praiseworthy in its ethical motives and in its goals. If it worked according to its proponents' hopes, it would correct injustices, raise the moral consciousness of psychotherapists, and increase the level of rationality attached to the whole psychotherapy enterprise. The health care system would be officially committed to a search for effective therapies, the effectiveness to be established by scientific criteria. Unsafe and ineffective treatments would be eliminated.

It is therefore noteworthy that the opposition encountered by this proposal has been powerful and apparently nearly unanimous. To our knowledge, everyone who has spoken publicly on the matter has opposed it. It will be interesting to briefly review the reasons for this opposition, both the stated reasons and those that may be inferred.

Some of the opposition arguments concern the inevitable practical difficulties in implementing the proposal. Parloff (1982) has pointed out that because of the large number of therapies and of disorders, the attempt to establish effectiveness data through adequate clinical trials would be impossibly difficult and expensive since each of the therapies would have to be tested against most of the disorders. It has also been claimed that the London/Klerman proposal would discriminate against psychotherapy because demonstrated effectiveness of treatment is not required for reimbursement for medical treatments.

Neither the proponents nor opponents of the London/Klerman proposal considered the special point of view of women in psychotherapy. When we do so, we encounter another possible complication, having to do with the difference between what is best for the whole population and what is best for subgroups. Suppose that the London/Klerman proposal were carried out and, through its system of selective approval, increased the rationality and effectiveness of the therapy received by the *average person*. Might there not be subgroups of clients who would suffer from centralized decisions about approved therapies? For example, for some women, psychotherapy is a corrective experience against the unfortunate effects of sex role socialization patterns. But such use of therapy might not win the support of a central agency that is sifting through treatments for what is considered the major mental health problems. Thus, the particular needs of a subgroup may be lost sight of in the bureaucratic machinery.

What we have described is part of an ongoing story that promises to be a long one and whose ultimate outcome is not apparent. But we believe that there are already certain conclusions to be drawn from these efforts to influence psychotherapy-related policy.

(1) There is unlikely to be general agreement on the existence of an inequity or at least whether it is serious enough to warrant strong action.

(2) There will be disagreement on what steps should be taken to correct it.

(3) The field of psychotherapy abounds with interest groups, each naturally opposed to any change that threatens its status.

(4) Even when good intentions have been translated into a government mechanism for implementing them, there is no guarantee that the implementation will actually be carried out; a change in policy may sweep away the machinery.

(5) Policy procedures that benefit the average client may not be beneficial to subgroups of clients, for example, women using therapy in a particular way.

POLICY RECOMMENDATIONS

Some attention should be paid to the rise and fall of fashions in women's issues. We note a pattern consisting of a sequence of phases: A woman's issue becomes "popular." This issue may be a problem prevalent in women such as eating disorders or trauma following rape; it may be a form of therapy (e.g., assertiveness training directed chiefly at women). Its popularity may attract funds for research projects, but mainly it attracts practitioners who become experts in the condition. After some time, the popularity fades, and interest shifts to another issue. Unfortunately, the fading usually occurs before much solid research on the condition or its treatment has accumulated. This pattern is not conducive to solid, permanent improvement in the therapy of women; it may predispose the issue to exploitation by some practitioners.

We would recommend attention to those areas previously discussed. First, psychotherapists, their teachers and their clients must be better educated about the idea of sex-fair therapy. Second, the examination of gender effects in all naturalistic psychotherapy studies should be encouraged. Third, more intensified efforts should be directed at helping women understand the social as well as the personal meaning of their difficulties with food and with drugs of all kinds. Finally, we would like to endorse the idea of educating clients and helping them to help themselves.

GIVING PSYCHOLOGY AWAY

In his 1969 presidential address to the American Psychological Association, George Miller exhorted us to use psychology as a means of promoting human welfare; he urged us to "give psychology away." These ideas were expressed at a time of high social consciousness, in a climate very different than that of the present. It has been said that, at present, there may be no takers if feminist psychologists try to give psychology away (Parlee, 1983); we do not feel so pessimistic. The feminist therapy movement certainly espoused Miller's ideas as did much of the self-help movement in which professionals served as consultants and facilitators (Kravetz, 1980). Miller emphasized that the means of giving psychology away would be through educating the public via offering help in response to their needs. He offered White's (1959) concepts of competence and effectance as the goals of this education. Self-help may be especially useful in providing women opportunities to develop a sense of effectiveness through helping themselves and through helping others.

We believe that it is important to focus more strongly on self-help groups because, as in traditional psychotherapy, women comprise the majority of these groups' membership. While some group members are also in psychotherapy (Lieverman, 1979), most are not. There are two points of view among self-help experts: one group believes that self-help is most effective when used in conjunction with professional help and the other group believes that self-help should replace much professional assistance. We would recommend that more careful research of self-help groups comparing these functions be conducted.

Lieberman has pointed to difficulties in analyzing process and outcome in self-help groups but believes he and Borman (1979) have demonstrated via studies of a number of different kinds of groups (widows, C-R groups, heart patient groups, etc.) that they *do* provide critical support. The factor that appears most salient across various kinds of groups is Yalom's (1975) universality factor, which embodies the idea that one is not isolated and unique but rather that one's pains and joys are shared and understood by many others. This realization, plus the support and acceptance of others in the group, is a critical curative element.

In addition to the need for more research, it is essential for clinicians to become informed about self-help groups to which they might refer clients or with which they might act as a resource (Rodolfa & Hungerford, 1982). This is sometimes a difficult task because of the proliferation of such groups but it can be done. It has been demonstrated that informed clinicians *do* make use of self-help groups as adjuncts or instead of their own services (Todres, 1982).

Professionals need (1) informative data about the efficacy of self-help groups; (2) information about groups in their area; and (3) a set of principles and practices for referring the right person to the right group. Several policy recommendations regarding self-help groups were made by Lieberman and his colleagues to the President's Commission on Mental Health (1978), including the development of clearinghouses of information about the groups. The self-help movement has become a worldwide phenomenon (e.g., the Canadian government provides financial assistance for developing clearinghouses and materials, the World Health Organization is promoting its importance, etc.). In the United States, 20 universities are currently creating self-help clearinghouses. The directory of self-help groups in Chicago (produced by the only free-standing national clearinghouse show a rise of 129 percent in the number of groups in that city in the past two years (Borman, 1983).

EDUCATION OR LEGISLATION?

We have distinguished between policy in the broader and in the more restricted sense. Corresponding to this distinction are two general ways of influencing policy, which may be called education and legislation. Our recommendations have been basically suggestions for education of therapists as well as clients. The notion of legislation is appealing because it promises a large-scale, logical attack on the problem with all the resources of government. For example, the London/Klerman proposal aspires to nothing less than a change in the basis of psychotherapeutic practice. It aims to weaken the principles that currently guide practice—authority, plausibility, fashion—and to substitute rationality and empirical grounding for them. If it worked, such a program would, among many other achievements, bypass the vagaries of fashion referred to above. However, we have given examples of the vicissitudes of plans and programs designed to change public policy, and these instances naturally qualify our optimism about what can be accomplished through legislation. What is needed—but what is very difficult to achieve—is to gain some understanding of the complex system in which psychotherapy is embedded. Some of the elements of this system are the following: the various psychotherapeutic professions and schools of therapy, with their competing interests; the great number of clients and potential clients, varying widely in their degree of pathology, personality structure, and attitude toward psychotherapy; policymakers with their prejudices, skepticism, and concern with issues other than the correction of inequities in psychotherapy; the psychotherapy research community, which has its own set of interests and ambitions; in short, all of the entrenched interests with a stake in preserving the status quo. If one had perfect knowledge of this complex system, she or he could, theoretically, exert leverage at the optimal point. In practice, knowledge is imperfect and the results of action are uncertain.

REFERENCES

Abramowitz, C., & Dokecki, P. (1977). The politics of clinical judgment: Early empirical returns. *Psychological Bulletin, 84,* 460-476.

American Psychological Association Division 17 (1981). *Report of the Division 17 Committee on Women Task Force on Training for Counseling Women* (Available from Mary Sue Richardson, Department of Counselor Education, New York University, New York, NY 10003.)

American Psychological Association Division 17 Committee on Women (1983). *Rationale and implementation of the principles concerning the counseling/psychotherapy of women.* Unpublished manuscript.

American Psychological Association (1978). Report of the Task Force on Sex Bias and Sex-Role Stereotyping in Psychotherapeutic Practice. *American Psychologist, 30,* 1169-1175.

American Psychological Association (1983). *Status report on the federal budget as it affects psychology, and behavioral and social science research, training, and services.*

Banta, H., & Saxe, L. (1983). Reimbursement for psychotherapy: Linking efficacy research and public policymaking. *American Psychologist, 38,* 918-923.

Bergin, A., & Garfield, S. (Eds.), (1971). *Handbook of psychotherapy and behavior change.* New York: John Wiley.

Birk, J., & Tanney, M. (Eds.). (1976). Counseling women II. *The Counseling Psychologist, 6*(2).

Borman, L. (1983). Personal communication, September 2.

Boskind-Lodahl, M. (1976). Cinderella's stepsisters: A feminist perspective on anorexia nervosa and bulimia. *Signs: Journal of Women in Culture and Society, 2,* 341-356.

Brodsky, A. (1977). Counter-transference issues and the woman therapist: Sex and the student therapist. *The Clinical Psychologist, 30,* 12-14.

Brodsky, A. (1980). A decade of feminist influence on psychotherapy. *Psychology of Women Quarterly, 4,* 331-344.

Brodsky, A. (1981). *Sex, race and class issues in psychotherapy research.* Master lecture presented at the annual meeting of the American Psychological Association, Los Angeles.

Brodsky, A., & Hare-Mustin, R. (Eds.). (1980). *Women and psychotherapy.* New York: Guilford Press.

Broverman, I., Broverman, D., Clarkson, F., Rosenkrantz, P., & Vogel, S. (1970). Sex role stereotypes and clinical judgments of mental health. *Journal of Consulting and Clinical Psychology, 34,* 1-7.

Bruch, H. (1983). *Eating disorders.* New York: Basic Books.

Chesler, P. (1972). *Women and madness.* Garden City, NY: Doubleday.

Collier, H. (1982). *Counseling women.* New York: The Free Press.

Cushey, W., Berger, J., & Densen-Gerber, J. (1981). Issues in the treatment of female addiction: A review and critique of the literature. In E. Howell & M. Bayes (Eds.), *Women and mental health.* New York: Basic Books.

Davidson, C., & Abramowitz, S. (1980). Sex bias in clinical judgment: Later empirical returns. *Psychology of Women Quarterly, 4,* 377-395.

DeLeon, P. VandenBos, G., & Cummings, N. (1983). Psychotherapy—Is it safe, effective and appropriate? The beginning of an evolutionary dialogue. *American Psychologist, 38,* 907-911.

Federation of Organizations for Professional Women (1981). *Women and psychotherapy: A consumer handbook.* Washington, DC: Author.

Fitzgerald, L., & Harmon, L. (Eds.). (1973). Counseling women. *The Counseling Psychologist, 4*(1).

Fodor, I. (1982). Behavior therapy for the overweight woman: A time for reappraisal. In M. Rosenbaum & C. Franks (Eds.), *Perspectives on behavior therapy in the eighties: Selected and updated proceedings from the First World Congress of Behavior Therapy.* New York: Springer.

Franks, V. (1979). Gender and psychotherapy. In E. Gomberg & V. Franks (Eds.) *Gender and disordered behavior.* New York: Brunner/Mazel.

Garfinkel, P., & Garner, D. (1982). *Anorexia nervosa: A multidimensional perspective.* New York: Brunner/Mazel.

Gomberg, E. (1979). Problems with alcohol and other drugs. In E. Gomberg & V. Franks (Eds.), *Gender and disordered behavior.* New York: Brunner/Mazel.

Hill, C. (1983, July). *Therapist's intentions in selecting interventions within psychotherapy sessions.* Paper presented at the meeting of the Society for Psychotherapy Research, Sheffield, England.

Hill, C., Birk, J., Blimline, C., Leonard, M., Hoffman, N., & Tanney, M. (Eds.).(1979). Counseling women III. *The Counseling Psychologist, 8*(1).

Kenworthy, J. (1979). Androgyny in psychotherapy: But will it sell in Peoria? *Psychology of Women Quarterly, 3,* 231-240.

Kiesler, D. (1966). Some myths of psychotherapy research and the search for a paradigm. *Psychological Bulletin, 65,* 110-136.

Klerman, G. (1983). The efficacy of psychotherapy as the basis for public policy. *American Psychologist, 38,* 929-934.

Klerman, G., London, P., Michels, R., & Sharfstein, S. (1983, May). *A scientific debate: Should third party reimbursement be reserved for treatments proven safe and effective?* Symposium conducted at the meeting of the American Psychiatric Association, New York City.

Kravetz, D. (1980). Consciousness-raising and self-help. In A. Brodsky & R. Hare-Mustin (Eds.), *Women and psychotherapy.* New York: Guilford Press.

Lieberman, M. (1979). Analyzing change mechanisms in groups. In M. Lieberman & L. Borman (Eds.). *Self-help groups for coping with crisis.* San Francisco: Jossey-Bass.

Lieberman, M., & Borman, L. (Eds.). (1979). *Self-help groups for coping with crisis.* San Francisco: Jossey-Bass.

London, P., & Klerman, G. (1982). Evaluating psychotherapy. *American Journal of Psychiatry, 139,* 709-717.

Loro, A., Fisher, E., & Levenkron, J. (1979). Comparison of established and innovative weight-reduction treatment procedures. *Journal of Applied Behavior Analysis, 12,* 141-155.

Mellinger, G. (1983). Personal communication, March 3.

Meltzoff, J., & Kornreich, M. (Eds.). (1970). *Research in psychotherapy.* New York: Atherton Press.

Miller, G. (1969). Psychology as a means of promoting human welfare. *American Psychologist, 24,* 1-13.

Minuchin, S., Rosman, G., & Baker, L. (1978). *Psychosomatic families: Anorexia nervosa in context.* Cambridge, MA: Harvard University Press.

Murray, J., & Abramson, P. (Eds.). (1983). *Bias in psychotherapy.* Los Angeles: University of California Press.

Office of Technology Assessment (1980). *The efficacy and cost-effectiveness of psychotherapy. Background paper 3: The implications of cost-effectiveness analysis of medical technology.* Washington, DC: U.S. Government Printing Office.

Orbach, S. (1979). *Fat is a feminist issue.* New York: Berkley Books.

Orlinsky, D., & Howard, K. (1976). The effect of sex of therapist on the therapeutic experiences of women. *Psychotherapy: Theory, Research and Practice, 13,* 82-88.

Orlinsky, D., & Howard, K. (1980). Gender and psychotherapeutic outcome. In A. Brodsky & R. Hare-Mustin (Eds.), *Women and psychotherapy.* New York: Guilford Press.

Parlee, M. (1983, August). The presidency of Division 35 from 1982-1983. In F. Denmark (Chair), *Division 35—Commemorating the first ten years of achievement.* Symposium conducted at the meeting of the American Psychological Association, Anaheim, CA.

Parloff, M. (1979). Can psychotherapy research guide the policymaker? A little knowledge may be a dangerous thing. *American Psychologist, 34,* 296-306.

Parloff, M. (1982). Psychotherapy research evidence and reimbursement decision: Bambi meets Godzilla. *American Journal of Psychiatry, 139,* 718-727.

Perry, S. (1983).The National Center for Health Care Technology: Assessment of psychotherapy for policymaking. *American Psychologist, 38,* 924-928.

President's Commission on Mental Health (1978). *Commission report* (Vol. 1). Washington, DC: U.S. Government Printing Office.

Richardson, M., & Johnson, M. (in press). Counseling women. In S. Brown & R. Lent (Eds.), *Handbook of counseling psychology.* New York: John Wiley.

Rodolfa, E., & Hungerford, L. (1982). Self-help groups: A referral resource for professional therapists. *Professional Psychology, 13,* 345-353.

Rogers, M. (1978). Fascinating womanhood as a regression in the emotional maturation of women. *Psychology of Women Quarterly, 2,* 202-214.

Smith, M. (1980). Sex bias in counseling and psychotherapy. *Psychological Bulletin, 87,* 392-407.

Stearns, B., Penner, L., & Kimmel, E. (1980). Sexism among psychotherapists: A case not yet proven. *Journal of Consulting and Clinical Psychology, 48,* 548-550.

Stephenson, P., & Walker, G. (1981). The psychiatrist-woman patient relationship. In E. Howell & M Bayes (Eds.), *Women and mental health.* New York: Basic Books.

Stricker, G. (1977). Implications of research for psychotherapeutic treatment of women. *American Psychologist, 32,* 14-22.

Stuart, R. (1967). Behavioural control of overeating. *Behavior Research and Therapy, 5,* 357-365.

Todres, R. (1982). Professional attitudes, awareness and use of self-help groups. In L. Borman, L. Borck, R. Hess, & F. Pasquale (Eds.), *Helping people to help themselves: Self-help and prevention.* New York: The Haworth Press.

Waskow, I. (1983). Personal communication, May 18.

Weisstein, N. (1971). Psychology constructs the female or the fantasy life of the male psychologist. In M. Garskof (Ed.), *Roles women play: Reading toward women's liberation.* Belmont, CA: Brooks/Cole.

White, R. (1959). Motivation reconsidered: The concept of competence. *Psychological Review, 66,* 297-333.

Whitley, B. (1979). Sex roles and psychotherapy: A current appraisal. *Psychological Bulletin, 86,* 1309-1321.

Wooley, S., & Wooley, D. (1980). Eating disorders: Obesity and anorexia. In A. Brodsky & R. Hare-Mustin (Eds.), *Women and psychotherapy.* New York: Guilford Press.

Yalom, I. (1975). *The theory and practice of group psychotherapy.* New York: Basic Books.

Zeldow, P. (1978). Sex differences in psychiatric evaluation and treatment. *Archives of General Psychiatry, 35,* 89-93.

4

THE RELATIONAL SELF IN WOMEN: DEVELOPMENTAL THEORY AND PUBLIC POLICY

Alexandra G. Kaplan
Janet L. Surrey

Until recently, one would search in vain for a theory of psychological development that consistently and explicitly explored developmental patterns for women. Previous theories of development were put forth to portray human development pertaining, so the theorists would argue, to women and men alike. However, even a cursory reading of such theories makes clear that, in fact, in every case basic assumptions about the course and goals of human growth derived from the perspective and experience of men (Gilligan, 1982). This had problematic consequences for attempts to assess women's psychological growth, in that women were understood within a context that did not quite "fit." It also meant that those qualities, aspirations, and motivating factors that are more typically found in women than in men did not figure prominently—if at all—in such theories. The loss, then, was not just in the understanding of women, but in understanding certain key elements of the human experience (Miller, 1976).

Perhaps the most central aspect of the human experience that becomes lost when theory derives from the male experience is the development, meaning, and utilization of one's capacity for relatedness—what we will term the *self-in-relation* (Surrey, 1983). We are using this concept in its broadest sense—to encompass not only one's attention to and capacities in enhancing and furthering connectedness with others, but more fundamentally in the way in which being a relational being evolves as a core component of women's psychological development. It is a primary factor in women's core sense of self, the conscious and unconscious identifications that shape her way of being in the world, her aspirations and longings, and her modes of achievement and sense of purpose. In turn, this implies that any model of psychological growth for women must include, as a major component, a careful consideration of relational development throughout the life span, including the changes in the quality and meanings of connectedness to others, and the changes in one's self-image as a relational being. Finally, it suggests that women's strivings and achievements are best fueled by a process of mutual empowerment—that self-enhancement occurs most fruitfully in a relational context where one's own growth is coexistent with and facilitative of the growth and fulfillment of another.

Such a model has major implications for public policy formulations. At base, it stresses that psychological development occurs *in context,* at the point of intersection of the individual and her social/psychological environment. Policy decisions based on a recognition of self-in-relation, then, would be oriented to creating contexts that would facilitate mutual empowerment and that would recognize the relational meanings and implications inherent in organizational structure.

CRITIQUE OF EXISTING THEORIES

Existing theories of psychological development, including the psychoanalytic and neopsychoanalytic theories of Freud (1925/1953), Sullivan (1953), Erikson (1950), and Mahler, and the more recent theories of adult development offered by Levinson (1978) and Gould (1978), all equate maturation and healthy adult functioning with some form of autonomy, separation, independence, or individuation from others. That is, development is portrayed as a sequential movement from fusion or enmeshment with the mothering one in the early months of life to a condition in which one is able to act independently and has evolved a core sense of self that is not "dependent on" or "in need of" others. Relationships with others are by no means ignored in these theories. In fact the theories do make important contributions to recognizing the significance of early mother-infant relations, and the processes of unconscious identifications that begin at this phase and that play a key role in one's evolving core sense of self. However, as Chodorow (1978) has elucidated, these theories paid insufficient attention to differences in maternal relationships with daughters and sons, and particularly the ways in which the mother-daughter relationship, even in its early phases, fosters a process of self-identification within a relational context, and of mutual attention to the affect of another.

A developmental theory that derives from women's experience, then, would need to pay much closer attention to these early precursors of mutuality and the early development of the self-in-relation.

Relationships per se are not ignored in theoretical portrayals of adolescent and adult development, especially in Sullivan's neoanalytic formulations (1953). However, for Sullivan it is primarily the specific impact of a particular relationship that is important (e.g., mother, playmates, "chum"), rather than a process of evolving and refining one's core sense of self as a relational being. Further, at the point of adolescent sexual identity formation, Sullivan clearly has men in mind, as in his assertion that the commonly held distinction between the "good" and the "bad" girl impairs boys' ability to simultaneously satisfy their needs for sexuality and self-esteem (Kaplan & Yasinski, 1980).

The absence of a developmental theory centered on the self-in-relation means that women do not fit the prescribed pattern. Unfortunately, it has been most often the woman and not the theory that was held to be inadequate. One variant of this pattern has been that women are seen as lacking something; the "deficiency" model. Freudian theory illustrates this perspective most clearly in his assertion that women's conscious and unconscious reactions to the "fact of her castration" (1931/1974) played a formative role in key aspects of her personality structure, including passivity, masochism and narcissism, and superego deficiencies.

Another major consequence of the nonrecognition of women's core self-in-relation is that her relational qualities and strivings tend to be seen as pathological. Qualities that a theory of self-in-relation might consider evidence of mutuality or contextual sensitivity are considered signs of "dependency" or "immaturity" (Stiver, 1983). This is especially true in descriptions of adult women, and particularly adult women in heterosexual relationships. Not only is the supportive and caring nature of these relationships ignored, but in addition there is no analysis of the social construction of marriage that might leave the women themselves out of touch with their own relational strengths (Miller, 1983). In a similar way, "too much relationship" between a mother and her child becomes labeled as "intrusive" or "overinvolved" and is held responsible for virtually every childhood psychological disorder. Again, what is lost is the benefit to mother and child of being in relation, of developing a sense of self that grows through connections with others and that gains sustenance as a relational being. Also lost is the context of isolation and devaluing in which mothering often occurs, and its detrimental impact on the evolving mother-child relationship.

It is essential, then, that major aspects of developmental theory be reformulated so as to take into account the meaning and evolution of the self-in-relation. This chapter will first turn to the initial dimensions of such a reformulation. With this new model in mind, we will then turn to potential implications for public policy, and the ways in which the social structure can serve to enhance and foster key aspects of women's psychological development.

SELF-IN-RELATION:
A THEORY OF WOMEN'S DEVELOPMENT

Before discussing the early development and core structure of the self-in-relation, it is important to clarify and describe the aspects of adult women's experience which these concepts are useful in explaining. As Jean Baker Miller (1976) has pointed out, women in our culture are the "carriers" of certain aspects of the total human experience (e.g., emotionality, acceptance of human vulnerability, and most important of all, the fostering of the growth and development of others). This last characteristic is sometimes called "nurturance" or "caretaking" when applied to the mothering of infants and children, but it is clearly a much broader aspect of woman's primary identification and relational experience. This interest in and ability to be closely involved in other's development and well-being are seen at all stages of life for women. Therapy research and clinical observation show, in general that women have a greater interest and capacity for relatedness, emotional closeness, and boundary flexibility than do men (Orlinsky & Howard, 1978). The capacity for empathy, again consistently found to be more developed in women (Hoffman, 1977), appears to be a good organizing concept to explain women's relational experiences.

Jordan (1983) has reexamined the concept of empathy in this light. She argues that the ability to experience, comprehend, and respond to the inner state of another person is a highly complex process relying on a high level of psychological development and ego strength. Accurate empathy involves a simultaneous balancing of affective arousal and cognitive structuring; an ability to build on the subjective, emotional experience of identification with the other person to forming a higher order cognitive assimilation of this experience. Kohut (1971) has emphasized the profound importance to the developing child of the experience of empathy from the early parental figures. He does not describe, however, the origins and development of the capacity for empathy which in the past have often been construed as a highly subjective, intuitive, slightly mysterious, and unexplainable phenomena. The concept of the relational self relies heavily on this new definition of empathy, stressing the growth of such capacity as primary in women's development.

Self-in-relation theory begins to sketch out a developmental model to account for the development of empathic competencies in women, beginning with the early mother-daughter relationship. The assumption is that the "self" in women is organized and developed through practice in relationships where the goal is toward increasing development of reciprocal and mutually empathic relationships. Such a theoretical framework must examine the following:

(1) What are the *motivational dynamics* of such relational development? How do women grow and change, and what is the motivation for this process?

(2) What are the *early precursors* of this relational capacity as developed within the mother-daughter relationship? What would be the core self-structure formed in this relationship? How does this early core sense of self relate to the development of the capacity for "mothering" in adult life? Winnicott (1965) has described the "good-enough" mother as essential for all human growth, but he does not specify the learned determinants of this essential characteristic nor its centrality as a primary component of women's identity and development.

(3) What are the key elements of this theory that would describe the development of this relational capacity throughout the life cycle? What would be the necessary experiences and relational contexts necessary for such development to proceed along healthy lines?

(4) What would be the strengths and weaknesses inherent in such a developmental pathway, especially given the structures and values of our current social, political, and educational organizations? How could those structures and values be modified to encourage women's participation and contribution?

EARLY ASPECTS OF
THE MOTHER-DAUGHTER RELATIONSHIP:
PRECURSORS OF THE SELF-IN-RELATION

The dynamics of the mother-daughter relationship are crucial in understanding the early precursors of relational development in women.

There are three key aspects of this relationship that influence the core sense of self as it develops throughout the life cycle. They are primary identification, mutual identification, and mutual reciprocity and empowerment.

PRIMARY IDENTIFICATION

It has been well established that the early mother-daughter relationship has important meaning in forming women's sense of self (Chodorow, 1978). Having a same or different gender parent as the primary caretaker is thought to have powerful impact on all later male and female development (Dinnerstein, 1978). Girls develop a basic sense of self through *primary identification* with their mothers. It is important to note that this primary identification with the mother for girls is a very early identification with mother *as* the mothering, caretaking person. Boys in our culture are encouraged to curtail this primary identification with mother, since developing a male identification requires a high degree of differentiation and emotional disconnection (separation) from the mother. Thus, girls seem to develop a capacity for a less conflictual identification with the other person that supports the formation of more open emotional connection and boundary flexibility.

MUTUAL IDENTIFICATION

The second key aspect of the early mother-daughter relationship is the relative ease and fluidity of mutual identification that appears to be significantly different from what is acceptable in our culture between mothers and sons. The mother more easily identifies with the daughter (an identification based on part on body likeness and supported by cultural norms), which leaves the daughter feeling more deeply understood and "recognized" for herself at a deep, emotional level. This early experience becomes the basis for the woman's sense of expectation of being affectively recognized, understood, and validated within relationship.

MUTUAL RECIPROCITY AND EMPOWERMENT

The emotional and cognitive connections based on shared feeling states and identification develop over time into a mutual reciprocal process where both mothers and daughters become highly responsive to the feeling states of each other. Both are energized to care for, respond to, or attend to the well-being of the other. Through this mutual sensitivity and mutual caretaking mothers already are teaching practices of mothering or caring to girl children. Again, by "mothering" I do not necessarily mean what has been traditionally labeled as one-directional mothering, but attentiveness and emotional responsivity to the other as an intrinsic, ongoing aspect of one's own experience. This perspective enriches existing theories of what constitutes mothering. Winnicott's idea of the "good-enough mother" who is capable of fusing in such a way as to be responsive to the feeling states and needs of the infant does not go far enough in elaborating the awesome complexity and skill involved in mothering behaviors. We can at least say that within the early mother-daughter relationship—certainly as it grows over the life cycle—we can begin to see the precursors of women's capacity and pleasure in relatedness: the ability to identify with the other, the sense of connectedness through feeling states, and the activation and energizing based on complex cognitive operations involving the awareness of the needs and/or reality of another person as well as one's own. This we have labeled *empowerment,* the mobilizing energy of relationship.

It is important to note that the development of accurate empathy involves a complex process that involves interactive validation of the differences between self and other and the recognition of the other as an individual with changing needs and growing and newly developing competencies. Within the early mother-daughter relationship, the daughter is thus encouraged to learn to take the role of both the provider ("mother") and the receiver ("daughter"), depending on the needs of the situation or the individual at any given time. Clearly, in problematic situations, both the daughter and mother can become overinvolved in feeling responsible for the other. But this model does suggest that a healthy degree of reciprocity is essential for woman's growth and development. The dynamics of such reciprocity establish in women the capacity to move from one perspective to another as the needs of the relational situation arise.

The basic elements of the core self in women can be summarized as follows: (1) a basic emotional connection and ability to identify with the other; (2) the expectation of mutuality and the sharing of experience leading to a heightening of self-awareness and sense of well-being; and (3) the expectation of relationship as a process of mutual sensitivity and mutual responsibility as an ongoing, intrinsic aspect of one's own growth and motivational framework. In adult women, we can surmise how these basic factors develop. Women experience a heightened, enhanced sense of their personal identity

and personal powers in the context of relationships. This early emotional sensitivity develops into complex cognitive and affective interactions that we later identify as empathy. The connectedness and the
capacity for identification is the basis for the later feeling that to
understand and to be understood are crucial for self-acceptance and
are fundamental to the feeling of existing as part of a unit or network
larger than the individual.

Kohut (1971) emphasizes the importance of empathy as a more
one-directional, parent-to-child phenomenon. We are broadening this
to a more two-way interactional model, where it becomes as important
to understand as to be understood. All of us probably need to feel
understood or recognized by others. It is equally paramount, but
not yet emphasized, that women all through their lives feel the need
to understand the other. Indeed, such understanding is desired as
an essential part of their own growth and development. Such a model
follows the usual and typical form of self-development. Some
problems that can follow in development based on such a model
in our own cultural context will be discussed later.

MOTIVATIONAL DYNAMICS OF
RELATIONAL DEVELOPMENT

A review of the way self-development has been defined in existing
developmental theory reveals the importance typically placed on
autonomous growth. The whole notion of *separation-individuation*
as the basis of human development implies that the person must first
disconnect from relationship in order to form a separate, articulate,
firm sense of self or personhood. The process of male development
is clearly defined as the disconnection and differentiation from the
mother early in childhood. Only much later in the life cycle, according
to Erikson (1950), do intimacy and generativity become "tasks" to
be "mastered competently." This intimacy, empathy, and relatedness
can be experienced as threats to autonomy, agency, and self-
determination.

To see beyond the limits of the model of separation-individuation,
our theory proposes a new construction: relationship-differentiation.
It is difficult to find the right language to describe such a developmental
growth process. By differentiation, we do not mean to suggest as
a developmental goal the assertion of difference and separateness,
but rather a dynamic process that encompasses increasing levels of

complexity, structure, and articulation within the context of human bonds and attachments. Such a process needs to be traced from its origins in early childhood relationships through its extensions into all later growth and development. What this new model does emphasize is that the *direction* of growth is not toward greater degrees of autonomy or individuation and the breaking of early emotional ties. This model defines development as a dynamic process of growth *within* relationship, where both or all people involved are challenged to maintain connection as well as foster, allow, or adapt to the growth of the other. This is the basic model inherent in parenting, but we are again broadening this to include a more generalized dynamic of mutual interactional growth within relationship. Such a construction does not diminish the significance of other lines of self-development (e.g., agency, initiative, or creativity). What is implied is that these other capacities are enhanced for women in the context of important relationships. It is probable that for women at all life stages, opportunities for *relational* growth are primary and healthy dynamic relationships are the motivating force that propels psychological growth.

ELEMENTS OF A NEW THEORY

The pathways of development of the self-in-relation are only beginning to be charted. The nature of the development of empathy needs to be further elaborated, and the relational opportunities for such development need to be more fully established. The actual application to other lines of self-development are only beginning to be understood, but it is clear that woman's basic sense of self-worth and self-esteem are closely linked to the establishment of mutually empathic and reciprocally empowering relationships.

We are beginning to develop a framework for studying the developmental pathway of the relational self. This framework contains a number of basic principles that form the rudimentary outline of a development theory. Some of the basic principles can be described as follows.

Critical relationships are seen as evolving throughout the life cycle in a *real* as well as intrapsychic form. As we know, one of the hardest developmental tasks is the challenge to grow into psychological adulthood in relationship with one's own parents, especially one's mother. The capacity to maintain relationships with tolerance, consideration, and mutual adaptation to the growth and development of each person needs to be accounted for. Such a system would validate developmental movement in many directions, recognizing the reality of the child and the adult in each human being, or perhaps recognizing periods of greater and lesser need and varying forms of need. All fruitful relationships need to accommodate to this cyclical and multifaceted movement, and this is a critical foundation for accepting such movement within ourselves. The ability to move closer to and further away from other people at different moments, depending on the needs of the particular individuals and the situational context, would be seen as crucial to development. We would explore the capacity for developing additional relationships based on broader, more diversified new identifications and corresponding patterns of expanding relational networks—including relationships with father, triangular relationships, preadolescent and adolescent friendship patterns, sexual relationships, marriage, mothering and family networks, teaching relationships, role modeling, women in work groups, and still broader reference groups. Such a female-centered theory would, therefore, trace the development of identity through specific relationships and relational networks. The theory would examine the nature of the cognitive and emotional internal capacities necessary for such growth, and the availability of appropriate relational networks to foster the development of such capacities, especially at critical developmental milestones. An example of this was the importance of the emergence of consciousness-raising groups in facilitating the women's movement of the 1960s and 1970s. Potential problems and vicissitudes inherent in the development of these relational capacities are examined. Our new theory does not talk about fixed states, developmental crises, or one-dimensional, unidirectional goals of development. Rather, it is multidimensional in nature.

STRENGTHS AND WEAKNESSES
OF RELATIONAL SELF-DEVELOPMENT

Many adult women who seek therapy experience difficulty in delineating, articulating, and acting directly on their own needs and perceptions. This is often conceptualized as a deficiency or a weakness in "individuation." Our theory offers a new perspective on this phenomenon in which the female client can be seen as not having sufficient relational experience and support in developing such competencies. Therapeutic interventions and strategies would work to provide such a relational framework to highlight and enhance a woman's experience of herself. Such an approach would validate and build on the client's relational capacities rather than help her become more separate or autonomous.

Many women today often experience anxiety, confusion, guilt, and conflicting value systems when they attempt to meet the challenges of new opportunities with traditional male self-definitions (for example the new assertive, competitive, managerial woman). It is important to explore how these more recent models of female identity may be incongruent or directly in conflict with the powerful aspects of early relational self-definition described in this model. This helps us better to understand some of the internal psychological obstacles to the expansion of self-definition and self-esteem. Further, women need to be encouraged to explore and develop new relational patterns and networks to support growth in new directions and into new contexts. Recognizing the significance of relational growth as a framework for self-development suggests new therapeutic interpretations, new forms of clinical intervention, and broader mental health policies specifically designed for women.

IMPLICATIONS FOR POLICY

At present, most social institutions—from the classroom to the corporate world—have evolved along lines consistent with traditional developmental models. There is an emphasis on individual action and achievement and on competitive rather than collaborative modes of endeavor rather than on the mutual realms of personal and institutional growth. Thus, if women are motivated by the self-in-relation, as this model proposes, it can be expected that women will experience a lack of fit between individualized demands of their setting and their own internal sense of well-being as fostered by reciprocal strivings and mutual goals. In the world at large, the qualities associated with the self-in-relation are rarely recognized or validated. The only contexts in which such qualities are supported are those that are explicitly defined as caretaking: wife and mother at home, and human services in the paid labor force. But even within human services, relational strengths are seldom directly linked with successful performance.

A fundamental policy consideration, then, would be the need to recognize and validate the self-in-relation as a mode for *simultaneously* enhancing women's own experience within an institutional structure and supporting the experience of the collective body. Without such changes, women will remain in the conflictual position of having to deny a part of themselves in order to conform to what is appreciated and rewarded in most settings. When women themselves are not aware of this inherent conflict, there is the added danger that they will identify the locus of the problem as within themselves rather than within the institutional structure and blame themselves for their discomfort and lack of fit (Miller, 1976).

A first step for translating the theory of self-in-relation into public policy would be that the theory, itself, be accepted as one viable and valid model of psychological development worthy of further study and exploration. For its implications to have any major impact on public policy such acceptance would have to be felt by those in positions of highest power and authority, men as well as women. Attention would have to be given at the highest levels to considerations of how and where the theoretical implications could be translated into meaningful and beneficial social change. Without such broad-based acceptance, the policy implications and their implementation would remain a "women's issue," probably resisted by those in power and able to make only small inroads into societal structure.

The theory as is presented here is still in rudimentary form, and many questions remain to be explored before specific policy changes should be suggested. Thus, the first area of policy change would involve those funding sources and academic institutions that influence the direction of approved and acceptable areas of inquiry. While there are a vast number of directions that such inquiry could take, one logical first step would be to explore the ramifications of self-in-relation for specific subgroups. One such group would be men. Although the theory is derived from a consideration of women's experience, it raises important questions about the relative importance and meanings to men of seeing themselves as relational beings—a topic that is downplayed in traditional theory. Such inquiry could provide new insights into some of the most pressing issues for men in contemporary society: their expanded roles as fathers, conflicts in relational styles between men and women (Chodorow, 1979; Rubin, 1983; Miller, 1981), and "humanizing" the work place. Such an inquiry could cover, among many other potential topics, the ways men perceive and integrate the needs of self and others, men's awareness of the nature and quality of relationships, the contexts that facilitate or inhibit men's abilities to take in the needs of others (empathy).

The meaning of self-in-relation to other subgroups, male as well as female, bears exploration as well. This would include variations based on differences in socioeconomic status, ethnic origin, race, and sexual preference. One major theme might be to understand the impact on sense of self if one is in a relatively dominant or subordinate social status. Earlier work (e.g., Miller, 1976) suggests that the condition of subordination enhances one's sensitivity to relational nuance. Further studies could address the ways in which relational concerns become increasingly devalued as they are expressed by subordinate groups. If indeed members of subordinate groups are especially developed along certain relational modes, it would be important to explore how this could be translated into economic gain. Such a line of inquiry could be of major importance in redressing the increasing "feminization of poverty," especially among women of color and older women.

Finally, if the theory of self-in-relation is to become a complete developmental theory, more attention would need to be given to evolution of the self-in-relation throughout the life span. Attention to the self-in-relation at specific age periods would contribute both to theory development and to policy formulation. Take but one example: the development of self-in-relation during early adolescence. It is well documented that during these years girls begin to decrease in their levels of academic achievement (especially in the areas of math and science) while simultaneously shifting their relational focus from same-sex peers to boys. (Frazer & Sadker, 1973). Self-in-relation theory would suggest that attention be given to possible changes in the classroom atmosphere and curriculum that would help girls expand rather than constrict their realms of connectedness that could then serve as a base for increased, rather than decreased, academic performance. Areas of exploration might include the possible advantages of collaborative work on projects, modes of positive student-teacher interaction that would affirm girls' successes, and ways of presenting material that would bring it closer to a relational mode of experience. Such endeavors would affirm girls' motivation toward enhancing relationships that would then include, rather than be in opposition to, the full development of their academic pursuits.

It would also be important to explore the facilitative quality of the self-in-relation across a variety of contexts—from psychotherapy to large business institutions, to the medical field, government agencies, and so on. The basic purpose here is to examine the extent to which a relational orientation enhances the goals of a particular endeavor in a way that remains congruent with the core self-structure of individuals involved. This admittedly broad quest would include collegial as well as management-worker and doctor-patient relationships; it would require a look at the reward structure and built-in avenues for relational considerations; it would consider the meaning and place of work for the individual in terms of broader aspects of the self. This line of inquiry, again, is consistent with suggested advances in various disciplines, from humanizing medicine to increasing collaboration within the work place, to the growing attention to the relational bond as a facilitator of growth in therapy (Kaplan, 1984).

The basic concept that self-identity evolves in relationships can be expanded for policy purposes to suggest a greater emphasis on learning and development within a relational context. Learning would thus become a collaborative, rather than competitive, endeavor in which a mutuality of concern enhances the experience of all. While group modes of learning are not new, they have not yet been grounded in a strong theoretical rationale, and tend to be considered "softer," "easier," more peripheral to the "real stuff," which is the individual working in a competitive mode on her or his own.

A shift toward collective modes of learning and doing would require that one consider carefully how and when such a mode should be adapted. In introducing a new structure into an ongoing system, such as a business corporation, careful thought must be given to how this new mode will blend with and impact on the existing structure. Certain tasks or processes might be more amenable to a collaborative mode than others. Individuals, as well, will vary in their proclivity toward and eagerness for such a form of work. Attention to all of these details is essential; without it, any difficulties then run the risk of being blamed on the model rather than on inadequate planning or poor implementation.

At essence here is the assumption that a collaborative mode provides a model of self-learning as well as task accomplishment. The manner of performance and the mutual facilitation of the work become indistinguishable from and enhance the final outcome. Thus, each individual can bring to bear a more personally meaningful commitment, and a sense of greater connectedness with the ultimate outcome and process of working with others toward its attainment. Such a structure probably involves more time for the implementation of projects, but it is assumed that the gains in the final outcome to the individuals and the agency will more than compensate for the additional expenditure of time. This assumption can and should be tested against specific institutional and individual goals. Factors to be looked for on the positive side would include increased work motivation, enhanced sense of one's own abilities, use of individual initiative and creative solutions to problems, increased capacity to make appropriate use of the resources of others, and a stronger sense that one's own growth is fostered by one's actions in the institution.

To illustrate, this model can be applied to the situation of women holding low income positions in the paid labor force. The numbers of such women have increased significantly in recent years: 10 percent of children school age or younger live with single mothers receiving low income and no additional adult support at home (Kamerman & Hayes, 1982). These women are working under conditions of high stress. In addition to their low wages, they typically have little opportunity for advancement or on-the-job training, and for the most part are in routinized or closely supervised positions such that they have very little control over or choice about how they will carry on their required tasks. These stresses in the work place are enhanced by the fact that they typically have major or sole responsibility for the daily care of their children, including responsibility for illnesses, changes in day-care arrangements, and all of the other unpredictable events associated with parenting young children.

Both the needs of these women and their usefulness to their corporations could be enhanced by steps suggested by a consideration of self-in-relation. Within the work place, programs could be developed that build on a recognition of the women's shared concerns and their capacity for mutual support and facilitation. It is noteworthy that while corporations have recently introduced programs to enhance physical fitness and Employee Assistance Programs (EAPs) for key problems such as alcohol, virtually no attention has been given to the parallel needs for sharing, support, and affirmation felt by low income women. The simple recognition of their shared concern and the agencies' willingness to offer a context in which this concern could be addressed could, in itself, be of major benefit.

In additon, corporations could recognize and support the total demands placed on these women's lives, including their responsibilities at home. Some choice in selecting the hours and days to work (flextime) is a useful beginning—a choice more often available to management than to low income employees. Time away from work required to tend to a sick or needy child could be considered as valid as sick leave. "Cafeteria" benefit programs could be instituted so that corporate contributions to the cost of child care would be an option. Importantly, the women, themselves, should be solicited for requests as to what additional options would facilitate their daily lives and hence their capacity to function more effectively at home and at work. Further, the very process of seeking their suggestions could lessen the sense of isolation and indifference from above that is felt by so many women in low income positions.

Self-in-relation theory, then, opens many new avenues for exploration regarding women and mental health policy. These range from the specifics of daily interaction to large-scale planning. But at every level, it invites us to consider the relational core of growth and development, and to think broadly about the individual and the social context in ways that promote the well-being of both.

REFERENCES

Chodorow, N. (1978). *The reproduction of mothering: Psychoanalysis and the sociology of gender.* Berkeley: University of California Press.

Dinnerstein, Dorothy (1978). *The mermaid and the minataur.* New York: Harper & Row.

Erikson, E. (1950). *Childhood and society.* New York: Norton.

Frazier, N., & Sadker, M. (1973). *Sexism in school and society.* New York: Harper & Row.

Freud, S. (1974). Female sexuality. In J. Strouse (Ed.), *Women and analysis.* New York: Dell. (Originally published in 1931.)

Freud, S. (1953). Some psychical consequences of the anatomical distinction between the sexes. In J. Strachey (Ed.), *The standard edition of the complete works of Sigmund Freud* (Vol. 19). London: Hogarth Press. (Originally published in 1925.)

Gilligan, C. (1982). *In a different voice.* Cambridge: Harvard University Press.

Gould R. (1978). *Transformations: Growth and change in adult life.* New York: Simon & Schuster.

Hoffman, Martin L. (1977). Sex differences in empathy and related behaviors. *Psychological Bulletin, 84* (4) 712-722.

Jordan, J. (1983). "Empathy and the mother-daughter relationship."

Kamerman, S., & Hayes, C. (1982). Dimensions of change: Trends and issues. In S. Kamerman & C. Hayes (Eds.), *Families that work.* Washington, DC: National Academy Press.

Kaplan, A. G. (1984). Female or male therapists for women: New formulations. Wellesley, MA : Stone Center Works in Progress, Wellesley College.

Kaplan, A. G., & Yasinski, L. (1980). Psychodynamic perspectives. In A. M. Brodsky & R. T. Hare-Mustin (Eds.), *Women and psychotherapy* (pp. 191-216). New York: Guilford Press.

Kohut, Heinz (1971). *The analysis of self.* New York: International Universities Press.

Levinson, D. J. (1978). *The seasons of a man's life.* New York: Ballantine.

Mahler, M. S. (1968). *On human symbiosis and the vicissitudes of individuation.* New York: International University Press.

Miller, J. B. (1981). Intimacy: Its relation to work and family. *Journal of Psychiatric Treatment and Evaluation, 3,* 121-129.

Miller, J. B. (1983). The construction of anger in women and men. Wellesley, MA: Stone Center Work in Progress, 83-01, Wellesley College.

Miller, J. B. (1976). *Toward a new psychology of women.* Boston: Beacon Press.

Orlinsky, D., & Howard, K. I. (1978). The relation of process to outcome in psychotherapy. In S. L. Garfield & A. E. Bergin (Eds.), *Handbook of psychotherapy and behavior change: On empirical analysis* (2nd ed.). New York: John Wiley.

Rubin, Lillian (1983). *Intimate strangers.* New York: Harper & Row.

Striver, I., (1983). *The meaning of "dependency" in female-male relationships* (Work in progress, 83-07). Wellesley, MA: Stone Center Working Papers Series.

Sullivan, H. S. (1953). *The interpersonal theory of psychiatry.* New York: Norton.

Surrey, J. (1983). The "self-in-relation": A theory of women's development. Wellesley, MA: Stone Center Colloquium Presentation, Wellesley College.

Winnicott, Donald W. (1965). The maturational processes and the facilitating environment. London: Hogarth Press.

5

WOMEN, SPIRITUALITY, AND MENTAL HEALTH

Maureen C. Hendricks

Once you start moving in depth in asking what it means to affirm the full personhood of women, then you start getting into other kinds of aspects. Not only opening up social/political access to the existing social order for women, but you begin to ask what kind of psychic price has been paid by both men and women through the centuries through the suppression of women. It seems that what has happened culturally with the suppression of women has also been a suppressing or distorting of whole dimensions of human affectivity. . . . What that really ends up doing is modeling a whole style of human relationships which makes everybody schizophrenic. It forces men to operate on one kind of line and women to cultivate another kind of line and nobody is really allowed to cultivate holistic humanity. . . . If you would think in terms of psychiatry and medicine. . .these are models based on making people dependent rather than empowering people. (Ruether, in Fox, 1983, pp. 7-8)

Ruether, a feminist Christian theologian, could well have included organized religion along with psychiatry and medicine in her preceding statement. What she is alluding to is the current religious and societal expectations of women upon which mental health policy is based. The manner in which mental health policy itself is oppressive to women has been discussed by Sturdivant (1980) in relationship to the failure of traditional psychotherapy to deal with the effects on women of sociocultural factors by (1) focusing on traditional female sex role behavior as most desirable, (2) reinforcing passivity and dependence in women, (3) relating to women as sex objects. The above behaviors on the part of mental health practitioners do not allow women to cultivate the "holistic humanity" to which Ruether refers.

Furthermore, spirituality as a dimension of the person in the holistic framework is frequently ignored in a discussion of mental health. Since mental health policy flows from such discussions, the current stance of omission is in reality a tacit policy of "hands off." When such a tacit policy is viewed in the light of the power that religious groups have in determining societal expectations of women, it becomes necessary to question the ethics of such a "hands off" policy. Expressed policies that relate to the handling of spiritual/religious issues in therapy need to be formulated. Therapists can deal with the spiritual dimension of the whole person in a manner that respects the client's chosen belief system without proselytizing. This chapter will attempt to give an overview of the major religions; their patriarchal oppression of women; the spiritual/religious issues that women bring to therapy; the need for established mental health policy about these issues in therapy; and finally, will suggest some approaches to therapeutic intervention.

RELIGION/SPIRITUALITY

Religion and spirituality are two dimensions of a belief system that follow one another. Religion may be described as a specific belief system that attributes to a being or beings of a higher order than humankind the creation and ordering of the universe from its beginnings through the present time. The deity or deities that a religion proclaims are usually acknowledged as having power over human beings in one or more specific areas of life. They are, therefore, to be respected and obeyed. In the early stages of the development of a religion, a certain person or persons proclaim that the deity has revealed to them norms of behavior for all believers. Laws that are based on the norms of behavior are proclaimed by the religious leaders as the will of the deity. From these initial laws many finely detailed rules and regulations may be developed. Penalties for failure to observe the laws, rules, and regulations are prescribed and attributed to the command of the deity. Reward for obedience may be defined as a happy life, prosperity or good fortune in this present life, or a life after death. Failure to obey may be said to result, conversely, in unhappiness, misfortune, and misery in the present life as well as in an afterlife.

Spirituality is the manner in which a person chooses to respond to a specific religion or to a nonspecific, broad understanding of the meaning and purpose of life. A spirituality continuum can be conceptualized as containing a broad spectrum of responses to a specific religion or to a nonspecific belief system. It is, therefore, possible that this response to religious values could result in a legalistic form of spirituality that would emphasize the adherence to the minutiae of religious rules and regulations or in a holistic form of spirituality that would look beyond the letter of the law to the sense or meaning of life as understood in light of the belief system. How spirituality develops among religious groups profoundly influences their basic attitudes toward the relationship to the members of the groups, especially the roles and position of women.

DIVERSITY OF RELIGIOUS TRADITIONS

Due to the diversity of religious traditions throughout the world, it is appropriate to mention the major contemporary religious groups and their characteristics. Goddess worship, however, the earliest form of religious tradition, will be discussed later in this chapter.

Judaism, a monotheistic belief system, is one of the most ancient world religions. Still vital and flourishing today, it has three main branches: Orthodox, Conservative, and Reform (Kertzer, 1978). Kertzer gives a practical definition of a Jew as "one who considers himself (sic) a Jew or is so regarded by his (sic) community" (1978, p. 3); he further states that there are about 14,000,000 Jews in the world today (1978, p. 221). Judaism focuses on home life rituals as well as temple or synagogue practices, all of which vary according to the branch to which a person belongs.

Christianity, which evolved from Judaism, is probably the world's largest religious group with about one-third of the world population, mainly in Europe, North and South America (Encyclopaedia Britannica, 1969, vol. 5, p. 693). A 1977 estimate puts the number at about 950,000,000 (World Book Encyclopedia, 1980, vol. 16, p. 210). Christian churches range from the oldest, the Roman Catholic, with centuries of theology and very specific dogma, rules, and regulations, to the Unitarian Universalist Association formed in 1961 by a merger of two church bodies with similar belief systems. Mainly Christian from their beginning, the association formed by the two churches has no set dogma and is not accepted as a Christian church by a part of Christiandom (Encyclopaedia Britannica, 1969, vol. 22, p. 553). Christians are subdivided into Catholic, Protestant, and Orthodox groupings with a great diversity of beliefs and practice.

Islam, with over 500,000,000 followers (World Book Encyclopedia, 1980, vol. 16, p. 210) is a major religion in the Eastern world. It honors elements of both the Judaic and Christian traditions but is primarily based on the writings of the Koran. It is a religion of very specific dogma, rules, and regulations (Encyclopedia Britannica, 1969, vol. 12, p. 663).

Buddhism, another predominantly Eastern religion, has about 245,000,000 followers (World Book Encyclopedia, 1980, vol. 16, p. 210). A diversity of schools and practices exist, often related to the culture of the country in which it is found. Japan is heavily Buddhist (Encyclopaedia Britannica, 1969, vol. 4, pp. 354-359).

Hinduism, an Eastern religion found mainly in India, has many diverse beliefs and practices and about 520,000,000 members (World Book Encyclopedia, 1980, vol. 16, p. 210). It also has a social caste system, which has a powerful effect on the life of the people, especially women (Encyclopaedia Britannica, 1969, vol. 11, p. 512).

Native American people have an ancient religion about a "high God" found in their mythology (Starkloff, 1974, p. 25). Although many have become Christian, the traditions of their ancient religion are still often a part of daily life. How this tradition is lived varies from tribe to tribe and little of it is shared with outsiders.

"Cults" is a word that in the United States has come to mean a variety of new religious movements, some from Eastern traditions, which the mainstream religions and many parents find to be suspect. Such groups are the "Moonies" (Unification Church), Hare Krishna, Divine Light Mission, and Children of God. The tactics used by these groups to attract and keep members have been highly criticized as akin to brainwashing. Some parents have requested psychological help to extinguish the effect of such conditioning in their children.

As can be seen from the preceding listing, religion is a dominant force in the world and is as diverse as are the peoples of the world. One common thread, however, runs through all the diversity. That thread is male oppression of women through the patriarchal systems of the varied religions. This commonality means that regardless of the ethnicity of the woman who comes for therapy, if she does or has belonged to an organized religion, she is most likely oppressed by the beliefs and practices of the religion. If mental health policy is to be appropriate for holistic care, the victimization of women by patriarchal religious practices, overt and covert, must be acknowledged and remedied.

PATRIARCHAL EVOLUTIONS OF RELIGIONS

Judaism and Christianity both evolved in patriarchal form for somewhat different reasons but are representative of the process in other religions. Judaism focuses more on the uncleanness taboo of women while Christianity focuses on labeling women the "sinful successors of Eve." Since these are the major religions in the United States and have influenced the status of women in this country, a review of their patriarchal evolutions will be presented first, followed by a synopsis of the other major world religions.

Judaism and Chrisitianity both reverence as the Word of God a series of books of Scripture that recount the early understandings of one God ("monotheism") and the evolution of the image of this God as both powerful and male. Genesis, the first book of the Bible, contains three traditions that have been and still are very important to its interpretation: (1) Yahwist, the earliest and most symbolic; (2) Elohist; and (3) Priestly, characterized by law, ritual, and theology (Hunt, 1960). The Yahwist and Priestly traditions each present a separate account of the creation of the world and of humankind. In the Priestly tradition, women and men are created equally at the same time "male and female he created them" (Genesis 1:27). In the Yahwist tradition, woman is created from the rib of man and then is named by him: "she shall be called woman for from man she has been taken" (Genesis 2:23). Hunt (1960, pp. 13-14) comments that the Yahwist, while trying to show woman equal to man by nature, also places the man in authority over the woman because he names her. The Yahwist account also tells us that the woman, Eve, is the cause of misery for all humankind to come, therefore, she is to bear children in pain and be under her husband's domination (Genesis 3:1-24).

From this early part of Scripture on, regardless of which tradition authored the content, the history of the Jewish people is told in terms of male relationship to God and the continuity of the tribes enumerated by male lineage. Women are named sporadically and usually in relationship to a man, either father, brother, husband, or son. The genealogy in the story of Moses clearly demonstrates this pattern (Exodus 6:14-25).

Further, male sacrifice, male priests, male elders, predominant male inheritance, and a God referred to as "He" demonstrate the early establishment of patriarchy in Judaism. However, as Rein (1979) comments in her book about the women's movement in Israel, there are two books of the Old Testament devoted to women: Ruth and Esther. Rein details the struggle of women in Israel to become liberated from sexism in a state which "became kosher" (1979, p. 11) to preserve a people and their tradition. Kertzer (1978) in his explanation of contemporary Jewish practice among Orthodox, Conservative, and Reform branches of Judaism gives repeated examples of how persistent, except among Reformed Judaism, the patriarchal pattern still is.

The Christian tradition, departing from or ignoring the feminist teachings of Jesus, slowly, through its first five centuries, evolved into a patriarchal mode similar to Judaism ("Report of the last three sessions," 1982). Along with the patriarchal-mode revival was the development of a theology based on the Yahwist Genesis tradition that has been and continues to be used to oppress Christian women. It is the most commonly used creation story in Christian churches. All Roman Catholic clergy and most Protestant clergy are male. God is referred to as "He" in the religious literature and acts of faith that Christians profess. The current Moral Majority Christians especially use the Yahwist account of creation and the fall to claim the need for male dominance over females in all aspects of life. Eve, the cause of the fall of humankind from the garden of Eden according to the Yahwist tradition (Genesis 3:1-24), apparently was not used in Jewish patriarchal tradition to oppress women. This may be because the Priestly tradition, which discontinues at Genesis 5 (Hunt, 1960), does not mention Eden or a banishment. It was Christian theologians who later capitalized on the Eve story in order to oppress women (Clark & Richardson, 1977, p. 29).

In Judaism it was the childbearing function of the women that led to oppressive rules and regulations about sexual behavior and menstrual uncleanness. McGrath (1976) reports the post-Mosaic times as those in which the connection was established between uncleanness and moral transgression. By the time of the Essenes, about the same time as the life of Jesus, "woman was both guilty and contemptible" (p. 17). Tong (1977) comments, "the Judaic and Christian Churches have sacralized, internalized and transformed cultural prejudices against women into dogmas and articles of faith" (p. 337).

In early Islamic tradition women were fairly independent and a matriarchal family system existed. That system was gradually replaced by patriarchy, especially when harems, veiling, and polygamy became part of the tradition. Menstrual uncleanness was also an Islamic issue, although to a far lesser extent than in Judaism (Parrinder, 1980).

The history is not too different for Buddhism, which "cut across caste divisions and gave more freedom to women (in its homeland of India), yet traditional male dominance remained" (Parrinder, 1980, p. 55). As in the Roman Catholic church, male Buddist monks are perceived of as more important than female Buddist nuns.

Child marriage, widow burning, and polygamy have all been part of the Hindu tradition (Encyclopaedia Britannica, vol. 11, p. 512). As in Christianity, women were honored on one hand for their childbearing and child-rearing responsibilities but were kept in subjugation by fathers and husbands (Parrinder, 1980).

Although diverse in their traditions, Native American tribes have a communality in the menstrual uncleanness taboo and a patriarchal society (Maynard & Twiss, 1970). Witt (1981), however, reports that these tribes, as agricultural peoples, were originally matriarchal, a pattern found in historical evidence of many early agricultural peoples. When the agricultural focus of these early peoples lessened due to hunting and warring, more physically powerful male activities, patriarchy crept in (Carmody, 1981). Interestingly, while Todd (1982) tells of a prepatriarchal Great Spirit that is "no more male than female" (p. 434) and Witt explains the religious role of women in various tribes, Starkloff (1974), a Jesuit priest, claims that the men are the usual mediators with the spirits while the women tend to the needs of the men. Native American women thus pay a costly price for the double patriarchy of colonization and Christianization.

CONTEMPORARY OPPRESSION OF WOMEN
BY RELIGIOUS BELIEF SYSTEMS

Porter and Albert (1977) report on the complexity of values within contemporary Judaism in regard to the role of women. "The religious role of women is to provide the proper home atmosphere for a Jewish life" (p. 347). Ritual and ceremonies clearly define the division of labor. Until 1983 Jewishness was considered to be by matrilineal descent and the woman was responsible to pass on the cultural aspects of the tradition. Now the American Reform Rabbis are supporting patrilineal descent and much controversy has ensued ("Conversion and Patrilineality," 1983). At the same time, women, like men, are encouraged toward the development of self, education, and effective means for coping with life. The Porter and Albert (1977) study found that Jewish women had the least adherence to the traditional role model of woman solely as a homemaker when compared with several groups of Christian women. Umansky (1979) documents the manner in which Jewish women have come to their present status in the several branches of Judaism as well as the growth of Jewish feminism, which will be discussed later in this chapter.

Christian women have not fared much better than their Jewish sisters in the patriarchal oppression their churches both allow and promote. As noted earlier, it was Christian theologians in the early church who promoted the Eve myth as a proof of women's inferiority, while imposing another mythological oppression on Christian women to control their "Eve-ness": Mary, the Mother of Jesus, is presented in traditional Roman Catholic teaching as a perpetual virgin. There is even a belief that she did not labor and deliver Jesus vaginally; he somehow miraculously exited her womb (a good example of the uncleanness taboo continuation). Perpetual virginity, especially for women, soon became an ideal and has continued to be so in the Roman Church.

Mary is the only acceptable role model for a Christian woman who is supposed to spend her life repenting her "Eve-ness." In the Roman Catholic Church a woman is either a celebate nun or married with children (childbirth helps to pay the Eve debt). The virgin nun has had higher regard and respect than the married woman. There is a belief in some Catholic circles that the woman who dies in childbirth goes straight to heaven! For both Catholic and Protestant churches, marriage is traditionally the only acceptable place where a woman is allowed sexual activity. This activity is allowed in order that she may pay her Eve debt through childbirth.

In explaining her understanding of Eve versus Mary myths, Janeway (1980) states "Mary is never going to let Eve enjoy herself without waking up to a guilty morning after" (p. 576). That statement illustrates her explanation of the Protestant Victorian attitude toward women, which was devised in a male-dominated society and persists to this day. The Protestant churches, some of whom denied the virginity of Mary as taught by the Catholic church, chose to focus on the motherhood of Mary. Marriage was the saving grace for sensual men. The wife provided a safe outlet for the husband's sexual appetite while serving as a role model of virtue for him. By having children the wife not only satisfied her husband but allowed both spouses to satisfy the command of God. Women were seen as void of passion and solely meant to serve as receptacles of male sperm and the children thus conceived.

Islam has had a resurgence of sexism in the recent years, and women are once more required to be veiled in some countries, notably Iran. Buddhism, diversely practiced in China, Japan, and other countries, has changed little though Western influences can be seen. Hinduism persists in having very oppressive roles for women. Parrinder (1980) gives much detail by country and culture of the persistence of oppression of women throughout the world by religion in general. True (1981) gives more specific detail by generation, regardless of religious background, of the variety of struggles of Asian American women.

Racism as well as sexism, both within and without religious groups, is an additonal form of oppression for black, Hispanic, and Native American women. Compared to the volumes written about white women, the literature of the oppression of these minority women is sparse although slowly growing. Murray (1981) presents a brief overview of the stereotypes and roles of black women while Smith-Penniman and Giles (1980) deal specifically and very briefly with black women in ministry. More details about black women in African religions is found in the work by Mbiti (1969), who reports on the function of women as both priests (p. 187) and religious "specialists" (p. 193) in African society. Black women's Goddess heritage has recently been revived in the United States as explained by Sojourner (1982). For Catholic Hispanic women in the United Sates there is a national organization known as Las Hermanas which is a source of support for dealing with both racism and religious oppression. Native American women who choose to adhere to Christianity have added the patriarchal oppression of Christianity to their already significant struggles with racism. As the "lowest paid, lowest ranked, most unemployed segment of the national workforce" (Witt, 1981, p. 152), these women are, therefore, in double jeopardy. Like black, Hispanic, and Asian women, the Native American woman is part of a minority and subject to both racism and patriarchal oppression in the Christian churches.

Streiker (1978) reports on the inferior position of women in the majority of contemporary cults. Childbearing and rearing, while catering to the needs and wishes of men, are characteristic of the role of women within these groups. This is not surprising, considering the origins of cults: The Hare Krishna movement is derived from an ancient Hindu sect (Johnson, 1976, pp. 31-51); the Guru Maharaj Ji of the Divine Light Mission claims he only wants people to be perfect in their Christianity, Buddhism, or Islam (Messer, 1976, p. 53); the Unification Church and the Children of God were started with a basis in Christianity although both have now gone beyond it (MacCollam, 1979, pp. 168-177). With their origins in patriarchal religions, cults continue and add to the already present religious oppression of women.

PATHOLOGICAL EFFECTS ON WOMEN

In today's society the Eve-versus-Mary myth is losing its power as women become more conscious of their personhood. The remnants of that myth, however, are still present and still wreak havoc on women's mental health as well as their spirituality. The male controlled Moral Majority in the United States contains a strong evangelical, fundamental Christian ideology that can be quite traumatic to women. Meadow (1980) details the harmful effects of the female subordination to male authority in marriage that these religious tenets require. In a study of depressed housewives, Stoudenmier (1976) found that many women who choose to adhere to the submissive wife doctrine became depressed. He sees their depression to be related to four factors: "suppressed anger, poor body image, an absence of reinforcing events in life, and an interpersonal anxiety that includes feelings of excessive dependency and inferiority" (p. 62). Given the Eve-versus-Mary myth with its negation of the woman as a person, it is not hard to see how such depression occurs. A woman who is socialized into the Eve-versus-Mary myth may believe she must choose submission yet may find it intolerable because it is an extrinsic male value. Persons with extrinsic religious orientations have also been found to be more anxious and to have decreased internal locus of control (Sturgeon & Hamley, 1979). If a woman is placed in a Catch-22 situation in her faith tradition, she cannot be both "a normal woman and a normal human being" (Janeway, 1980, p. 575) for her submissive stance does not allow for growth and individuation. An example is the high psychological price that hispanic women pay for their Catch-22 traditional role (Senour, 1981). Stoner and Parke (1977) also report on the demeaning and sometimes brutal treatment of women in the Hare Krishnas. Since degree of religious involvement is no guaranty of safety, a deeply depressed, submissive wife or nun might commit suicide (Beit-Hallahmi, 1975).

Although these data are primarily based on studies of Jewish and Christian women, they can be applied to the other religious groups discussed. Wherever women are oppressed, pathology will most likely follow. However, when women are able to resist the patriarchal system, they are healthier: A study of religion and American women demonstrated that those women with a high degree of religiousness who did not follow religious tenets that they did not believe also had a high degree of health and reported happiness (Shaver, Lenauer, & Sadd, 1980). Due to the lack of available material on all the religious belief systems cited earlier, the ways in which women respond to patriarchal oppression will be discussed primarily in relationship to the Jewish and Christian traditions.

RELIGIOUS/SPIRITUALITY ALTERNATIVES FOR WOMEN

As Jewish and Christian feminists come to terms with the reality of the powerful patriarchy of their faith traditions, two main avenues of response are being chosen by those who do not abandon all forms of spiritual life. The first avenue is working for liberation of the tradition from all oppression and restoration to a balance of sexual equality as stated in the Priestly tradition of Genesis 1:27: "male and female [God] created them"; the second avenue is reviving and recreating the Goddess as a focus of spirituality.

Jewish feminists focus on revising ritual through change in God language, balancing the forms of address to God with female terms to make the language nonoppressive (Gross, 1979). Sabbath prayers have been rewritten with reference to God-She (Janowitz & Wenig, 1979). Rituals to celebrate the birth of a female child and her initiation into the covenant community of Israel have been developed (Plaskow, 1979), as well as a revised Haggadah that reflects the importance of Jewish women in the history of Israel (Cantor, 1979).

Although the patriarchial tradition of Judaism has grown in Israel, so has feminism. As reported by Rein (1980), feminism in Israel has gained a small but sure foothold. Unlike their Israeli sisters, many American Jewish women can now aspire to rabbinical ordination. Reform Judaism has ordained women for 11 years and in 1983 ordination for women in American Conservative Judaism was accepted (Austin, 1983). Orthodox Judaism remains against women's ordination but Greenberg (1981) has questioned it about its treatment of women.

Christian feminism is based more on theology than ritual and seeks to restore full humanness to Christianity. Christian feminist spirituality deals with "Enablement, empowerment, and mutuality. . .[and the issue of] the bonding of women across barriers of color, sexual preference and life style" ("Spirituality, Prayer, Call," 1982, pp. 4-5). It "understands the Spirit in the biblical sense of the divine power and dynamic enabling us to live as Christians. . .[in] enabling love, inclusive community, and service for all humankind" (Fiorenza, 1979, pp. 137-138). Christian feminists attest to the feminist messages of Jesus that presented women as equal to men, especially in religious matters: (1) Jesus taught women, (2) sent them as his religious messengers to men, (3) insisted on their rights in marriage as equal to that of men, (4) cured women of infirmity even on the sabbath or when ritually unclean, (5) chose a woman as the first witness to his resurrection (McGrath, 1976, pp. 26-32).

Other feminist concerns such as changes in sexist language have been an issue for almost a decade in the Roman church and most other churches as well; these changes are slowly coming about, frequently with a great deal of resistance. Ministry is denied women in varying degrees throughout the Christian church. Roman Catholicism denies women ordination to the priesthood because they are not male and therefore do not look like Jesus. Other denominations admit women to various levels of ministry, even ordination, yet tend to keep them in teaching rather than management positions.

Within the Roman church women in religious orders (nuns) have been kept segregated from other women. The Women's Ordination Conference of the Roman church is working to break down those separation barriers as is a newly formed group called the Association for the Rights of Catholics in the Church. All Christian feminists are attempting to bond with women of color and diverse ethnic backgrounds. The Daughters of Sarah is an evangelical feminist publication that has also attempted to facilitate this bonding.

Grapevine reports within the Roman church claim that even some nuns have stopped participating in regular services because of sexism. Throughout the United States some groups of people are meeting to celebrate a nonsexist Eucharist which is also noncultic. The present clerical system is not the kind of priesthood that many of these women wish to be part of. These small groups are evolving the new priestly ministry where all the church members share their gifts.

Both Christian and Jewish feminists are developing the "healthy-minded" religion, which according to Shaver, Lenauer, and Sadd (1980) consists of placing value on religious experience and fashioning a belief system that includes both the religious experience and a variety of interpretations of its meaning (p. 1564). They are doing this at the risk of excommunication as the story of Mormon Sonia Johnson reveals (1981).

However, in order for women to be free of "patriarchal policemen," Christ (1979, p. 197) claims that they need to abandon the Judeo-Christian traditions altogether and turn to the Goddess, to proclaim their long denied power, beauty of body, will, and heritage. The Goddess is seen as a symbol of affirmation of the female power to be independent and competent in being and acting without men. In the Goddess belief system the cyclical function of the female body is revered for its life-giving ability in contrast to the uncleanness attributed to it by patriarchal beliefs, while the affirmation and assertion of female willpower overcomes the sin of self-negation of women in these systems. "This feminist spirituality proclaims wholeness, healing love, and spiritual power not as hierarchical, as power 'over', but as power 'for', as enabling power. It proclaims the Goddess as the source of this power" (Fiorenza, 1979, p. 137). Finally, the bonding of women to share their common heritage is encouraged, especially that of mother and daughter, where the mother can pass to the daughter the "herstory" of their heritage (Christ, 1979, pp. 273-286).

Janeway (1980) sees the Goddess as just another form of the Mary myth and a way of keeping women's identity focused on their reproductive capacity. Wilson-Kastner (1982) reports on the concern of Christian feminists that the Goddess focus will simply promote a form of reverse sexism where females are superior and males are inferior. Collins (1981) sees this form of feminist spirituality as dealing only with white, middle class women and causing a further division of women among themselves as well as between women and men. The role of men in Wicca is explained by Farrar and Farrar (1981), while a detailed history of Goddess religions can be found in a work by Stone (1976).

One segment of religiously oppressed women, overwhelmed by the negation of their personhood, choose to reject their religious faith tradition. Korman (1983) found that women with no religious preference had a higher percentage of commitment to feminism, and 83 percent of feminists report little or no church or synagogue attendance (p. 435); of those feminists who expressed a religious preference, only 10 percent attended services regularly (p. 435). The ability of a woman to reject the tradtion is closely tied into her ethnicity and social class. A minority woman, who would alienate herself from a support system by such a choice and thus find herself more isolated in a racist and sexist culture, is probably the least likely to do so. A white, middle class professional woman who has many resources open to her is far more likely to "chuck it all!" Although each one would bring different issues to therapy, the basis for both would be a lack of wholeness directly related to religious oppression.

IMPLICATIONS OF RELIGIOUS/SPIRITUALITY ISSUES FOR MENTAL HEALTH POLICY

As noted earlier, a state of limbo exists in mental health policy about dealing with religious and spiritual issues in therapy. With the practice of separation of Church and State in the United States a sense of "walking on egg shells" seems to exist about religious issues in any institution that receives federal funding. Mental Health agencies, schools, most psychiatric hospitals, and various other agencies that provide psychotherapy usually receive some form of federal monies. In the absence of established policy, a melange of approach/avoidance practices probably exist in regard to dealing with client's religious issues in these institutions. As demonstrated earlier, to neglect the spiritual dimension is not only to deny caring for the whole person and prevent healing in some, it is also denying the very real oppression of women in society through the influence of organized religion. There is a vast difference between proselytization and respect for a women's faith while affirming her as a person. With affirmation and growing self-respect, a women becomes able to choose for herself how she will nourish her spirituality.

Graduate schools have the optimal situations for the formulation of mental health policy about religious/spiritual issues in therapy. The time and resources are more available to them to discuss, debate, and experiment with the subject. Their findings of the most useful and appropriate methodologies could then be shared with the mental health community that is actively involved in practice. What these programs will be developing will be a more holistic approach to client needs rather than the current somewhat phobic approach to spiritual issues that often exists. An example of such attempts can be found in the collaboration of the University of Denver School of Professional Psychology with Iliff School of Theology and the Institute for Judaic Studies.

Policy issues that may arise and would need to be carefully addressed in mental health policy formulation are the following: (1) What is the difference between proselytization and affirmation of a client's spiritual choices? (2) What guidelines can be developed to allow clients to receive therapeutic support and guidance for spiritual issues in publicly funded institutions? (3) What differentiates therapeutic support and guidance from pastoral counseling and/or spiritual direction? The reader will probably think of several other questions; those listed are basic. Therapists need to define for themselves both their level of comfort and their level of competency to deal with religious/spiritual issues. The primary focus of therapy is to foster wholeness in the person: Spiritual wholeness is fostered as a part of psychological wholeness in the context of whatever theoretical approach the therapist uses. Most therapists are competent to some degree to deal with the issues but many lack the comfort in doing so. A therapist can usually collaborate with a client's spiritual guide if it would be indicated. The approach I often use with deeply religious women struggling over the conflicts mentioned will be discussed to demonstrate one method of incorporating religious/spiritual issues in therapy. This approach is applicable to other faith traditions.

ISSUES IN THERAPY

The focal point of therapy with women dealing with religious issues is, as I see it, affirmation of her personhood by a feminist therapist. Role modeling of female ability to be of service to others, which these women frequently feel called to, while not being male dependent or submissive, is another function of the feminist therapist and very important for the client's growth (Miller, 1976).

Women who present themselves for therapy to deal with current religious conflict or the impact of past religious conflict are similar only in the harmful impact that patriarchy has had on them. Some have abandoned religious practice in their late teens or early twenties and come to therapy in their early thirties to find meaning in life and heal the wounds of patriarchal oppression. Others are active in ministry in their church and are trying to deal with their sexist experiences and/or decide whether or not to resign their ministry. A third group are women who are active members of a patriarchal religion and are in conflict because of its oppressive tenets.

One of the first assessments I make in the initial stages of the therapeutic process is the woman's God-image. It is almost always male, usually an old man, who has very conditional love: a "perform or else" love where the "or else" is harm to the person. One client imaged God as an old man dealing a deck of cards and giving her an ace of spades, telling her that she was creating her own hell. This client had long ago abandoned the faith of her childhood but the impact on her current life was precipitating panic attacks.

An assessment of the most significant male in the woman's childhood (father or grandfather, etc.) usually reveals a connection between their behavior and her God-image. Much can be worked through simultaneously as this connection becomes clearer to the client. Depression and acute anxiety over God-wrath is found regardless of the woman's current religious affiliation. Those women in ministerial positions who feel externally controlled or oppressed by men are usually growing in feminism and experiencing a great deal of conflict. McClain

(1970) reports study findings that demonstrate that feminists are either less religious than women who are not feminists (as has Korman, 1983) or anti-religious. Actively religious women become acutely anxious when thoughts of abandoning their faith arise as patriarchal oppression becomes more apparent. What I have termed the "zapping-God" phenomenon can be quite powerful, especially for women in ministry. This phenomenon is based on fire and brimstone teachings about God's punishment, which could strike at any time, and a final judgement at which the unfaithful will be cast into eternal punishment. Once these teachings are firmly believed and a woman begins to question her faith tradition, her fear of God's punishment can be overwhelming.

The "Mary syndrome" in Catholic women, especially nuns and ex-nuns, is one in which the woman can never let herself be affirmed as a person because she can never meet the perfection criteria of Mary who has been given to her as a role-model. When a Catholic woman has both the zapping-God fear and the Mary syndrome, her anxiety and depression can be quite intense. Nuns and ex-nuns are the women most likely to have had the least affirmation and can experience great conflict (Hart, Ames, & Sawyer, 1974). If a nun has let herself become sexually active—and Halstead and Halstead report that only 32 percent of the resigned priests and nuns they studied have been celibate while in their communities (1978, p. 86)—then she not only is conflicted about her sexual activity but may also be at risk for pregnancy. These clients need to be affirmed as sexual beings, be helped to look at what choices are available to them, and then be allowed to decide what the choices are with which they can live. The process is usually fraught with both anxiety and depression as old powerful messages of Eve versus Mary complicate it. These myths need to be acknowledged and then demythologized by the client with the support of the therapist and good Christian feminist literature. Dream work in which the client's conflict and growth can be seen and utilized for the work of therapy and for client affirmation, is very helpful.

Obviously the issues are diverse but all are powerful. Whether the client is a distressed housewife, an oppressed minister or a nonpracticing (of religion) woman, the commonality of patriarchal oppression and/or the zapping-God syndrome results in varying degrees of anxiety and depression. Unless these oppressive issues of spirituality are acknowledged and carefully worked through, they will continue to disturb the client, for they are often at the core of her distress.

It is essential to comment on several complicating factors for minority women. There is in Christianity a deep and ancient pattern of anti-Semitism, which the Christian therapist needs to be aware of when working with Jewish clients. Ruether (1982) is a Christian feminist theologian who has written about this issue in a scholarly and competent manner. Letty Cottin Pogrebin and others have also prepared material on this subject for the American Jewish Committee. Racism in the churches, especially in regard to black women, has been discussed comprehensively by Hooks (1981). Since the majority of feminist therapists are white, middle-class women of Judeo/Christian heritage, we have a responsibility to learn about the double jeopardy oppression of our minority sisters of color while dealing with whatever degree of latent racism we harbor within ourselves. Lastly, the homophobia in the vast majority of religious groups, especially the Moral Majority Christians, leaves many lesbian women virtually without a spiritual home unless they stay in the closet. Within some mainline Christian churches there are support groups for gay people (Dignity for Catholics; Integrity for Episcopalians) but the official church positions tend to be for celibacy as the only acceptable gay life-style.

Support groups for women dealing with religious/spiritual issues are an almost necessary adjunct to the therapy process. As an oppressed group, women have been pitted against each other for centuries. Support groups not only provide support, they also help women learn how to bond with each other in a healthy way. Feminist literature for both Jewish and Christian women, as cited in this chapter, is available and very useful to clients. Referral to appropriate spiritual guides can also facilitate the healing process. The woman who chooses to disaffiliate herself from a religious tradition will need to be supported in her grief process, especially if she would choose Goddess spirituality. That choice is probably less socially acceptable than is no religious affiliation at all. The therapist can then facilitate the client's search for whatever new meaning in life or spirituality will promote wholeness and healing. The new spiritual path can be a lonesome journey and the client will benefit from the therapist's support and affirmation of the client's growth in wholeness.

SUMMARY

The absence of established mental health policy in regard to dealing with clients' religious/spiritual issues deprives clients of a holistic approach to therapy. Women are especially victimized by this tacit hands-off policy due to the impact of patriarchal religious attitudes toward women in society. The need for established policy, focused on promoting wholeness while healing the wounds of patriarchy, is evident. Graduate schools have the most resources available to them for development of such policies. Since wholeness and healing, not proselytizing, is the purpose of the therapeutic work, conflicts about separation of Church and State and third-party payment need not be an issue. The most important issue is the therapist's own level of comfort and skill in meeting the client's needs. Referral to and collaboration with spiritual guides can facilitate the therapy work.

The therapeutic work about religious/spiritual issues is integrated into the therapy process. Virtually all women seeking therapy have some amount of distress relating to these issues because patriarchal religions have fostered conflict in many contemporary women. Feminists often feel that they must abandon the faith of their childhood, and many do so. Jewish feminists choose to revise ritual and God language. Christian feminists choose to affirm the unpreached feminist teachings of Jesus. Some feminists are choosing the Goddess as a source of spirituality rather than abandon all religion. Women who are not yet feminists can also experience a great deal of mental anguish while trying to adhere to an oppressive religious belief system that negates their personhood.

The most important affirmation the woman in these situations needs is that whatever choice she makes in regard to her spirituality that contributes to her personal growth is supported by the therapist. If the working through process has been done at the client's pace, with respect for her belief system, she will usually make a choice that is most livable for her at that point in time. Affirming her choice, which may still keep her in an oppressive situation, can be done with a summary of her growth and an offer of availability for future work on further growth. A feminist therapist is most likely to be able to provide the therapy and role model that women with religious/spiritual conflicts need. The therapist can also suggest appropriate feminist reading material for the client.

To conclude this chapter I will use the words of Rosemary Radford Ruether (1980, p. 8) that emphasize the importance of the topic:

> The religious sacralization of patriarchy means that religions shaped by and shaping patriarchal cultures give religious validation to patriarchy, not just within the religious institution, but within the whole society.

We must remember that, until modern liberal revolutions separated Church from State, religious law functioned as part of general social law for the whole society. In classical Judaism and Islam, religious law and social law were identical, i.e. the law code for all social matters was regarded as given by God. Even today, when patriarchal law is largely dismantled, religion functions as a prime legitimizer and socializer of patriarchal norms.

REFERENCES

Association for the Rights of Catholics in the Church, P.O. Box 3932, Philadephia, Pa. 19146. (215) 623-0590.

Austin, C. (1983). Women rabbis approved. *The Denver Post,* October 28, p. 10C.

Beit-Hallahmi, B. (1975). Religion and suicidal behavior. *Psychological Reports, 37,* 1303-1306.

Cantor, A. (1979). Jewish women's Haggadah. In C. P. Christ & J. Plaskow (Eds.), *Womanspirit rising.* New York: Harper & Row.

Carmody, D. L. (1981). *The oldest God.* Nashville: Abingdon.

Christ, C. P. (1979). Why women need the Goddess: phenomenological, psychological, and political reflections. In C. P. Christ & J. Plaskow (Eds.), *Womanspirit rising.* New York: Harper & Row.

Clark, E., & Richardson, H. (1977) The Old Testament. In E. Clark & H. Richardson (Eds.), *Women and religon.* New York: Harper & Row.

Collins, S. D. (1981). Feminist theology at the crossroads. *Christianity and Crisis, 41*(20), 342-347.

Conversion and patrilineality (1983). *Intermountain Jewish News,* December 2.

Daughters of Sarah, 2716 W. Cortland, Chicago, IL 60647.

Encyclopaedia Britannica (1969). (vols. 4, 5, 11, 12, 14, 22). London: Encyclopaedia Britannica.

Farrar, J., & Farrar, S. (1981). *Eight sabbats for witches.* London: Robert Hale Ltd.

Fiorenza, E. S. (1979). Feminist spirituality, Christian identity, and Catholic vision. In C. P. Christ & J. Plaskow (Eds.), *Womanspirit rising.* New York: Harper & Row.

Fox, M. (1983). Interview with Rosemary (Radford) Ruether. *Bear and Company, 2*(3), 7-9, 23-24.

Greenberg, B. (1981). *On Women and Judaism.* Philadelphia, PA: The Jewish Publication Society of America.

Gross R. M. (1979). Female God language in a Jewish context. In C. P. Christ & J. Plaskow (Eds.), *Womanspirit rising.* New York: Harper & Row.

Halstead, M. M., & Halstead, L. S. (1978) A sexual intimacy survey of former nuns and priests. *Journal of Sex and Marital Therapy,* 4(2), 83-90.

Hart, A., Ames, K. A., & Sawyer, R. N. (1974). Philosophical positions of nuns and former nuns: A discriminate analysis. *Psychological Reports, 35,* 675-678.

Hooks, B. (1981). *Ain't I a woman: Black women and feminism.* Boston: South End Press.

Hunt, I. (1960). Commentary. *Genesis* (Vol. 2). New York: Paulist Press (Pamphlet Bible Series).

Janeway, E. (1980). Who is Sylvia? On the loss of sexual paradigms. *Signs, 5*(4), 573-589.

Janowitz, N., & Wenig, M. (1979). Sabbath prayers for women. In C. P. Christ & J. Plaskow (Eds.), *Womanspirit rising.* New York: Harper & Row.

Johnson, G. (1976). The Hare Krishna in San Francisco. In E. Y. Block & R. H. Bellak (Eds.), *The new religious consciousness*. Berkeley: University of California Press.

Johnson, S. (1981). *From housewife to heretic*. Garden City, NY: Doubleday.

Kertzer, M. N. (1978). *What is a Jew?* New York: Collier Books.

Korman, S. K. (1983). The feminist: Familial influences on adherence to idealogy and commitment to a self perception. *Family Relations, 32*(3), 431-439.

Las Hermanas, P.O. Box 31, Tucson, Arizona, 85702.

MacCollam, J. A. (1979). *Carnival of souls*. New York: Seabury Press.

Maynard, E ., & Twiss, G. (1970). *That these people may live*. (DHEW Publication No. HSM 72-508) Washington, DC: U.S. Government Printing Office.

Mbiti, J. S. (1969). *African Religions & Philosopshy*. New York: Praeger.

McClain, E. W. (1979). Religious orientation the key to psychodynamic differences between feminists and nonfeminists. *Journal for the Scientific Study of Religion. 18*(1), 40-45.

McGrath, A.M. (1976). *Women and the church*. New York: Image Books

Meadow, M. J. (1980). Wifely submission: psychological/spiritual growth perspectives. *Journal of Religion and Health, 19*(2), 104-120.

Messer, J. (1976). Guru Maharaj Ji and the Divine Light Mission. In C. Y. Glock & R. H. Bellak (Eds.), *The new religious consciousness*. Berkeley: University of California Press.

Miller, J. B. (1976). *Toward a new psychology of women*. Boston: Beacon Press.

Murray, S. R. (1981). Who is that person? Images and roles of black women. In S. Cox (Ed.), *Female psychology*. New York: St. Martin's.

Pamphlet Bible Series. (1960). *Exodus* (Vol. 4). New York: Paulist Press.

Parrinder, G. (1980). *Sex in the world's religions*. New York: Oxford University Press.

Plaskow, J. (1979). Bringing a daughter into the covenant. In C. P. Christ & J. Plaskow (Eds.), *Womanspirit rising*. New York: Harper & Row.

Plaskow, J. (1979). The coming of Lilith: toward a feminist theology. In C. P. Christ & J. Plaskow (Eds.), *Womanspirit rising,* New York: Harper & Row.

Porter, J. R., & Albert, A. A. (1977). Subculture or assimilation? A cross-cultural analysis of religion and women's role. *Journal for the Scientific Study of Religion, 16*(4), 345-359.

Rein, N. (1980). *Daughters of Rachel*. New York: Penguin Books.

Report of the last three sessions of the dialogue between Women's Ordination Conference and the bishops committee on women in society and in the Church. (1982). *New Woman, New Church,* (July) pp. 4-6.

Ruether, R. R. (1980) *The religious sacralization of patriarchy*. Paper commissioned for the dialogue between the Bishop's Committee on Women in Church and Society and the Women's Ordination Conference, Spring, 1980.

Ruether, R. R. (1982) *Disputed questions: On being a Christian*. Nashville: Abingdon.

Senour, M. N. (1981). Psychology of the Chicana. In S. Cox (Ed.), *Female psychology, New York: St. Martin's.*

Shaver, P., Lenauer, M., & Sadd, S. (1980). Religiousness, conversion and subjective well-being: The "healthy-minded" religion of modern American women. *American Journal of Psychiatry, 137*(12), 1563-1568.

Smith-Penniman, A., & Giles, C. (1980). Black women in ministry, Boston Theological Institute. In the Cornwall Collective (Ed.), *Your daughters shall prophesy*. New York: The Pilgrim Press.

Sojourner, S. (1982). From the house of Yemanja: The Goddess heritage of black women. In C. Spretrak (Ed.), *The politics of women's spirituality*. Garden City, NY: Doubleday.

Spirituality, prayer, call, renewed priestly ministry, bonding. (1981). *New Woman, New Church,* (March), pp. 4-5.

Starkloff C. (1974). *The people of the center.* New York: Seabury Press.

Stone, M. (1976) *When God was a woman.* New York: Harcourt Brace Jovanovich.

Stoner, C., & Parke, J. A. (1977)*All God's children.* Radnor, A Chilton Book Company.

Stoudenmier, J. (1976) The role of religion in the depressed housewife. *Journal of Religion and Health, 15*(1), 62-67.

Streiker, L. D. (1978). *The cults are coming.* Nashville: Abingdon.

Sturdivant, S. (1980) *Therapy with women.* New York: Springer Publishing Co.

Sturgeon, R. S., & Hamley, R. W. (1979). Religiosity and anxiety. *Journal of Social Psychology, 108,* 137-138.

Todd, J. (1982). On common ground: Native American and feminist spirituality approaches in the struggle to save Mother Earth. In C. Spretnak (Ed.), *The politics of women's spirituality.* Garden City, NY: Doubleday.

Tong, P. K. (1982). A cross-cultural approach to women's liberation theology. In R. M. Gross (Ed.), *Beyond androcentrism.* Missoula, MT: Scholars Press.

True, R. H. (1981). The profile of Asian American women. In S. Cox (Ed.), *Female Psychology.* New York: St. Martin's.

Umansky, E. M. (1979). Women in Judaism: From the Reform movement to contemporary Jewish religious feminism. In R. Ruether & E. McLaughlin (Eds.), *Women of spirit.* New York: Simon & Schuster.

Wilson-Kastern, P. (1982). Christianity and new feminist religions. *New Woman, New Church,* (January), pp. 4-5.

Witt, S. H. (1981). The two worlds of Native women. In S. Cox (ED.), *Female psychology.* New York: St. Martin's.

Women's Ordination Conference, P.O. Box 29124, Washington, D.C. 20017.

World Book Encyclopedia (Vol. 16). Chicago: World Book - Childcraft International, Inc., 1980.

6

REPRODUCTIVE ADVANCEMENTS: THEORY, RESEARCH APPLICATIONS, AND PSYCHOLOGICAL ISSUES

Carol C. Nadelson
Malkah T. Notman

Recent social changes have affected women's lives in major ways and have resulted in greater equality in employment and in public and private life; but women's biology and reproductive capacity continue to be subjects of discussion and concern. Future generations are dependent on the health of today's women and on the choices they make about personal goals and fulfillment. The choices must be balanced with societal expectations, needs, values, and policies. Because of their reproductive roles, women's lives are intimately affected by the concerns of society.

In recent years, values that emphasize the rights of individuals to self-fulfillment have become prominent. These values are also affected by technological advances. In the past, it was necessary to bear many children to ensure the survival of future generations. Pregnancy was also frequent because, except for celibacy, effective birth control methods were not available. Medical advances have substantially reduced maternal and infant mortality, and increased health and longevity. Together with the contraceptive revolution, they have created new reproductive options. Women now have the potential to determine the number of children they will have, the timing and spacing of their pregnancies, and the ways in which they will combine childbearing with other life goals. The development, availability, and safety of contraception and abortion are examples of the results of enormous advances in technology, which in turn are affected directly by public funding, policy, and support. They are also vulnerable to opposition fueled by political or religious arguments and policy that reflect these views.

Conflict between family control and involvement and individual rights has come into sharp focus. The conflict is particularly intense around issues such as a teenager's right to obtain contraception privately when family values prohibit premarital sexuality. Supporters of effective contraception have opposed legislation that demands disclosure of teenagers' birth control prescriptions to parents since this disclosure would interfere with the use of contraceptives and reproductive choice. This constitutes a challenge to traditional areas of parental control and influence. Similar concerns apply to a husband's right to decide about his wife's reproductive life in decisions about abortion and future childbearing. These concerns reflect the ongoing tension between secular and religious values and present policymakers and lay people alike with more challenging ethical and moral dilemmas.

Policy regarding contraception also has important forensic interest, particularly with regard to the definition of "informed consent." Early research on contraception occurred in an era when many of the legal and ethical considerations currently debated were not formally questioned, and, in some cases , technologic advances were not yet sophisticated enough for the issues to emerge. Early researchers did not obtain "informed consent," with near disastrous results for some subjects. Many women who participated in the original studies of contraceptive effectiveness did not know what they were given; those given placebos did not know that they were vulnerable to pregnancy. Since most were women whose religious and ethical values opposed abortion, they were not only exposed to the risk of unwanted pregnancy but they were also exploited by not being informed about the nature of their participation.

There have been many changes in the ethics of research and in regulations involving procedures, responsibilities, boundaries, restrictions, and cautions for conducting research. Enforcement of these regulations is variable, and the pendulum often swings from one extreme to the other, at one time requiring protective disclosure that may interfere with research and be unduly restrictive, and at another time not requiring adequate information and perhaps insufficient surveillance. The roles of subjects, patients, pharmaceutical companies, consumers and researchers, and decisions about who determines the cautions and restrictions to be enforced are yet to be defined. Dialogue on these issues must take place in the context of changing knowledge, and include the recognition that all advances have their costs. Recent publicity about DES effects illustrates this point. DES appeared to offer the promise of preventing spontaneous abortion. At the time of its original use there was no information about what subsequently emerged as the DES syndrome, which can result in cancerous changes in the offspring. Similarly, the use of oxygen in the care of premature infants was widely practiced before its potential for causing blindness was known. It is clear then that there are constant tradeoffs between risks and responsibilities.

In order to make the best possible choices, current information must be made available to both patients and practitioners. Over medicalization and unnecessary intervention presents risks; likewise there are risks inherent in assuming that no intervention is necessary when one is in fact indicated. Examples of this are the widespread use of estrogen as a treatment for menopausal symptoms, the "over use" of hysterectomy, or the use of a single treatment approach for all forms of premenstrual syndrome.

The issue of sterilization also raises concern and debate. New surgical techniques have made such procedures as tubal ligation simpler and more available. In general, studies suggest that women who elect sterilization instead of temporary contraception are not individuals with particular psychopathology leading them to make impulsive decisions. However, some women who are sterilized are not fully aware of the permanent effects of the procedure to which they give written consent.

Values and norms concerning family size, parenting ability, and appropriateness of career or family choice have clearly influenced medical recommendations concerning contraception, sterilization, abortion, and other surgical procedures. Legislation has been enacted to prevent exploitation and inappropriate recommendations for those who may be vulnerable; however, subtle social and personal influences that cannot be legislated affect these decisions and also determine what may be considered a "problem." Research priorities are also matters of policy. Decisions about where to invest financial and intellectual efforts and resources have major implications for women, since there has been insufficient research in many of the areas affecting women's health. Pressure arising from health crises has generated rethinking of some priorities. The investigations of toxic shock syndrome, the effects of DES, and the carcinogenicity of estrogens are examples of problems that come to attention in the aftermath of such crises. There is concern that insufficient attention has been devoted to prevention.

Policy regarding research into reproductively related problems also reflects judgments about whether a particular condition or state is considered "normal" or physiological, or whether it is seen as a pathological or disease state. Pregnancy and menopause, for example, are conditions where there has been sharply divided opinion about how much medical intervention is appropriate and what is normal and what is pathological in these conditions.

The questions raised in connection with these reproductive concerns are serious, and decisions have important implications for the future. This chapter will address only a few of the areas of public policy that affect women. These examples provide an introduction to the larger areas of concern.

MENSTRUAL CYCLE

Knowledge of the physiology and psychology of menstruation still suffers from past limitations of research methods and techniques, and reflects older beliefs about femininity, reproduction, and the psychology of women.

Research has suffered from methodological problems such as difficulties in accurately determining the hormonal status of subjects, the reliance on self-reports, selection bias toward women with regular cycles, and confounding of objective with subjective data (Koeske, 1981). Results obtained with objective measures differ from those using subjective methods. Results also differ when the subject is aware of the hypotheses, goals, and design of the research. Further, correlational data have been gathered to indicate causal relationships.

The extent to which women are subject to mood and other fluctuations and thus thought of as unreliable has affected policy and economic decisions (Brooks, Gunn & Ruble, 1980). Women have been excluded from jobs on the grounds that they are too strongly affected by cyclic changes. Past discussions of "raging hormones" and the stereotype of women as unpredictable have been echoed in current claims about the effects of "premenstrual syndrome," with major implications for policy regarding women. Certainly if women were for periods of time irrational or unable to perform in work or other activities, they could not be counted on as stable members of a community. This would be consistent with the stereotypical view of women as childlike. Therefore the prevalence, epidemiology, and symptom pictures of what is now a grab-bag term, "premenstrual syndrome," need to be more firmly established.

The view of premenstrual syndrome as a manifestation of an affective disorder represents another aspect of the problem and further underscores the need for careful research in this area. The history of medicine is replete with disorders, even syphillis and tuberculosis, that have been known as great "imitators" or that have had complex symptom manifestations attributed to them without establishing the symptoms as related to the specific disorder.

The symptoms considered as part of the "premenstrual syndrome" are nonspecific, vague, and overinclusive. Tension, irritability, anxiety, feeling bloated, headaches, depression, and a host of other symptoms are reported variably by 30-90 percent of the women surveyed (Parlee, 1973). However, the severity and specificity of symptoms or their effects on the individual are difficult to document. Crimes committed, suicide attempts, misbehavior of school girls, psychiatric admissions in emergency rooms, and visits to clinics have been correlated with the premenstrual period (Morton, Addition, Addison et al., 1953; Parlee, 1973; Sommes, 1973).

The important role of social and psychological expectations in producing symptoms has been emphasized; when a women expects that her behavior and responses will be affected by her menstrual cycle, and the social setting supports these expectations as normal, it is likely that her perception of her function will reflect this (Brooks-Gunn & Ruble, 1980). Cross-cultural studies indicate that women in different societies report different symptoms.

It has been suggested that between 5-10 percent of women experience severe symptoms, but there is as yet no single causal factor. Premenstrual symptoms have been ascribed to fluid retention, shifts in fluid balance, excessive secretion of prostaglandins, elevated prolactin, estrogen deficiency, disturbed progesterone/estrogen balance, vitamin B_6 deficiency and other nutritional factors, as well as emotional state. The fact that emotional state affects ovulation and menstruation has long been known, but regulatory mechanisms are not clear.

At this time, a number of treatment approaches have been proposed, but no one treatment has been shown to be "the" effective one. It is likely that both dysmenorrhea and premenstrual syndromes are not specific syndromes but represent sympton clusters with a number of causal factors. In considering treatment, it is important to emphasize the danger that inadequate evaluation may lead to inappropriate treatment. The "weak women" paradigm can result in overaggressive therapeutic approaches and the assumption that a larger percentage of women than is probably accurate belongs in the seriously symptomatic group.

PREGNANCY AND CHILDBIRTH

Psychosomatic concepts in the past have also postulated a connection between difficulties in pregnancy, labor and delivery, and conflicts with ambivalence concerning motherhood. Those women who had difficulties with pregnancy were frequently labeled as immature or emotionally disturbed. From more traditional psychoanalytic and societal viewpoints, the choice not to seek motherhood was seen as necessitating developmental compromises (Deutsch, 1945). Pregnancy can be thought of as a developmental experience providing maturational potential but also accompanied by ambivalence and conflict.

Symptoms that occur during pregnancy such as fatigue, nausea, and vomiting, and problems with labor and delivery, including anxiety and pain, have been regarded as expressions of "excessive" conflict about pregnancy. There are no conclusive data supporting this view, nor establishing what can be seen as excessive. Research confirms what has been known clinically: Lack of social or family supports has been linked with symptom severity and even with some cases of difficulty in labor and delivery. It is possible that hormonal responses are mediators of cortical stimuli. The emotional lability, anxiety, and depressive feelings that are not uncommon in the first trimester of pregnancy can be traced to biological changes, and in part these symptoms may be emotional expressions (Benedek, 1970).

Policy issues potentially affect every aspect of pregnancy. The amount of time taken for rest and other children, and the balance of responsibilities and work, are influenced by concepts of pregnancy and expectable symptoms or disruption. Care considered necessary, support for that care, and measures to provide it are also affected by these views.

Labor and delivery is another phase of pregnancy where understanding reciprocal psychobiological interactions can contribute to care and where changes in medical practice have played an important role. Women experience varying degrees of anxiety in response to labor and delivery. Some reactions are based on expectations formed while listening to the experiences of others. Some are derived from individual fantasies evoked by the process in the context of the individual's personality style. For example, a woman who feels herself to be a victim in life may expect to feel "torn apart" by the experience while another woman may expect to view it as a challenge to be controlled and mastered. Approaches to birth that maximize safety and offer optimal care need to allow for the variety of individual and cultural meanings. Families are also variably involved. Sometimes young children want to be involved or parents want them to be. Their wishes and those of their families need to be assessed. One cannot make a blanket statement that one should or should not include children in the labor or delivery room.

There is little doubt that the information provided in childbirth preparation has been effective in alleviating pain. This diminishes the anxiety due to ignorance and fosters self-confidence and mastery. Preparation also results in the need for less anesthesia for many women (Enkin, Smith, et al., 1972). The progress of labor itself is also affected by cultural and psychosocial factors, including support systems and beliefs about pregnancy and delivery (Rosengren, 1961).

"Natural childbirth" instruction, which is aimed at reducing fear and tension, leads not only to pain reduction but can promote an enhancement of the birth experience and of the development of the mother and child relationship, (Enkin et al., 1972). However, since there are multiple and often interconnected reasons for difficulty in childbirth that may be physiologically and/or psychologically based, there is no clear, single determinant of the course of labor and delivery, and it is difficult to predict the course for an individual, particularly in a first pregnancy.

Neuroendocrine and child developmental research indicates that behavior influences biological processes in complex ways and may also suggest a basis for the different experiences of mothers as compared to those of fathers with infants. For example, eye contact with the infant may be a critical biological releaser, affecting lactation as well as bonding (Mead & Newton, 1967; Shereshefsky & Yarrow, 1973). Thus, the sources of women's nurturance may derive in part from the experiences originating in pregnancy, the capacity to lactate, as well as their identifications. Parenting for fathers possibly has different sources. The extent of these has not been fully explored. Biological variables, socialization, personal expectations, and exposure to newborns all contribute. Social and health care policy decisions will affect the time mothers and fathers have to spend with young infants if the parents also work. Day care, flexible work hours for both parents, and the possibility of less rigidly stereotyped parental roles are some of the mediating conditions.

The increased number of late first pregnancies that are occurring in women in their thirties, who are often established in careers or jobs, places pregnancy in another part of the life cycle for these women, and is accompanied by different expectations and realities. Those in policymaking positions need to consider the needs of families where both parents work, where facilities for child care may be necessary, and where patterns are examined that implicitly suggest that women are at home while the children are young.

POSTPARTUM REACTIONS

The etiology of postpartum reactions has also been a subject in which myths and stereotypes have substituted for knowledge. Symptoms were among those formerly attributed to ambivalence about motherhood or inadequate feminine identity. The implications of the high incidence of some symptoms, such as the "blues" and the extensive physiological changes that occur including disturbances of sleep/wake cycle in the postpartum period, were rarely acknowledged as relevant.

Currently, we differentiate between mild, early (two to three days) transient depressive reactions or "blues," which occur in between 60-80 percent of women, depressive reactions that may be precipitated by the pregnancy as one factor but not a unique one, severe postpartum psychiatric disorders precipitated by the particular events of childbirth, which occur far less frequently (about one to four per 1000 births), and psychiatric disorders that occur in the postpartum period but may not be specifically linked to the physiological experience of childbirth (Normand, 1967; Pitt, 1973). For example, "postpartum" depressions have been reported in adoptive parents. Severe emotional disorders and postpartum psychoses are more often associated with obstetrical abnormalities, but there is no specific association of these obstetrical abnormalities with other emotional disturbances.

There has been considerable controversy as to whether postpartum psychosis is a specific syndrome or a nonspecific reaction to the psychological and physiological changes of childbirth. While there is no resolution of this question at present, some investigations do distinguish postpartum reactions from other responses to stressful experiences. There does not seem to be a specific relationship between antepartum emotional disorder and postpartum psychosis. In fact, it is unusual to find them both occurring in the same pregnancy. However, one-third of the women who experience puerperal psychosis have been reported to develop similar difficulties in subsequent pregnancies. Etiological factors include biochemical, endocrinological, genetic, as well as psychological variables. Obviously pregnancy also occurs in women with psychiatric illness, and the pregnancy may precipitate symptoms, as can any stressful or meaningful life event. Of all the conditions in which endocrine changes and mood or emotional responses seem connected, the most accepted relationship between these is in postpartum reactions (Herzog & Detre, 1976; Nilsson & Almgren, 1970; Norman, 1967). Clearly, there is a need for research on postpartum syndromes and attention to the possibility of their occurrence when considering employee benefits and insurance coverage.

ABORTION

Recent controversy about ethical issues related to abortion and challenges to access to abortion have provoked new arguments and renewed claims that abortion should be considered as a psychologically damaging procedure, in addition to having other detrimental consequences. In the past, physicians and other health professionals opposed abortion because it seemed to violate the Hippocratic oath and because it was not a safe medical procedure, especially compared with the risks of childbirth. Before the 1960s, many professionals believed that guilt and shame resulting from abortion would lead to serious depression and disturbance in relationships.

As medical techniques improved and resulted in changes in mortality rates so that childbirth carried a greater risk than abortion, medical risk could not be cited as a possible argument. Currently, for a pregnancy under 16 weeks, the risk of death from a legally performed abortion ranges between 1:25,000 and 1:400,000. The estimated mortality to be expected in childbirth is 1:10,000, the same as the abortion risk for a pregnancy over 16 weeks. The risk of maternal death from illegal abortion is estimated to be 1:3,000.

Prior to 1973, in most states, abortions were legally performed only for "therapeutic" reasons. The indications permitted were to preserve the life and/or health of the mother. Most states differed on grounds and indications, and hospitals as well as physicians accepted different criteria. For example, in one hospital a woman would have been required to have made a suicide attempt in order for the pregnancy to be considered a danger to her life, whereas in another hospital a statement of suicidal intent was sufficient. There were few abortions performed for purely medical reasons because over the past several decades the technical ability to preserve life through pregnancy had improved to the extent that life-threatening disorders during pregnancy were rare. Thus, the vast number of therapeutic abortions were performed for psychiatric reasons, although guidelines and criteria were vague.

The myth that psychological damage was inevitable or frequent following abortion persisted despite the results of Ekblad's 1955 study of 479 women who had legal abortions in Sweden for psychiatric reasons. Of the 1 percent of women who demonstrated emotional consequences following abortion, all had had previous histories of emotional disorders. Ekblad concluded that there was little evidence that abortions had serious effects on the mental health of women.

This report did not evoke much interest until the 1960s when other studies began to challenge pervasive views about sequelae to abortion, and to develop methodologies for more systematic investigation. In fact, Peck and Marcus (1966) found that some women who had already been diagnosed as psychologically ill benefitted from the procedure.

Gradually the medical literature noted the lack of serious post-abortion complications and recommended that the physician explore the motivation for the decision with the woman. Following the changes in their law that made abortion more easily available, studies from Britain refocused the issue on the stress of bearing an unwanted child (Pare & Raven, 1970). They reported that psychiatric symptoms were more likely to occur in the overburdened multipara and the single woman without support, and found that women who had a pregnancy terminated had little overt psychiatric disturbance. The attitude that has gained greatest clinical acceptance holds that an abortion may certainly be stressful for an individual but assessment of the psychological effects must be related to the significance of the pregnancy and the abortion for the individual with regard, as well, for the values and beliefs of her culture.

A study of the history of abortion suggests that attitudes tend to be more conservative and practices more restrictive when there are politically expedient reasons; for example, when population is low, or when there is economic need for more or fewer people. In fact, abortion has been practiced throughout history and has been either aboveground or underground depending upon the context.

From the perspective of social policy, one cannot discuss abortion without considering the unwanted child, its impact on the mother, the family, and the community, and available alternatives. Restricting abortions does not address the human or societal problem. Although earlier studies made it clear that psychiatric risks of abortion must also be considered concomitantly with preventative gains, for a time there was little attention paid to this recommendation. In 1954, Caplan reported that special problems were apt to develop between mother and child when an unsuccessful attempt at abortion had been made during the pregnancy. Hook (1963) studied 213 children born to women who had been refused therapeutic abortion and found that unwanted children were both physically and mentally impaired, compared to controls.

In a classic study by Forssman and Thuwe (1966), 120 Swedish children who were born after an application for a therapeutic abortion was refused were followed for 21 years and compared with matched controls. The results indicated that the unwanted children fared worse in almost every way. Subsequent studies of child abuse and neglect repeat warnings about the fate of unwanted children.

THE EFFECT OF LEGALIZATION OF ABORTION

As the climate of opinion about abortion began to change and some states liberalized their laws, investigations began to focus on counseling and crisis intervention in the decision-making process. Research has indicated that for most women abortion was indeed therapeutic when they had made a decision that this was the best course of action for them. One study pointed out that under legal conditions requiring severe prior psychiatric illness, one would find a group least likely to respond favorably to abortion as a therapeutic procedure since these were likely to be a more emotionally disturbed group of women (Partridge, Spiegel, Rouse et al., 1971). While apparently contradictory reports concerning the effects of previous psychiatric history on predicting postabortion problems can be found, differences in criteria and categories of mental illness probably account for these data. In any case, history of emotional disturbance does not always imply postabortion symptoms.

Although in 1973 the United States Supreme Court eliminated the "reason" for abortion and the necessity for psychiatrists to "approve" a "therapeutic" abortion, the belief that abortion was psychologically damaging persisted. While the evidence runs counter to this view, it is also clear that abortion cannot be seen as a minor procedure without significance to the individual. The decision for abortion is an important one, requiring careful consideration, which may be facilitated with counseling. For many women this may extend into the postabortion period. When counseling is provided in an atmosphere where a woman's decision is respected and her right to make that decision is not interfered with, fewer adverse reactions are to be expected. Here, too, public policy has often followed prevailing points of view that often do not take account of available data.

MENOPAUSE

Menopause has been considered a major transition point in women's reproductive and emotional life. While its reproductive significance is clear, its emotional implications have been confused with cultural expectations, life cycle concerns, and the particular implications of aging for an individual woman. Although many of the symptoms that appear in women in midlife have been attributed to menopause, most of them are not directly connected with physiological processes. Life cycle developmental changes of the midlife period and midlife stresses must be differentiated from menopausal effects.

Symptoms that have been attributed to the menopause include depression, irritability, insomnia, headaches, dizzy spells, palpitations, weight increases, hot flashes and flushes, night sweats, sleep disturbances, and a variety of other disturbances. Vasomotor instability has been attributed to the instability of balance between hypothalamic, pituitary, and ovarian hormones, which has an effect on the heat regulating mechanism. These symptoms and sleep disturbances that may accompany the vasomotor changes do appear to be the consistent symptoms accompanying menopause (McKinlay & Jeffreys, 1974). These have been reported in up to 75 percent of women, but vary considerably with culture and population studied. Other symptoms described do not actually show a direct relationship to the menopause.

Among the symptoms that can be troublesome are those attributed to changes in the vaginal and other mucosa. These changes may affect vaginal lubrication and sexual functioning. While sexual interest does not appear to diminish at menopause, if there is a drying of vaginal mucosa, discomfort may occur. Many women report increased sexual satisfaction as they are freed from anxiety about pregnancy. Masters and Johnson (1966) and others have documented that full sexual activity continues in middle-aged and older women, particularly if they have had active sexual lives previously. Although changes in patterns of sexual response occur with age, particularly for men, they believe it is a myth that sexual functioning inevitably diminishes with age.

Osteoporosis is a particularly distressing postmenopausal problem for some women. The mechanisms of calcium metabolism and the relationship to ovarian estrogen and to estrogen converted from adrenal hormones is not cleary delineated. Osteoporosis does not usually become a problem until well after actual menopause, when hormones from nonovarian sources also diminish.

Those women who experience most emotional distress at the time of menopause seem to be those who have relied most on their childbearing role as a source of self-esteem and status (Zilbach, 1982). Women who have had children and have invested heavily in their childbearing and rearing, or who live in a society rewarding these, are more likely to experience depression. Those who have not had children do not necessarily have the most difficulty with menopause. Cross-cultural studies indicate that in those cultures where there is improved status at middle age and a clear role for the middle-aged woman, there are greater feelings of well-being at midlife. Family experiences are important in determining the outcome of this period (Neugarten, Wood, Kraines et al., 1968; Zilbach, 1982).

Anxiety experienced in anticipation of menopause appears to be greater than that experienced during the actual menopausal period. Postmenopausal women are reported to take a more positive view than premenopausal women, with higher proportions agreeing that the menopause creates no major discontinuity in life and that, except for the underlying biological changes and their concomitant symptoms, menopause need not inevitably cause difficulties. However, ignoring distress—whether related to hormonal, life cycle, or other determinants—does not serve a woman better than holding the expectation that manifestations of stress are inevitable. Depression does not appear to be as clearly associated with the endocrine changes of the menopausal period as with psychosocial variables (Neugarten et al., 1968; Zilbach, 1982).

The treatment of menopausal symptoms has been controversial. The view that menopause is a "deficiency disease" and requires replacement of estrogen is one that reflects a bias in favor of "medicalized" intervention. However, symptom relief may be very important to individual women at particular times. Estrogens have been used clinically to relieve hot flashes for many years. Recent data suggest that there may be an increased risk for endometrial carcinoma with prolonged estrogen use and current practice recommends a conservative approach. Vaginal estrogen creams have been successful in alleviating some of the specific symptoms related to vaginal lubrication. If necessary, sequential treatment using estrogens with progesterone in small doses has been advocated, although this does cause cyclic bleeding.

Osteoporosis following menopause constitutes a potentially serious problem, with treatment still controversial. Since some estrogen is converted from adrenal hormones, low levels are not reached and severe osteoporosis is a problem that occurs after the immediate menopausal years. Current approaches include considering diets rich in calcium and encouragement of physical activity. Recommendations must be made by carefully weighing risks and benefits.

The concept of normal life transition in a culture that devalues aging and that relates women's self-esteem with reproduction and sexuality raises important health policy concerns. These must address the unresolved problems of seeking the best preventive and therapeutic approaches and must support further careful research into menopausal symptomatology and normative development.

HYSTERECTOMY

The number of hysterectomies performed in the United States is greater than that of any other major operation performed on women. The National Center for Health Statistics estimates that in 1981 571.3 per 100,000 women were performed, which has remained stable in this country since 1973 (National Center for Health Statistics, 1984).

The indications for hysterectomy have not been universally agreed upon and often seem to be subjective. A Canadian study revealed a 32.8 percent drop in the total number of hysterectomies done when it was suggested that cases would be reviewed (Dyck, 1977). There have been accusations that hysterectomies are performed as practice for surgeons, especially where poorly educated women, who are not fully informed about the alternatives, are the patients. On the other hand, some women who are themselves ambivalent about contraception or for whom contraception causes conflict with religious beliefs or cultural practices may seek a hysterectomy essentially for contraceptive purposes. While this has not been an accepted medical indication, there is a subtle interplay between a physician's attitudes toward women and childbearing and a patient's pressure. Careful research on indications and outcome is essential. Policy regarding this procedure reflects values as well as health concerns.

The impact of a hysterectomy is variable and is difficult to assess out of context. It is a stressful procedure, but it is important to separate the response to the underlying disease, such as whether it is benign or malignant, from the response to the procedure, or the loss of the uterus. The consequences in a premenopausal woman involve the ending of reproductive possibilities and menstruation. For a postmenopausal woman the presence of a uterus may continue to play an important role in her self-concept and body image. Social and cultural factors as well as the symbolic and unconscious significance of the uterus for an individual woman must be considered (Martin, Roberts & Clayton, 1980; Polivy, 1974).

For some women a hysterectomy is perceived as ending the era of "youth," and beginning undesirable middle age. Because of changes in social roles and opportunity and the current increase of nonreproductive options, a hysterectomy may have different current implications than in the past. Even though a woman may know rationally that a hysterectomy will not affect her day-to-day life or her sexual function, she may continue to be concerned since femininity, sexuality, and motherhood have for so long been related to the uterus. Women often reveal this when they say about a hysterectomy, "Everything was taken out" or "I lost my nature."

Research in this area has also suffered from methodological and conceptual problems. Variables have been inappropriately grouped or eliminated, resulting in problems in differentiating the effects of surgically induced menopause from those of hysterectomy. Many studies that reported serious psychological consequences from hysterectomy were retrospective and did not assess the premorbid state. Assessment of effects and outcomes were further hampered by not differentiating those patients with preexisting psychopathology from those without such problems. Further, the particular procedure performed may affect physical recovery and possible sexual response.

A number of studies report a higher incidence of depression following hysterectomy compared with other surgical procedures. Although sampling and methodological problems complicate these studies, they do suggest the vulnerability of some women to posthysterectomy depression (Turpin & Heath, 1979). Recent better designed studies do not report a higher posthysterectomy incidence of depression (Polivy, 1974). This suggests either that better delineation of variables provides different and possibly more valid information or that changes in attitudes and expectations regarding hysterectomy may decrease the trauma for many women. It is clear that a rigorous search for criteria and delineation of outcome factors are essential.

CONCLUSION

Reproduction related events may be regarded as illness because medical interventions are expected, often without recognition of the full meaning of these experiences or implications of "treatment." Any process involving reproduction or reproductive organs is emotionally significant and the potential for adaptive resolution or maladaptive responses may be greatly affected by the kind of intervention and its effects. In obstetrics and gynecology there has been particular danger of overreading symptoms, drawing premature and exclusionary conclusions as to their "psychogenic" or "biologic" nature, and treating patients inadequately because of still prevalent stereotyped views regarding women. On the other hand, new data continue to suggest that many symptoms must be taken seriously and treated. The equation of psychogenic and, therefore, not serious or treatable cannot be accepted. Values, attitudes, and preconceptions as to appropriate family styles and sexual and social choices can color objectivity.

Newer observations have changed concepts of normality and increased understanding of universal experiences such as menstruation, pregnancy, menopause, and of conditions such as sterility. Of enduring importance is the maintenance of an integrated approach to women's health care with the goal of empathic understanding of processes, symptoms, and communications rather than fitting these rigid categories. In this chapter we have chosen to exemplify some of the areas of current preventive and therapeutic concern in relation to reproductive issues and suggest areas for inquiry and policy.

REFERENCES

Andersch, B., Hahn, L. Anderson, M. et al. (1978). Body water and weight in patients with premenstrual tension. *British Journal of Obstetric Gynaecology, 85,* 546.

Benedek, T. (1970). The psychobiology of pregnancy. In J. Anthony & T. Benedek (Eds.), *Parenthood: Its psychology and psychopathology.* Boston: Little, Brown.

Brooks-Gunn, J., & Ruble, D. (1980). Menarche: The interaction of physiological, cultural, and social factors. In A. Dan, E. Graham, & C. Beecher (Eds.), *The menstrual cycle* (vol. 1). New York: Springer.

Caplan, G. (1954). The disturbance of the mother-child relationship by unsuccessful attempts at abortion. *Mental Hygiene, 38,* 67.

Deutsch, H. (1945). *The psychology of women* (vols. 1 and 2). New York: Grune & Stratton.

Dyck, F. (1977). Effect of surveillance on the number of hysterectomies in the province of Sasketchewan. *New England Journal of Medicine, 296*(23), 1326.

Ekbald, N. (1955). Induced abortion on psychiatric grounds. *Acta Psychiatrica, Scandinavian Supplement, 99.*

Enkin, M., Smith, S., Dermer, S., et al. (1972). An adequately controlled study of the effectiveness of p.p.m. training. In M. Norris (Ed.), *Psychosomatic medicine in obstetrics and gynecology: Proceedings.* Basel, Switzerland: S. Karger.

Forssman, H., & Thuwe, I. (1966). 120 children born after application for therapeutic abortion refused: The mental health, social adjustment and education level up to the age of 21. *Acta Psychiatrica, Scandinavian Supplement, 42,* 71.

Herzog, A., & Detre, T. (1976). Psychotic reactions associated with childbirth. *Disorders of the Nervous System, 37*(4), 229.

Hook K. (1963). Refused abortion: A follow-up of 249 women whose applications were refused by the National Board of Health in Sweden. *Acta Psychiatrica, Scandinavian Supplement, 168,* 39.

Koeske, R. (1981). Theoretical and conceptual complexities in the design and analysis of menstrual cycle research. In P. Konmenich, M. McSweeney, J. Noack et al. (Eds.), *The menstrual cycle* (vol. 2). New York: Springer.

Martin, R., Roberts, W., & Clayton, P. (1980). Psychiatric status after hysterectomy: A one-year prospective follow-up. *Journal of the American Medical Association, 244*(4), 350.

Masters, W., & Johnson, V. (1966). *Human sexual response.* Boston: Little, Brown.

McKinlay, S., & Jeffreys, M. (1974). The menopausal syndrome. *British Journal of Preventative Social Medicine, 28*(2), 108.

Mead, M., & Newton, N. (1967). Cultural patterning of prenatal behavior. In S. Richardson & A. Guttmacher (Eds.), *Childbearing: Its social and psychological aspects.* Baltimore: Williams & Wilkins.

Morton, J. Addition, H., Addison, R., et al. (1953). A clinical review of premenstrual tension. *American Journal of Obstetric Gynecology, 65,* 1182.

National Center for Health Statistics. (1984). Personal communication.

Neugarten, B., Wood, T., Kraines, R., et al. (Eds.). (1968). *Middle age and aging.* Chicago: University of Chicago Press.

Nilson, A., & Almgren, P. (1970). Paranatal emotional adjustment. A prospective investigation of 165 women. II: The influence of background factors, psychiatric history, parental relations and personality characteristics. *Acta Psychiatrica, Scandinavian Supplement, 63.*

Normand, W. (1967). Postpartum disorders. In A. Freedman & H. Rapkin (Eds.), *Comprehensive textbook of psychiatry.* Baltimore: Williams & Wilkins.

Pare, C., & Raven, H. (1970). Follow-up of patients referred for termination of pregnancy. *The Lancet, 635* (March 28).

Parlee, M. (1973). The premenstrual syndrome. *Psychological Bulletin, 80,* 454.

Partridge, J., Spiegel, T., Rousse, B., et al. (1971). Therapeutic abortion: A study of psychiatric applications at North Carolina Memorial Hospital. *North Carolina Medical Journal, 32,* 132.

Peck, A., & Marcus, H. (1966). Psychiatric sequalae of therapeutic interruption of abortion. *Journal of Nervous Mental Disorders, 143,* 417.

Pitt, B. (1973). Maternity blues. *British Journal of Psychiatry, 122,* 431.

Polivy, J. (1974). Psychological reactions to hysterectomy: A critical review. *American Journal of Obstetric Gynecology, 118,* 417.

Ramey, E. (1982). The endocrinologist's approach. In C. Debrovner (Ed.), *Premenstrual tension: A multidisciplinary approach.* New York: Human Sciences Press.

Rosengren, W. (1961). Some social psychological aspects of delivery room difficulties. *Journal of Nervous Mental Disorders, 132,* 515.

Shereshefsky, P., & Yarrow, L. (1973). *Psychological aspects of a first pregnancy and early postnatal adaptation.* (NICHD Monograph). New York: Raven

Sommer, B. (1973). The effect of menstruation on cognitive and perceptal motor behavior: A review. *Psychosomatic Medicine, 35*(7), 515.

Turpin, R., & Heath, D. (1979). The link between hysterectomy and depression. *Canadian Journal of Psychiatry, 24*(3), 247.

Zilbach, J. (1982). Separation: A family development process in mid-life. In C. Nadelson & M. Notman (Eds.), *The woman patient* (vol. 2). New York: Plenum.

7

INEQUALITY AND MENTAL HEALTH: LOW INCOME AND MINORITY WOMEN

Deborah Belle

If one main objective of the War on Poverty has been to achieve racial and sexual equality of opportunity, we are losing—and losing badly. (National Advisory Council on Economic Opportunity, 1980, p. 9)

Certain groups of women in our society have a significantly greater than average risk of suffering from depressive conditions. To the extent that the unequal distribution of such risk is the result of more widely recognized inequalities within our society, and our findings certainly point in this direction, we believe that it constitutes a major social injustice. (Brown, Bhrolchain, & Harris, 1975, p. 248)

The mental health needs of low income and minority women cry out for attention from those who provide mental health services and from those in many other sectors of our society. While poor women experience a particularly high incidence of mental health problems, they are often reluctant to use mental health services. Among those who do seek professional help many are so dissatisfied that they drop out of treatment. Minority women particularly are likely to be poor, to find their opportunities limited by discrimination, and to discover that potential therapists do not share basic knowledge and values with them.

This chapter discusses the environmental context that precipitates so much emotional distress among low income and minority women, the experiences of those women who do seek out treatment services, and several recommendations for the prevention and treatment of mental health problems among low income and minority women.

Author's Note: The author is grateful for helpful comments on an earlier draft from Weining Chang, Dana Jack, Maureen Reese, Lenore Walker, and Barbara Wolf.

WOMEN AND POVERTY

We are often told that women and minority members have come a long way toward equality. Yet economic conditions have actually deteriorated for many women over the past decade. Women and their children have come to constitute an increasingly large proportion of America's poor, a phenomenon that has been called the "feminization of poverty" (Pearce, 1979). The poverty population has also become increasingly minority as it has become more female.

Divorce has pushed many women who once were economically secure into poverty. Few families receive regular child support payments from the noncustodial father over the years following a divorce, and even those who do typically receive only a small fraction of what it costs to support a family (Pearce, 1979). Almost 1 female-headed family in 3 is poor, in comparison to 1 in 18 families headed by a man. In 1977 the median income of female-headed families was only $340 above the poverty line, and among black and Hispanic single mothers it was about $1000 below it. In 1967 a black woman heading a family was 7½ times more likely to be poor than was a white man; 10 years later she was 10½ times more likely to be poor. Among Hispanic women heading families the incidence of poverty is 11 times that of white men heading families, and among Puerto Rican female family heads the rate is almost 15 times that found among white male family heads (National Advisory Council on Economic Opportunity, 1980).

While women have moved into the paid labor force in great numbers, their earnings relative to those of men have actually declined in recent years. Women college graduates earn less than male high school graduates and about as much as male high school dropouts (Barrett, 1979). Female full-time, year-round workers earn less than 60 percent of what male full-time, year-round workers earn in the same fields (Barrett, 1979). Nor do government welfare payments often raise families out of poverty. Virtually all families receiving Aid to Families with Dependent Children (AFDC) benefits would have incomes below the poverty line if they did not have additonal income from other allowable sources such as employment. Three-fourths of all families receiving AFDC benefits have poverty-level incomes even after adding their legally allowed earnings to their welfare checks. AFDC benefits have not come close to keeping pace with inflation in the last decade, and recent regulations have made it increasingly difficult for women to add earnings from employment to their minimal welfare checks.

The lack of decent affordable child care prevents many women from holding regular jobs and leads them to part-time and at-home jobs that are typically poorly paid and lacking in benefits and advancement opportunities (Tebbets, 1982).

POVERTY AND MENTAL HEALTH

These social and economic realities are destructive to women's mental health because poverty is associated with a high incidence of mental health problems (Brown, Bhrolchain, & Harris, 1975; Pearlin & Johnson, 1977; Radloff, 1975). This association is particularly strong among women who are responsible for young children (Brown et al., 1975; Pearlin & Johnson, 1977; Radloff, 1975). In the study by Brown and his colleagues, for instance, the rate of affective disorders among a sample of women living in central London was 5 percent among middle-class women, 25 percent among working-class women, and an astounding 42 percent among working-class women with at least one child of preschool age. While the mothers in Brown's study were married, other evidence suggests that the single parent woman is at greater risk than her married counterpart (Pearlin & Johnson, 1977; Radloff, 1975).

STRESS

The high rate of mental health problems among low income and minority women becomes much more understandable when we examine the stressful contexts of their lives. Stress research indicates that rapid life change can be threatening to mental health, particularly when changes are unexpected, negative in overall impact, and beyond the control of the individual who experiences them. Those who experience a rapid succession of changes may not have adequate opportunities to recuperate after each life event or to integrate the new experience into their sense of what their lives are about. Too rapid an experience of change can lead to anxiety and to the belief that life is not coherent or predictable. This can erode the self-esteem that comes when one can predict and control one's future. Specific events may also produce intense sensations of loss or lead to undeserved feelings of guilt and worthlessness, which are often precursors of depression.

Low income and minority women experience more frequent, more threatening and more uncontrollable life events than does the general population, and this excessive rate of change appears to be responsible for some of their heightened risk of mental disorder (Brown et al., 1975; Dohrenwend, 1973; Makosky, 1982). Crime and violence occur disproportionately to the poor. Belle et al. (1981) found, for instance, that a sample of 42 urban low income mothers had experienced a total of 37 violent events during the preceding two years, and these same women reported an additional 35 events that had happened to close friends and relatives. Merry (1981) discovered that at one small urban housing project almost half of the surveyed households had experienced a robbery, burglary, or assault against one of their members. Poor women are also more likely to experience the illness or death of children (Children's Defense Fund, 1979) and the imprisonment of husbands (Brown et al., 1975). Women in minority groups are frequently exposed to painful incidents of discrimination in their everyday lives and are also at risk for discrimination-provoked violence (Steele, et al., 1982). Many minority women are also immigrants to this country and thus must adjust to a dramatically different way of life. Moreover, poor women are likely to have experienced severe losses in childhood, such as parental death, which may still reverberate in adulthood, especially at the time of new losses (Brown et al., 1975; Langner & Michael, 1963; Reese, 1982).

While rapid, uncontrollable change is one important source of stress, many stresses occur in the absence of change, from persisting, undesirable conditions that must be endured daily. While moving from one home to another may be stressful and require readjustment, remaining in the same cramped, dilapidated apartment in an unsafe neighborhood may also be stressful. Recent studies indicate that chronic life conditions such as inadequate housing, dangerous neighborhoods, burdensome responsibilities, and financial uncertainties can be even more potent stressors than acute crises and events (Brown et al., 1975; Makosky, 1982; Pearlin & Johnson, 1977). Furthermore, low income women are at very high risk of experiencing just such noxious, long-term conditions (Brown et al., 1975; Makosky, 1982). Thus, low income women are more likely to experience both chronic stressful conditions and acute stressful events.

For many low income women life consists of a succession of threatening, stressful events woven into a fabric of ongoing, chronically stressful life conditions. As one woman expressed it, "My life has always been a matter of coping with one thing or another. I get through one crisis to find another coming up. Sometimes it feels as if everything is caving in all at once" (Dill & Feld, 1982, pp. 184-185).

SOCIAL SUPPORT

When stressful life events and conditions threaten mental health, the woman who can share her troubles with a supportive confidant or circle of friends is less likely to be overwhelmed by them. Timely material and instrumental assistance can often prevent a crisis from becoming a catastrophe and can prevent a stressful event from becoming a chronically stressful condition. Many poor and minority women create mutual aid networks through which they care for and sustain each other in times of stress. Such support networks are truly "strategies for survival" in a hostile world (Stack, 1974).

Yet poverty often exacts a toll on a woman's support system, just as it directly subjects her to stress. One of the greatest sources of social support is the intimacy of the marital bond (Brown et al., 1975; Pearlin & Johnson, 1977), which poverty often threatens. Parents living below the poverty line are less likely to be happily married than those above the poverty line (Zill, 1978), and low income women are less likely than middle-class women to turn to their husbands as confidants, particularly during the phase of the life cycle when there are young children at home and when low income women are thus at highest risk for depression (Brown et al., 1975). Men who provide very low or sporadic income for their families are likely candidates for marital dissolution and divorce (Cherlin, 1979), and husband-wife families are dramatically underrepresented among families living at or below the poverty level. Half of all families living in poverty do not include a husband-father (U.S. Bureau of the Census, 1980).

Extensive involvement in a social network may also threaten the mental health of women heavily committed to the traditional woman's role of "kin keeper." Cohler and Lieberman (1980) studied the social networks and psychological well-being of ethnic women, many of whom were highly involved in sociable and helping relationships with others. The researchers found, in contrast to their own hypotheses, that the women who were more involved with relatives and friends experienced more psychological distress than their less involved peers. Apparently the recurrent demands to provide care to others were more stressful than supportive overall.

A woman's sense of connection to and responsibility for others may make her more vulnerable to what has been called the "contagion of stress" (Wilkins, 1974), when stressful events and conditions afflict those close to her. Such stress contagion can result from emotional identification with the suffering of another and from the added practical burdens that another's misfortune may create if one takes responsibility for providing assistance oneself. Since the relatives, friends, and neighbors of a low income woman are themselves likely to be poor and stressed, the low income woman often experiences considerable stress contagion from her social network. Eckenrode and Gore (1981) found, for instance, that women whose relatives and friends experienced stressful life events such as illnesses and burglaries reported finding these events personally stressful and even reflected this vicarious stress in their own poor health.

Among middle-class women and men social ties often bring with them access to substantial material resources, information, and political power. The relative who can loan a vacation home, the acquaintance who can help a child find an after-school job, or the colleague who can make a referral to the best medical specialist offer resources and help to solve problems without extensive personal effort of their own. The social networks of poor women, particularly of those who are second or third generation poor, generally lack such resources. Each woman's friends, relatives, and acquaintances are approximately as powerless and vulnerable as she.

COPING

In the face of much stress and with limited economic, social, and political resources at their disposal, low income women attempt to cope with their problems and to keep their families going. Many exchange child care assistance so that they can hold jobs and raise the family income. They budget carefully to use their incomes as effectively as possible. Some even confront officials who have unreasonably denied their requests for needed welfare benefits, housing, or job training. Dill and Feld (1982) have chronicled some of the "persistent, energetic and imaginative strategies" that low income black and white women use to cope with the threatening situations they face.

Yet in spite of their best efforts, many such efforts at coping do not achieve their original goal or do so only at the cost of considerable inconvenience, humiliation, or pain. Dill and Feld describe one woman whose apartment in public housing was being ruined by leaking water. Public health officials declared the apartment unsafe, but the public housing authority never came to make repairs. The woman appealed to everyone she could find to listen to her case and even called in the local television station for an exposé. At the time she was interviewed her suit was pending in court, while water continued, years after her efforts began, to leak into her apartment. Another woman waited six months to get welfare approval of a furniture voucher and assistance with her utilities bills, both of which had been promised her. During the six-month period she repeatedly visited the welfare office but could not receive any information on her case. She hired a lawyer who finally determined that her caseworker had been laid off several months before. Another woman was worried about her son who was dyslexic and emotionally disturbed. She tried and failed to get him an early learning abilities evaluation through his school and tried and failed to have him placed in a Big Brother program, in after-school day care, and in a special school for the learning disabled. Unable to obtain the help she needed, through no failure of effort or imagination on her part, she felt guilty and inadequate as a mother and increasingly concerned that her son's problems, left untreated, would only get worse.

These coping failures occurred not because of any fault in the woman's coping strategy but simply because powerful institutions declined to respond. One of the salient facts of low income life is utter dependence on such institutions (welfare, health care, criminal justice) and lack of clout with them. Poor women who seek change through personally confronting such institutions often experience repeated failures.

To fail repeatedly at active coping can lead to the (often veridical) perception that one is indeed powerless to remove the major stressors from one's life. In such circumstances one may be moved to adopt palliative forms of coping that do not attempt to change the stressful situation itself but merely to dull the pain of its persistence. Self-medication with alcohol and drugs can have such palliative intent as can overeating, sleeping during the day, and repressing thoughts of the problem (Pearlin & Radabaugh, 1976; Wolf, 1983; Fine, 1983-1984). Sometimes the choice of one palliative method of coping reflects a highly self-conscious decision-making process. As one woman interviewed by Wolf (1983) explained it,

I ain't gonna worry myself about everything that happens—you crazy? I'd be *dead* from worryin' if I did that, or be in the nut-house, either one. No, not me! Might sound funny but know what I do when I got trouble? I get in the bed and go to sleep. Now I know that doesn't solve my problem, but it's better than worryin' till you get yourself crazy like all these other mothers. I will admit I been sleepin' too much in the daytime, though, and I know that ain't good for me—can't get anything done that way, your housework, shopping. But it's better'n always hollerin' or beatin' up the kids. It's better than takin' dope and pills, that's for sure. (pp. 41-42)

While most commentators have decried the apparent helplessness represented by the choice of such palliative strategies, Fine (1983-1984) argues that such behaviors are also ways of taking control, given the impracticality and even the danger of more "active" problem-solving techniques for low-income and minority women in many situations. In her conversations with a low income black woman who had survived a rape, Fine found that while the woman rejected several coping strategies which Fine (as rape counselor) offered her (e.g., pressing charges against the assailant, confiding in friends and counselors), the woman did find ways to take control of her situation.

Unable to trust existing institutions, for Altamese self-disclosure would have exposed wounds unlikely to be healed. Responsible for a network of kin, Altamese could not rely on but had to protect her social supports. Resisting social institutions, withholding information and preserving emotional invulnerability emerged as her strategies for maintaining control. . . . Expecting God to prosecute, loss of memory to insure coping and fantasy to anesthetize reality, Altamese is by no means helpless. (p. 256)

Yet no form of coping can offer protection from demoralization if stressors continue to multiply and to defie solution. Another of Wolf's respondents graphically described how her inability to remedy the threatening problems of her life led her to hopelessness and depression:

You have to understand, for fifteen years I had been trying to stop my husband's drinking, and I couldn't, and to pay my bills, which I couldn't. Then, with Joey [her son], I'd been banging my head against the wall, trying to keep him out of trouble, and *I couldn't do that either*. My husband was a drunk, my financial situation was a shambles, my son was beating up little kids, he was practically killed in a fight and was becoming a drunk himself, and *there was nothing I could do about it*. I couldn't even get my son the treatment he desperately needed. It just got to the point, after trying and trying to pay the bills, to take care of my husband and my five kids—six, really, because my husband was really a child—that I just *stopped. Literally*, I realized,

I *can't*. God knows I tried, but I *couldn't*. And I became a very depressed lady. It got to the point, I didn't get up at all—I stayed in bed. The house got so bad you couldn't walk through it—you can imagine, with five kids. And I had no idea what was happening to me—I just knew I was exhausted, I couldn't try anymore; I couldn't *feel* anymore. (pp. 42-43)

Many women arrive at such a condition, in spite of their intelligence, ego strength, and energy, worn down by unremitting stress and repeated, undeserved coping failures. Their problems are often further compounded by stress-related physical ailments. Many also experience difficulties in the parenting role, which requires so much energy, frustration tolerance, and self-denial (Longfellow, Zelkowitz and Saunders, 1982; Zelkowitz, 1982). Such difficulties are themselves guilt producing, which further exacerbates feelings of stress and depression.

MENTAL HEALTH SERVICES

While many women attempt to solve their emotional, physical, and environmental problems on their own, others do seek help. Some turn to professional mental health services or to community-based services such as mothers' groups that provide mental health care. Others seek help through the general medical system for relief of the physical ailments that accompany their emotional distress. Many women first contact service providers about parenting difficulties or the emotional or behavioral problems of their children.

Clinicians do help many women to resolve their difficulties and overcome their emotional distress. Yet all too often a woman's attempt to find help from a professional service provider becomes simply another punishing coping failure. When my colleagues and I interviewed low income black and white women about their experiences with mental health services (Belle et al., 1982) we learned that women were likely to receive only drug therapy when they wanted a chance to discuss their problems with a therapist. Others experienced themselves as blamed by therapists for their children's problems without receiving any help in solving these problems.

In many instances therapist and client hold such disparate world views and understandings of the causes of the client's emotional distress that there is little shared vision that could serve as a starting point for therapy. Many low income women experience their environment as the cause of their own emotional distress and their children's problems. (In this, of course, they agree with a vast amount of published research!) Lurie (1974, p. 133) found, for instance, that the mothers she studied often attributed their children's problems to the "pathogenic conditions of their lives" such as inadequate income, poor health, substandard housing, and run-down and unsafe neighborhoods. My colleagues and I found that the low income mothers we interviewed often mentioned such environmental stresses when we asked them what kinds of problems they would view as emotional problems. As one respondent stated, "Welfare, you know, is emotional strain," or as another said, "No money or food would cause emotional problems."

Yet when these women seek professional help they often find that clinicians ignore these realities. Without ever inquiring about the stressful life events and conditions the woman is experiencing or the history of her active and palliative coping efforts, such clinicians instead limit their attention to intrapsychic issues. Such a limitation renders the therapist worse than useless, for by offering such a view of the woman's mental health problems the therapist misrepresents the realities of the woman's life and offers her a damaging view of herself. As one of our respondents told us, "I avoid it [treatment] because they make me feel *more* fucked up."

Race, ethnicity, and class differences between therapists and clients can pose barriers to understanding if therapists do not make a great effort to understand life experiences they have not shared. Boyd (1979) discovered that only 7.7 percent of the white psychologists he interviewed believed that socioeconomic or system problems were among the most common problems experienced by the black families with whom they worked, while white social workers and black clinicians (social workers and psychologists) were likely to view such issues as pervasive. At worst, clinicians may come to hold negative stereotypes about low income and minority women, attributing stress-related emotional problems to class or culture. As one woman we interviewed observed, "I've run into mental health workers who have a real bad attitude, and it's not so much an attitude of hostility or anything. . .they equate being poor with being stupid." Such experiences are in part responsible for the refusal of many low income and minority women to use mental health services and for the extremely high rates of "premature withdrawal" from treatment by low income and minority clients (Acosta, 1980).

Additional barriers to the use of services by low income and minority women include the cost of services, difficulties with transportation to and from services, and the difficulty of arranging child care so that a mother can keep her appointments. In addition, many women fear that revealing emotional problems or problems in the parent-child relationship may lead to their children being taken from them. When my colleagues and I began our interviews with low income women we began to hear from many women about the dangers involved in revealing one's vulnerability to anyone in a position of authority. We found a pervasive fear that children would be taken away. Several of the women we worked with had lost custody of their children, either temporarily or permanently, and others were threatened with such a loss. When we began our work with low income women I regretted the excessive fear of having a child removed and wished that our respondents could come to take a calmer, less fearful view of social agencies. After more experience in the field and after observing one incident that verified our respondents' worst fears, I came to wish that several of our respondents would show even more caution in their dealings with those in authority. While many judgments about a mother's fitness are made in the genuine best interest of the child and with consideration of the parent(s) as well, powerful social agencies sometimes do intervene to break families apart without justification.

PREVENTING MENTAL HEALTH PROBLEMS

The mental health of low income and minority women cannot be separated from the environmental contexts of their lives, and these contexts are shaped in important ways by social and economic forces beyond the control of any single individual. Women will continue to be overrepresented among the depressed as long as they are over-represented among the poor. Minority women will continue to pay emotionally for the racism of our society.

Passage of the Equal Rights Amendment and the enforcement of existing laws that promise equality of opportunity to women and members of minority groups must be a high priority. Prevention efforts must aim to halt the feminization of poverty and to increase women's opportunities.

Since economic difficulties are at the root of so many of the emotional problems of low income women, and since many women regard paid employment as the best escape from poverty and depression, programs that help women to find and keep decent employment could have a powerful impact on mental health. Since most traditional

"women's work" is poorly paid and offers little possibility of advancement, training programs that help women enter nontraditional employment areas are essential. Pay scales for traditional women's jobs must
also be upgraded so that women can actually support their families
when they work at jobs such as waitressing, human service work,
and clerical work. The lack of high quality affordable child care prevents
many women from entering the labor force and prevents many more
from holding well-paying, full-time jobs. This country can learn from
the successes of virtually every other Western industrialized nation
that societal support for the nation's children strengthens individuals
and families.

However, recent efforts to force poor women into the labor force
as the price of continuing to receive their meager welfare benefits
are extremely dangerous. Surviving on a poverty-level income is already
a full-time job that demands carefully planned shopping expeditions,
effortful networking with relatives, friends, or neighbors to ensure
against the inevitable financial crises, and continual attention to the
safety of the children. With all its stigma and frustrations, welfare
dependency is a highly undesirable option, and women who choose
it do so out of great need. If they could safely combine employment
with their childrearing responsibilities almost all would already do
so. Coercing women into humiliating job searches or essentially punitive
jobs will not improve the mental health of women. Ironically, this
rush to force unemployed women who do not want employment into
the work place comes just at the time that government actions are
denying needed resources such as child care, education, and training
to women who desperately want to work. Such misguided actions
create further frustration, stress, and feelings of helplessness for in-
numerable women today.

Another preventive strategy is to help girls and young women develop
the marketable skills that will enhance their employability as adults.
Female students are not now sufficiently encouraged to study
mathematics and science, to pursue technical skills, or to enroll in
government-sponsored apprenticeship programs that will lead to well-
paying jobs. This implicit sexism results in the impoverishment of
many women, often at the point when a marriage ends and a husband's
paycheck is no longer available. Education and counseling efforts
to help girls and young women prepare for well-paid employment
should be taken just as seriously as similar efforts with male students.
If anything, work with young women should receive a higher priority,
as it is needed to overcome the pervasive societal myth that most

women do not need to work and thus to develop their own earning capacity.

TREATMENT ISSUES

Mental health services for low income and minority women will improve as clinicians overcome their own classism, racism, and tendency to blame the victim by coming to see the low income or minority client within the context of her own life experiences and current options. If mental health professionals are knowledgeable about the relationship between women's psychological well-being and environmental circumstances they can incorporate this perspective into their treatment efforts. If therapy is properly oriented, in combatting depression women can also gain control over other areas of their lives. However, if environmental realities are ignored while therapist and client search for the intrapsychic flaw at the root of an emotional problem, a woman is likely to sink more deeply into passivity, guilt, and depression while losing the chance to overcome both environmental problems and emotional problems.

Since social and economic stress are often the root cause of emotional disorders, alleviating such stresses can often alleviate the mental health problems as well. Furthermore, the experience of successful active mastery (even with the assistance and clout of a professional helper) can be a gratifying, esteem-building experience. For once, the system did respond and acknowledge one's legitimate needs. Such experiences can offer not only a respite from overwhelming life stresses; they can also begin a "benign cycle" of new hope, new efforts, and new successes. Thus, advocacy efforts to help women resolve legal problems, gain the welfare benefits to which they are entitled, or secure job training can be a therapy in itself. Clinicians who cannot undertake such work might ally themselves with other service providers in a close working relationship so that all of a client's pressing and interlocking problems can receive attention as part of an overall treatment plan. Referrals to other, unknown providers should be an option of last resort. If a client is already demoralized she may reasonably not wish to squander her remaining hope and energy on the uncertainty of an unfamiliar professional helper.

Visits to clients' neighborhoods and homes can be important learning experiences for clinicians and can help them to understand their clients' stresses and coping struggles. Such experiences may be particularly important for male, middle-class, and majority clinicians, but may also be useful to those who have already shared to some extent in the life experiences of their clients. Home visits also demonstrate powerfully to a client that she is valued and that others will make special efforts to work with her. While financial cutbacks at most public mental health facilities make such visits quite difficult, they still remain of great value if they can be undertaken.

Women who are experiencing emotional problems or problems in their relationships with their children must not be kept away from professional help by the very real threat that they will be judged unstable and have their children taken away from them. Supportive services should be available to mothers to enable them to resolve their problems and keep their families together. Families that can be helped should not be torn apart.

Many members of racial or ethnic minorities find that the realities of their lives are best understood by someone from their own ethnic group. It is important, therefore, that opportunites and support are available to train minority mental health professionals.

Mutual help groups can also be powerful resources for women in emotional distress and in the midst of oppressive life conditions. In such groups women meet with others who have similar experiences, provide and receive emotional support, and work together toward solutions to problems. The realization that one is not alone in experiencing difficulties and failures, and the concomitant recognition that systemic rather than individual forces are responsible for many of these difficulties, can be a powerful antidote to guilt and depression. Similarly, the chance to be helpful to others by sharing experiences and providing reassurance can go a long way toward restoring a woman's lost self-esteem. Mental health care providers can play an extremely important role in helping to initiate and sustain such groups. If such efforts can be extended to community-based political action to address shared concerns, the chance of improving mental health is even greater.

The consciousness raising that mutual help groups can begin must also extend to the larger society, and particularly to those who come into contact with women at major institutions that affect their lives, such as the welfare office, children's schools, and mental health and medical care services. Such consciousness raising could enable us to stop blaming the victims of overwhelming life circumstances and could help us work together toward removing some of these stresses from their lives. Psychologists can play key roles by studying the connections between environmental stress and mental health, designing therapies that address these connections, and alerting the society at large to the bitter price low income and minority women pay for inequality.

REFERENCES

Acosta, F. (1980). Self-described reasons for premature termination of psychotherapy by Mexican American, Black American, and Anglo-American patients. *Psychological Reports, 47,* 435-443.

Barrett, N. (1979). Women in the job market: Occupations, earnings, and career opportunities. In R. Smith (Ed.), *The subtle revolution: Women at work* (pp. 31-61). Washington, D C : The Urban Institute.

Belle, D. (1980). Who uses the mental health facilities? In M. Guttentag, S. Salasin, & D. Belle (Eds.), *The mental health of women,* pp. 1-20. New York: Academic Press.

Belle, D., Dill, D., Feld, E., Greywolf, E., Reese, M., & Steele, E. (1982). Mental health problems and their treatment. In D. Belle (Ed.), *Lives in stress: Women and depression* (pp. 197-210). Beverly Hills, CA: Sage.

Belle, D. with Longfellow, C., Makosky, V., Saunders, E., & Zelkowitz, P. (1981). Income, mothers' mental health, and family functioning in a low-income population. In American Academy of Nursing, *The impact of changing resources on health policy* (pp. 28-37). Kansas City: American Nurses' Association.

Boyd, N. (1979). Black families in therapy: A study of clinician's perceptions. *Sandoz Psychiatric Spectator, 11*(7), 21-25.

Brown, G., Bhrolchain, M., & Harris, T. (1975). Social class and psychiatric disturbance among women in an urban population. *Sociology, 9*(2). 225-254.

Cherlin, A. (1979). Work life and marital dissolution. In G. Levinger & O. Moles (Eds.), *Divorce and separation: Context, causes and consequences,* (pp. 151-166). New York: Basic Books.

Children's Defense Fund (1979). *American children and their families.*

Cohler, B., & Lieberman, M. (1980). Social relations and mental health: Middle-aged and older men and women from three European ethnic groups. *Research on Aging, 2*(4), 445-469.

Dill, D., & Feld, E. (1982). The challenge of coping. In D. Belle (Ed.), *Lives in stress: Women and depression* (pp. 179-196). Beverly Hills, CA: Sage.

Dohrenwend, B. S. (1973). Social status and stressful life events. *Journal of Personality and Social Psychology, 28,* 2, 225-235.

Eckenrode, J., & Gore, S. (1981). Stressful events and social supports: The significance of context. In B. Gottlieb (Ed.), *Social networks and social support* (pp. 43-68). Beverly Hills, CA: Sage.

Fine, M. (1983-1984). Coping with rape: Critical perspectives on consciousness. *Imagination, cognition and personality, 3*(3), 249-267.

Langner, T., & Michael, S. (1963). *Life stress and mental health.* New York: Free Press.

Longfellow, C., Zelkowitz, P., & Saunders, E. (1982). The quality of mother-child relationships. In D. Belle (Ed.). *Lives in stress: Women and depression* (pp. 163-176). Beverly Hills, CA: Sage.

Lurie, O. R. (1974). Parents' attitudes toward children's problems and toward use of mental health services: Socioeconomic differences. *American Journal of Orthopsychiatry, 44*(1), 109-120.

Makosky, V. (1982). Sources of stress: Events or conditions? In D. Belle (Ed.), *Lives in stress: Women and depression* (pp. 35-53). Beverly Hills, CA: Sage.

Merry, S. (1981). *Urban danger.* Philadephia: Temple University Press.

National Advisory Council on Economic Opportunity (1980). *Critical choices for the 80's.* Washington, DC: U.S. Government Printing Office.

Pearce, D. (1979). Women, work, and welfare: The feminization of poverty. In K. W. Feinstein (Ed.), *Working women and families* (pp. 103-124). Beverly Hills, CA: Sage.

Pearlin, L., & Johnson, J. (1977). Marital status, life-strains and depression. *American Sociological Review, 42,* 704-715.

Pearlin, L., & Radabaugh, C. (1976). Economic strains and the coping functions of alcohol. *American Journal of Sociology, 82*(3), 652-663.

Radloff, L. (1977). Sex differences in depression: The effects of occupation and marital status. *Sex Roles: A Journal of Research, 1,* 249-266.

Reese, M. (1982). Growing up: The impact of loss and change. In D. Belle (Ed.), *Lives in stress: Women and depression* (pp. 65-80). Beverly Hills, CA: Sage.

Seligman, M. (1975). *Helplessness.* San Francisco: W. H. Freeman.

Stack C. (1974). *All our kin.* New York: Harper & Row.

Steele, E. Mitchell, J., Greywolf, E., Belle, D., Chang, W., & Schuller, R. (1982). The human cost of discrimination. In D. Belle (Ed.), *Lives in stress: Women and depression* (pp. 109-119). Beverly Hills, CA: Sage.

Straus, M. (1980). Social stress and marital violence in a national sample of American families. *Annals of the New York Academy of Sciences, 347,* 229-250.

Tebbets, R. (1982). Work: Its meaning for women's lives. In D. Belle (Ed.), *Lives in stress: Women and depression* (pp. 83-95). Beverly Hills, CA: Sage.

U.S. Bureau of the Census. (1980). *Money income and poverty status of families and persons in the United States: 1979 (Advance Report)* Current Population Reports, Series P-60, No. 125. Washington, DC: U.S. Government Printing Office.

Wilkins, W. L. (1974). Social stress and illness in industrial society. In E. K. E. Gunderson & R. H. Rahe (Eds.), *Life stress and illness.* Springfield, IL: Charles C Thomas.

Wolf, B. (1983). *The impact of socio-environmental stress on the mental health of low-income mothers.* Unpublished qualifying paper, Harvard Graduate School of Education, Cambridge, MA.

Wortman, R. (1981). Depression, danger, dependency, denial: Work with poor, black, single parents. *American Journal of Orthopsychiatry, 51*(4), 662-673.

Zelkowitz, P. (1982). Parenting philosophies and practices. In D. Belle (Ed.), *Lives in stress: Women and depression* (pp. 154-162). Beverly Hills, CA: Sage.

Zill, N. (1978). *Divorce, marital happiness and the mental health of children: Findings from the OCD National Survey of Children.* Unpublished report.

8

LESBIAN WOMEN
AND MENTAL HEALTH POLICY

Del Martin
Phyllis Lyon

Muriel Sivyer and Mari Gunn, students at a Palo Alto, California, high school conducted a three-week experiment to test the tolerance of other students to displays of affection between two women (Bess, 1973). They greeted and touched one another affectionately like warm friends: They held hands frequently as they walked across campus, put their arms around each other's shoulders, and sometimes exchanged kisses on the cheek. They emphasized that they did not try to give the impression that their feelings were sexual. Their behavior was nonetheless interpreted by other students as lesbian behavior.

The two young women were snubbed, harassed, taunted, insulted, and threatened. Their friends walked across the street to avoid them. Both were dropped by the young men who had been dating them, and no one invited either of them to the school prom. The experiment proved to be a vivid experience of what it is like to be a lesbian in this society and why so many stay in the closet.

That same year trustees of the American Psychiatric Association (APA) voted to remove homosexuality from the organization's Diagnostic and Statistical Manual. The resolution that was ratified by the membership stated that "homosexuality per se implies no impairment in judgment, stability, reliability, or general social or vocational capabilities"—the exact wording later adopted by the American Psychological Association.

At the same time the APA introduced a new category, *sexual orientation disturbance,* for individuals "whose sexual interests are directed primarily toward people of the same sex and who are either disturbed by, in conflict with, or wish to change their sexual orientation." The press release pointed out, however, that this diagnostic category is distinguished from homosexuality which, by itself, does not constitute a psychiatric disorder.

In effect, however, the new category served to keep homosexuals in a holding pattern of mental illness despite the disclaimer. If lesbians have positive self-esteem and are well adjusted, they are no longer considered ill and no longer a concern of the psychological professions. But every lesbian, in the process of self-acceptance and coming out, has to deal with the *sexual orientation disturbance* of heterosexuals in her life who are either disturbed by, in conflict with, or wish to change her sexual orientation. The period of self-discovery that has the potential of being a positive growth experience of joy and comfort thus often becomes one of pain, anger, isolation, fear, and conflict, which the APA would label a psychiatric disorder. There is no escape.

By 1978 the APA had found another way to dilute its 1973 bill of health for homosexuals. In its new list of psychiatric disorders (DSM III), a new category emerged: *ego-dystonic homosexuality*. This disorder is defined as the desire of a homosexually behaving person "to acquire or increase heterosexual arousal." Psychiatrists continue to dwell on the effects of heterosexual bias and the stigma attached to homosexuality to promote heterosexuality as the only viable and healthy sexual orientation. Ironically, should a lesbian succumb to the hard sell and seek help in the acquisition of heterosexual arousal, she is immediately labeled mentally ill.

Considering previous training and long-held views about homosexuality as a mental illness, perhaps it was too much to expect an immediate reversal on the part of mental health professionals. Seven years after the psychiatric and psychological associations' expressed change in policy, Dr. Terri Levy (1980) tested 106 graduate clinical psychology interns on their attitudes toward lesbians. Levy, who completed her study at the California School of Professional Psychology, had the interns view a 20-minute videotape of a therapy session with a woman who had just ended an intimate relationship. Instructions to the interns were the same, except that half of them were told that she had broken up with a woman and identified herself as a lesbian. Interns were asked to rate the woman client according to personal adjustment, personality characteristics, sexual identity, self-control, and attitudes toward men.

Interns who thought the client was heterosexual rated her "way above normal" and were impressed with the way in which she handled the stress of breaking up. Those who were told she was lesbian, however, gave her an overwhelming negative rating. They saw her as having a low personal adjustment, negative personality characteristics, poor sexual identity, poor self-control, and negative attitudes toward men.

The results illustrate that what lesbians and gay men had perceived as a major breakthrough in psychological theory and practice had little effect on what students are being taught. The observations of these interns reflect the negative stereotypes of lesbians that the psychological professions have held historically, despite numerous research studies to the contrary. Obviously, little attempt has been made to incorporate these new findings in course material or to stimulate students to challenge worn-out concepts and stereotyped attitudes.

The problem is that many mental health workers were raised like most of us in this society to believe in various myths and stereotypes about homosexuals and often interpret recent research on human behavior—particularly sexual behavior—on the basis of cultural values rather than the evidence. But parents, the police, and other members of society tell us that homosexuals are sick because trained psychiatrists and psychologists who are privy to the latest scientific research have said so. Professionals are the opinion makers in our society and should be held responsible as agents of change to correct erroneous and outdated assumptions about women and homosexuals.

The results of Levy's study also illustrate why lesbians are leery of seeking help from mental health specialists, why they have developed their own self-help networks, and why, when they realize they may need more professional help, they seek out lesbian, gay, or feminist therapists.

Despite the contradictions and confusions and the pressure to conform, the self-image of lesbians has changed dramatically (Martin & Lyon, 1983). Lesbians today have a sense of pride in themselves that was virtually nonexistent in 1955 when the Daughters of Bilitis was founded in San Francisco as a self-help organization. Through a network of similar organizations, peer counseling, and consciousness-raising groups across the country, lesbians have achieved higher levels of self-acceptance. Now they have more options, more social outlets, more publications, more communication, more advocates, more access to government and social institutions, and more freedom.

A study of 162 lesbians by Fleener (1977) shows that a substantial number (42 percent) had come out to their parents, 41 percent belonged to a lesbian or gay organization, and nearly 60 percent identified with the feminist movement. None of Fleener's respondents thought lesbianism was wrong, immoral, or dirty. An overwhelming 95 percent credited the women's movement with making life easier for lesbians, and 47 percent the gay movement for giving them more pride in themselves.

By 1977, in the face of Anita Bryant's burgeoning religious crusade against homosexuals and false pronouncements by the New Right political action network that passage of the Equal Rights Amendment would be tantamount to legalizing same sex marriages, the National Women's Conference in Houston passed overwhelmingly a resolution against discrimination on the basis of affectional or sexual preference.

GENDER IDENTITY, SEX ROLES, AND SEXUAL ORIENTATION

Women have been learning that women's liberation depends upon changing attitudes about gender identity, sex roles, and sexual orientation. What gains have been made over the last 10 years in unraveling the confusion around the reality of one's gender as female or male, definitions of feminine and masculine behavior, and the expression of one's sexuality is due largely to feminist scholars, often psychologists.

Jean Strouse (1974) discovered this quote from Freud (1905):

> "It is essential to realize that the concepts of 'masculine and feminine,' whose meaning seems so unambiguous to ordinary people, are among the most confused in science. . . Activity and its concomitant phenomena (more powerful muscular development, aggressiveness, greater intensity of libido) are as a rule linked with masculinity; but they are not necessarily so, for there are animal species in which these qualities are on the contrary assigned to the female. . . In human beings pure masculinity and femininity is not to be found in the psychological or biological sense. Every individual on the contrary displays a mixture of character-traits belonging to his own and to the opposite sex; and he shows a combination of activity and passivity whether or not these last character-traits tally with his biological ones." (pp. 219-220)

Yet mental health professionals, including Freudians, have been largely responsible for maintaining rigid gender stereotyping that assigns preferred dominant roles to men and inferior passive roles to women. The Broverman study (1970) demonstrated the sexist notions held by therapists as to what constitutes mental health in the adult male, the adult female, and the adult per se. In this study clinicians were asked to describe male and female behavior and also to indicate what they considered to be "normal, adult behavior" (sex unspecified). Not surprisingly, their descriptions of typical male and female behavior matched commonly accepted sex role stereotypes. Also, the therapists equated characteristics of the male with what is "normal" and "adult."

Women were viewed as "more emotional," "less objective," "more submissive," and "less competitive" than men. The "typical" behavior of women was not considered to be consistent with that of "normal adults."

It is no wonder that the woman who expresses her personhood and tries to act like a "normal adult" is often called unfeminine, masculine, or a lesbian if she succeeds. Feminist therapists Ruth Pancoast and Lynda Weston (1974) say that men experience no dichotomy between adulthood and manhood because society says that the two are identical. "Women, however, have two conflicting ideals: woman and adult. . . . A woman who tries to be a healthy adult does so at the expense of being a healthy woman, and vice versa. . . . Society then has constructed a no-win situation for women."

Letty Cottin Pogrebin (1980) states, "The woman who is called a 'dyke' not because she's wearing man-style clothes but because she lives her own life, owns her own time and earns her own keep, understands that this culture's definition of lesbian is 'autonomous woman.' Our fear of lesbianism for our daughters may simply be fear of female freedom and selfhood" (p. 290).

In early psychoanalytic literature homosexuals were called inverts because they displayed characteristics that were in opposition to their biological sex. Lesbians were perceived as masculine and male homosexuals as effeminate. Lesbians and gay men are presumed to be heterosexual at birth and are trained as other children are to emulate prescribed feminine and masculine roles. Somewhere in their development, however, many become aware of feelings and attitudes that are *both* feminine and masculine. Some tend to exaggerate the characteristics of the opposite sex, first as a means of finding others like themselves and, second, as an act of defiance against society's constraints on what we consider to be human traits (which all women and men possess to one degree or another) rather than nonconforming gender traits. In time, many homosexuals—particularly lesbians—find their insights and capacity to express their androgynous nature an enrichment in their lives.

Charlotte Wolff (1971) in her study of lesbians in England observed, "The retention of the capacity to change feminine into masculine feelings and attitudes, and visa versa, is one of the assets of female homosexuality, because it makes for variety and richness in personal relationships" (p. 46).

According to statistics from the early works of the Institute for Sex Research (Kinsey, Pomeroy, Martin, & Gebhard, 1953), some females were conscious of specifically erotic responses to other females when they were as young as 3 and 4. Of the women studied, 28 percent had recognized erotic responses to other women at some time in their lives. By age 40, however, only 19 percent had actually experienced sexual contact with another woman. We daresay that the figures today would be significantly higher. While the sexual revolution of the sixties and seventies has made little difference in the sexual behavior of the male, it has had a noticeable impact on women. There is now more information on female sexuality, and women are becoming increasingly aware of their bodies and how they function.

They are also more aware that sex role stereotyping is a means by which women have been controlled and exploited in patriarchal society economically, socially, intellectually, emotionally, and sexually. Consequently many women, who would otherwise identify as heterosexual but who are frustrated in their attempts to establish egalitarian relationships with men, have opened themselves up to lesbianism: to the possibility of finding sexual satisfaction, emotional and spiritual fulfillment, and human understanding with a woman.

"In short, women have two tasks before them," Janis Kelly (1972) concluded.

> They must bring their minds and bodies back together, and they must use them to change the society which now cripples them. For both, the ability to love themselves and others is prerequisite. Due to the openness and vulnerability required, they can develop this ability only in relationships free of power struggles. Because a real imbalance of power exists between the sexes, the conditions for their learning to love fully and without fear are at present met only in a homosexual setting. (Kelly, 1972, p. 107)

Indeed, studies of lesbians (Bell & Weinberg, 1978; Gundlach & Reiss, 1968; Jay & Young, 1977; Peplau, Cochran, Rook, & Padesky, 1978; and Schaefer, 1976), indicate that close to 80 percent of lesbians have had sex with men at some point in their lives. The number of lesbians in these studies who had married ranged from 14 percent to 35 percent. When asked to compare their experiences with men, lesbians in Schaefer's study said that sex with women was more tender, intimate, considerate, partner related, exciting, diversified, and less aggressive.

The theory behind sex role stereotyping is that opposites attract, that heterosexuality is necessary to perpetuate the human race, and that nonprocreative homosexuality can be deterred by conditioning girls and boys to conform to proper feminine and masculine behavior. But the practice often separates and divides the sexes and may, indeed, create a climate for hostility between them and may inadvertently encourage homosexuality.

Parents who fear sexual experimentation between girls and boys are apt to encourage sex-segregated activity and promote fear of the opposite sex (Greenberg, 1979). Girls are taught not to let boys touch them and are encouraged to shun boys as playmates and to develop deep friendships with other girls. Boys are admonished to stay away from little girls and are taught to exhibit aggressive *manly* behavior that inhibits emotion or displays of affection.

HOMOPHOBIA: SOCIETY'S SEX ROLE DYSFUNCTION

"Homophobia" is a term popularized by George Weinberg (1972). Although the term has appeared in dictionary supplements for 10 years and is now in common usage, it has been omitted in standard lexicons. An exception is the 1982 Second College Edition of the *American Heritage Dictionary.* "Homophobia" is defined as the fear, dislike, or hatred of gay men and lesbians. By popular usage, homophobia also encompasses negative attitudes toward homosexuality, prejudice, and discrimination against lesbians and gay men.

A bizarre example of homophobia was described by psychiatrist John Jameson, director of the Behavior Therapy Institute in Toronto (Soiffer, 1981). A 32-year-old male student was so terrified of being contaminated by homosexuals that he would shower for 10 hours after being in the same room with a gay man. If an effeminate man came into a restaurant and was seated at a table near him he would change his table to another waiter's station, fearing that if the same waiter served both of them he would be the carrier and expose him to the disease. He refused to seek help because he worried that if the doctor who treated him also had gay clients it might make him homosexual. The man was so overwhelmed by his fears that he became immobile. He sat on the sofa in his apartment for a year and a half and didn't move except to eat and go to the bathroom.

Except for extreme cases such as this, homophobia is a socially determined prejudice much like sexism and racism rather than a medically recognized phobia. It is used as a technique of social control to enforce norms of sex role behavior. Gregory Lehne (1976) states, "The male role is predominantly maintained by men themselves. Men devalue homosexuality, then use this norm of homophobia to control other men in their male roles" (p. 78).

Homophobia can lead parents to perpetrate irrational, cruel, and abusive behavior against their children who may exhibit signs of non-conforming gender behavior or attraction to members of their own sex. In one such case, the suspicion that their daughter was having a lesbian relationship with her roommate drove her parents to the extreme of hiring cult deprogrammers to kidnap and employ their techniques to change her life-style. When the daughter brought criminal charges for kidnapping and rape against her parents and the deprogrammers, a homophobic court compounded her victimization by rendering a verdict of not guilty. Her parents had been depicted as altruistically motivated, and the alleged rapist had testified that the young woman had willingly engaged in sexual intercourse with him. It was the victim's word against his. The court chose to ignore the fact she had been abducted and held captive for a week in a locked bedroom with her alleged assailant.

Aside from psychological put-downs and the discrimination with which all lesbians and gays must cope, homophobia is the motivating force and the justification for violent attacks—even murder—perpetrated against gay men and lesbians. The vast majority of offenders are youth who indulge in *gay bashing* sprees. Arson is another form of the violence. In New Orleans 32 people attending Sunday services of the Metropolitan Community Church were trapped and burned to death in an arson fire. In other cities millions of dollars have been lost because homes, businesses, and social clubs belonging to lesbians or gay men have been deliberately torched.

In a study of 161 gay male victims of murder, Brian Miller and Laud Humphreys (1980) noted,

> That intense rage is present in nearly all homicide cases with homosexual victims is evident. A striking feature of most murders in this sample is their gruesome, often vicious nature. Seldom is a homosexual victim simply shot. He is more apt to be stabbed a dozen or more times, mutilated, *and* strangled. In a number of instances, the victim was stabbed or mutilated. (p. 179)

Patterns of anti-lesbian violence include verbal and sexual harassment, beatings, and rape. Many of the incidents occur after the women are seen leaving a lesbian bar. Sometimes a man or group of men lie in wait for a vulnerable-looking woman. They drag her into a car or follow her home and attack her there. Lesbians who are afraid to travel alone on mass transit late at night may grab a cab, only to find that the cab driver parked in front of the bar was looking for more than a fare. Many men believe that all a lesbian needs is "a good lay." Others wish to punish and humiliate her because they perceive lesbianism as a threat to heterosexual marriage and the family. In patriarchal society the lesbian's heinous crime is that she doesn't need a man at all.

Lehne (1976) says that homophobia is not primarily directed at homosexuals, although it certainly affects them. Homophobia is not based on personal experience with homosexuals or any realistic assessment of homosexuality. It is a device to maintain the status quo and enforce the sex role structure of society that has been defined by men. Homophobia is an effective technique to reinforce male supremacy and keep women and homosexuals in their place—inferior and devalued.

Mothers are more apt to treat their sons and daughters simply as children. It is usually the father who insists on sex-differentiated training. So controlling is the patriarchal value system that many fathers spurn the natural love and affection of their sons. The kissing and hugging of males in so repugnant to these fathers that they hold their sons—even toddlers—at arm's length with a male handshake. Boys soon learn that they must take control and be aggressive if they are to achieve their manhood. They also learn to avoid behavior that could in any way be construed to be womanly or feminine (homosexual).

Girls are trained to be opposites, to modify their behavior so as to be complementary to the male: passive, submissive, self-sacrificing, dependent, and home-loving. Young girls may be tomboys, but in adolescence they soon learn to repress characteristics or interests that are presumed to be male prerogatives. Otherwise they will lose their femininity and will not be attractive to the opposite sex. The message is abundantly clear that nonconformity means lesbian.

Beverly Harrison (1981) analyzes the dualism of body/mind and of male/female concepts of dominant Christianity and its influence on Western culture to make the connection between homophobia and misogyny. "The depth of the revulsion toward women is clearly reflected in the projection of the female stigma onto any males who do not fit the dominant norms of 'real manhood' " (p. 9).

Pogrebin (1980) points out, "What sex-role stereotypes tell children and the rest of us is this: *Boys are better. Girls are meant to be mothers.* These two messages—male supremacy and compulsory motherhood—are the raw essentials of a patriarchal system" (p. 40).

Adrienne Rich (1980) says the fact that heterosexuality has to be imposed, managed, organized, propagandized, and maintained by force suggests to her that for women heterosexuality may not be either innate or a preference.

> The lie [of compulsory female heterosexuality] keeps numberless women psychologically trapped, trying to fit mind, spirit, and sexuality into a prescribed script because they cannot look beyond the parameters of the acceptable. . . The lesbian trapped in the "closet," the woman imprisoned in prescriptive ideas of the "normal," share the pain of blocked options, broken connections, lost access to self-definition freely and powerfully assumed. (Rich, 1980, p. 657)

Through the human potential movement of the 1970s many men began to get in touch with their feelings and began to recognize how compulsive masculinity controlled and robbed them of their humanity. Some men began to form men's liberation consciousness-raising groups and to hold conferences on men and masculinity. At the same time family violence surfaced as a national social issue, revealing the extent of male rage resulting from the socialization of men to be powerful and their limited opportunities to exercise power in society.

Anne Ganley and Lance Harris (1978) started a model program for batterers at the American Lake Veterans Hospital in Tacoma, Washington. They learned that these men's experiences of fear, anxiety, frustration, hurt, irritation, guilt, or disappointment get lumped together and are expressed as anger. Usually this anger is misdirected against women who may have nothing to do with their distress. The real culprit is the impossible image of masculinity that stunts emotional growth in men. The real dysfunction of the patriarchal design is that it is as controlling and harmful to heterosexual men as it is to homosexual men.

A household member was the victim of assault in more than 3.5 million American homes in 1980, according to a National Crime Survey of the U.S. Bureau of Justice Statistics, which admits the figures tend to be understated.

R. Emerson Dobash and Russell Dobash (1979) suggest that the way to dramatically reduce the number of violent marriages is to overcome the subordination, isolation, and devaluation of women and to change the hierarchical family structure. Lehne (1976) argues that homophobia must be eliminated before there can be a change in sex roles. Pogrebin (1980) says parents should stop worrying about how to raise a heterosexual child. By using stereotypes as a vaccine against homosexuality, parents try to mold children into ill-fitting behavior patterns that can be psychologically damaging. "In large and small ways, boys are actually conditioned against heterosexuality because society is so relentlessly *for* 'masculinity' '' (p. 298).

Homophobia is the disease, not homosexuality. It is a social disease that affects everyone. Homophobia does not deter the incidence of homosexuality—it may, indeed, contribute to its manifestation. Homophobia does not enhance the quality of life for heterosexuals—it polarizes the sexes and makes it more difficult to love the other sex.

PSYCHOLOGICAL THEORY AND THE REALITIES OF LESBIANISM

Early psychoanalytic theory about lesbians was based on small samplings of clinical patients. The literature was rife with assumptions of mental illness based upon strong mother fixations, father fixations, dominant mothers, passive fathers, penis envy, castration complex, narcissism, inability to accept one's womanhood, regression to the mother-child relationship, escape from fears of mutilation and destruction by pregnancy and childbirth, extreme oral eroticism, and extension of auto-eroticism to cooperative masturbation.

In psychoanalysis, it should be noted, the strong early attachment to the mother, the castration complex, penis envy, and the wish to be a male were attributed to *all* women, whether they became heterosexual or homosexual. Not until the clinical psychological theory became free of psychoanalytic dominance could women be seen as healthy no matter what their lifestyle. Lesbian women under psychoanalytic theory were seen as having no redemption as penis envy could only be cured by marrying and having a boy child with the highly coveted penis.

That was the state of the art in 1958 when the Daughters of Bilitis (DOB) decided to conduct its own survey on lesbians from among its membership, subscribers to *The Ladder*, and others with whom DOB had contact. It was the first attempt to gather data that was not patient centered and to stimulate further research on this heretofore unknown population. The effort was successful and for a number of years DOB members and other lesbians willing to act as guinea pigs were given a barrage of psychological tests and compared with control groups of heterosexual women.

Using Rorschach and Figure Drawings, Armon (1960) found that judges were unable to identify the homosexual from the heterosexual woman significantly better than chance. Hopkins (1969) used Cattell's 16 Personality Factor Questionnaire and found an .01 significance level. If anything, the lesbians were more independent, more resilient, more reserved, more dominant, more bohemian, more self-sufficient, and more composed than heterosexual women. Freedman (1971) gave a battery of psychological tests and found no significant differences. He noted that lesbians are either initially more independent and inner directed or become that way in reaction to societal pressures. Thompson, McCandless, and Strickland (1971) administered the Adjective Checklist and a Personal Adjustment Measure to matched samples of male and female homosexuals and heterosexuals. Of the four groups lesbians measured highest in self-confidence. Siegelman (1972), using the Scheier and Cattell Neuroticism Scale Questionnaire, failed to find lesbians more neurotic than their heterosexuals counterparts, but added that lesbians are better adjusted in some respects. Oberstone (1974) looked at psychological adjustment and current life-styles, finding no significant differences in adjustment, although lesbians expressed greater satisfaction in their relationships emotionally, sexually, in friendships, and in common interests.

Cotton (1975), who researched social and sexual relationships of lesbians, indicated they are as likely as heterosexuals to form long-lasting and committed relationships, particularly after the age of 30. Alan Bell, of the (Kinsey) Institute for Sex Research, observed in a letter (1973; see also Bell & Weinberg, 1978) that "large numbers of lesbians enjoy relationships which are more satisfying and stable than many heterosexual marriages." Tanner (1975) said the similarities between lesbian marriagelike dyads and heterosexual married dyads in her sample significantly outnumber the differences. She added that a child could fare just as well in either household if the only variable is sexual orientation.

Despite the volume of studies (we have mentioned only a few) on lesbians that provide evidence that they can and often do have stable, loving, and satisfying relationships, the myth of mental illness persists. It is due partly to cultural lag in the mental health professions and partly to the media. Psychiatrists who take an extremely orthodox "gay is sick" position and who are particularly articulate and aggressive get the publicity because they stir controversy—a media hype.

Richard Pillard said in an interview (Mass, 1979): "All sciences have to deal with the problem of new evidence which contradicts established views... [I]t's the test of a science whether it can absorb new ideas. If not, the discipline is more like a religion or a cult than a science."

THE TABOO OF HOMOSEXUALS HAVING CONTACT WITH CHILDREN

Because research findings are published primarily in professional journals and academic papers filed in university archives, the public is rarely apprised of changing data and professional attitudes. Parents thus continue to believe that acceptance of homosexuality as a way of life invites the danger of child molestation, of homosexual seduction of youth, of homosexual teachers proselytizing their students, of lesbian mothers rearing their children to be lesbian or gay.

In testimony before the California Commission on Crime Control and Violence Prevention, Hank Giaretto, director of the Child Sexual Abuse Treatment Program in San Jose, said that in a six-year period they had handled less than half a dozen cases of a homosexual nature out of a total of 700. By our math that is less than 1 percent.

In 1972, more than a decade ago, the Board of Education of the District of Columbia barred discrimination on the basis of sexual orientation in the hiring of school teachers. Two years later, in a telegram to Dr. Bruce Voeller, Marion Barry, Jr., then president of the Board of Education of the District of Columbia, stated that the change in policy met with limited community opposition and no opposition within the public school system itself. Nor had any problems occurred in the schools.

Dr. Benjamin Spock, who has been outspoken in recent years on scapegoating homosexual teachers, stated the following at a 1977 press conference in San Francisco: "The overwhelming majority of seductions and molestations of children are carried out by heterosexuals—and mostly by members of the family circle. Yet we would not recommend the firing of all heterosexual teachers because a few heterosexuals are unprincipled, nor the breakup of all families because of the culpability of an occasional family member."

CHILD CUSTODY AND LESBIAN MOTHERS

In 1972, for the first time to our knowledge, custody was awarded to admitted lesbian mothers in contested court cases. The courts added a proviso that the women could not live together with their lesbian partners. One judge additionally restricted the mother from seeing her lover unless the children were in school (they both worked) or visiting their father (two weekends a month). She was not even permitted to hire a babysitter in order to spend an evening with her lover outside the home. We have never heard of this happening in the case of a heterosexual mother's new male friend. The implication is that lesbians should devote their lives solely to mothering.

Weinberg (1972) says there is nothing wrong with a lesbian raising children, provided that she does not feel guilty about her lesbianism. But judicial decisions that inhibit a lesbian mother's adult love relationship not only presume her guilt but also prescribe the punishment. Expecting a mother to sacrifice her own needs for a satisfying and fulfilling adult relationship could have detrimental effects upon the parent-child relationship. What began as a loving and healthy parent-child relationship could be destroyed by the mother's self-denial, loneliness, guilt, self-pity, bitterness, or martyrdom.

While a significant number of lesbian mothers have since won custody without such conditions, the odds are still overwhelmingly against a lesbian mother, even if she is the primary caretaker and psychological parent. Once she is identified in open court as a lesbian the onus is on her to prove that she is not an unfit parent. Appeals courts have repeatedly held that custody decisions should not be based solely on the parent's sexual orientation, but rather on *the best interests of the child*. Judges indulge in speculation, however, that children (particularly sons) of lesbian mothers without a male model in the home will grow up to be gay, exhibit improper sex role behavior, and suffer stigmatization and conflicts with their peers. These fears serve to bolster the contention that only a heterosexual environment serves best interests.

A growing body of research on childrearing and lesbian mother-headed families tends to refute these assumptions. Stack (1978) studied children who did not have a father figure in the home but were exposed to a series of men over several years. They exhibited no difficulty in assuming appropriate gender behavior. Evelyn Hooker followed a number of gay families after therapy and reported to the National Gay Task Force that she had found no maladjustment of the children, no evidence of proselytizing on the part of the gay parent, and no untoward effects of growing up knowing the parent was gay.

Bryant (1975) found that lesbian mothers are just as concerned about raising a well-adjusted child as society claims to be. Their children usually have many male role models: the father, friends, relatives, teachers, babysitters, neighbors, and church members. These mothers generally let their children know they are lesbians, are open and honest with them, do not hide affection for a partner from them, and do not push any kind of sexual preference on them. The number of grown children in Bryant's sample was small, but the number who appeared to be lesbian, gay, or bisexual was no larger than estimates for the general population. Sons of lesbian feminists were apt to learn that their manhood does not depend upon the subjugation of women.

Kirkpatrick, Smith, and Roy (1977) found that there is no direct correlation between whatever problems the children have and the sexual orientation of the mother. Nor was there a direct connection between these problems and the presence or absence of the mother's lesbian partner. The problems related more to the parents' divorce, the trauma of separation, and the events leading up to it. The mother's sexual orientation was more easily taken in stride than the divorce or separation itself.

In a survey of child psychiatrists and their attitudes on a range of child custody issues, Byron Nestor (1977) found that 82 percent of the respondents felt that custody should be awarded to the best parent irrespective of their sexual orientation. What was of primary importance to them in determining the most competent parent is how stable and predictable they are in providing love, support, and protection for the child. Whether the child can count on the parent in good times and bad far outweighed the importance of unsubstantiated conjectures about the child's future sexual development.

Mandel, Hotvedt, Green, and Smith (1979) said their data showed far more similarities than differences in families headed by homosexual and heterosexual mothers. In areas of nurturance, attention to the children, relationships with fathers and other males, difficulties encountered as female heads-of-household, and mother-child relationship, the two groups were similar. Further, the study did not reveal any sexual identity conflict or homosexual interest in the children of lesbian mothers. Thus, concerns raised in child custody cases about the fitness of a lesbian to parent is not supported by the data.

The problem is that courts have not yet developed a fair procedure for determining this (Martin, 1979). Neither the biology of motherhood or fatherhood, nor the homosexuality of the mother or the heterosexuality of the father, proves or disproves either parent's childrearing capabilities. Where a court requires a psychological evaluation of the lesbian mother, the same requirement should be made of the father. Motivation of accusatory fathers should be examined by mental health professionals sensitive to and knowledgeable about homosexuality and men's proclivity to use violence—psychological or physical—to get what they want, including revenge.

Our experience shows that many cases where the father was awarded custody on the basis of his *avowed* heterosexuality have met with disastrous results. In some instances the fathers wanted only to get back at their wives and did not really want the children; they turned over responsibility for care of the children to relatives or eventually sent them back to their mothers. In one case the children kept running away to their mother until the court finally gave in. A grown daughter complained bitterly that her own wishes were not considered by the judge, that she was not apprised directly by the court of its decision, that her father lied to her saying her mother didn't want her, that she had always been close to her mother and suffered severely by her supposed rejection, that her father didn't really care for her and placed her with an aunt. Years later, when she found her mother and learned the truth, it was too late. Her mother had become a guilt-ridden alcoholic, was seriously ill, and soon died.

Lesbian mothers must be highly motivated parents to undergo the scrutiny of their personal lives in open court, a fact judges overlook. Openness and honesty on the part of lesbian mothers appears to affect their children far more favorably than the courts currently comprehend—an important factor that is often overlooked, too, in professional expert testimony.

In a contested custody case, emotional and psychological trauma is inevitable for the mother, her children, and, if she has one, her lesbian partner. The San Francisco-based Lesbian Rights Project, through a grant from the Rosenberg Foundation, pioneered in hiring a counselor to work with lesbian families (mother, children, partner) involved in custody cases. It is of utmost importance that where lesbianism is a factor in such a case, the children are apprised of what is happening so they know they are not to blame for the divorce and can begin to understand and cope with their changed circumstances, including Dad's anger and rage. The support of a knowledgeable and sensitive counselor can be invaluable. In custody suits where there is great publicity (usually because the mother must raise public money to pay her legal costs) the stress is often intolerable and has ended many relationships. So is the extraordinary stress from forcing the partner into a mental evaluation by insensitive court-assigned evaluators.

If custody is not a concern the question of telling the children about one's life-style will still arise, especially when and how to tell. Lesbian mothers' groups can usually be found in women's centers as a resource.

Attorneys and mental health professionals participating in the California Women Lawyers Child Custody Project (Ramey, Stender, & Dunn, 1977) stated, "Where the homosexual parent has custody of the child, the presence or absence of a supportive community can make a great deal of difference. If the parent and child can rely on a supportive network of friends, family and neighbors, the child's emotional development will generally be much smoother." This need has sparked the emergence of many support systems: lesbian mother rap groups; picnics and other social events arranged for lesbian families to give the children positive reinforcement by socializing with other children who have lesbian mothers; and extended families of friends who babysit and share responsibility for care of the children (Wolf, 1979).

LESBIAN COUNSELING ISSUES FOR THERAPISTS

When the Daughters of Bilitis began as a secret social group in 1955 we had no idea that it would become a self-help organization and that we would become peer counselors. Once DOB came out with *The Ladder* in 1956 the intensity with which lesbians called, wrote, and came to San Francisco to talk with other lesbians illuminated the vacuum in the larger society of any peer resources or known therapists who were knowledgeable about, and nonjudgmental of, lesbians and their concerns. For instance, a lesbian in Iowa called DOB and, when she found no one was in the office, talked for 45 minutes to the man at the answering service. The need to be able to express oneself honestly and openly—usually for the first time—was overwhelming.

Finding suitable referrals for lesbians in need of professional counseling was virtually impossible then. Their experience of therapy was more disastrous than helpful. Lack of knowledge or adherence to the sickness theory was most evident. The client often spent her money and her time educating her therapist about lesbians. The best she got in return was pity and attempts to help her change her sexual orientation. The *withered arm* syndrome—adjustment to one's disability—was pervasive among the more liberal practitioners. More common, however, was the male therapist who knew, without a doubt, that all a lesbian needed was intercourse with a man—and he was that man. Most lesbians dropped all thoughts of therapy at that point and developed hostile attitudes toward mental health professionals. Some lesbians, who had internalized homophobia and hoped their feelings for other women would go away, gave in to "a good lay." All they got, if they were lucky, was more confused.

Although some therapists were lesbians, few would risk revealing themselves to us. In the early seventies a lesbian therapist telephoned Phyllis to offer her services to lesbians in need of counseling. She wanted referrals, but was not willing to give Phyllis her name. She thought a phone number would suffice—and she had no intention of coming out to her clients. She could not be sure that they would observe confidentiality. Somehow it did not seem very therapeutic to refer a lesbian struggling with her own self-image to a lesbian therapist who obviously had not accepted herself. Over and over again lesbians expressed their preference for a lesbian therapist who has empathy and understanding of lesbian life-styles, thereby eliminating the necessity for explanations of lesbianism. As lesbians became more clear about the kind of counseling they wanted, the mental health profession made some responses.

It is a tribute to the toughness, commonsense, and innate awareness of lesbians that so many managed to accept themselves before the advent of the lesbian/gay and women's movements. While mental health professionals were convinced lesbians were mentally ill, most lesbians worked toward a different goal, that of mental health. Considering the pervasiveness of heterosexual propaganda, social conditioning, negative treatment, and moralistic value judgments, it is a wonder any women recognized their lesbianism, let alone were able to accept it in a positive way.

Many women who knew their feelings for women were different than those of other women did not have a word for those feelings. When they did find a word—homosexuality or lesbianism—they found scant comfort in the so-called scientific literature then available. Because of the conspiracy of silence at that time, the prevailing feeling of many lesbians was, "I am the only one." The overwhelming response to the first issues of *The Ladder* from throughout the country was relief that there are others like myself out there. Publication of Alfred C. Kinsey's groundbreaking study of female sexuality was the first book to provide scientific and nonjudgmental data on lesbians (Kinsey, Pomeroy, Martin, & Gebhard, 1953).

During the McCarthy era of the fifties many people lost their jobs because they were lesbian or gay—or were suspected of being so. Very few gay or lesbian therapists were open either to their coworkers, their boss, their discipline, or their clients. It was the late sixties before a few brave souls made tentative steps to bring the discrimination against lesbians and gays by the helping professions to the attention of their professional organizations. It has been a long process, which is not yet completed, to change attitudes of nongay mental health professionals toward their colleagues and their clients who happen to be lesbian or gay.

San Francisco, under the leadership of Pat Norman, Coordinator of Lesbian/Gay Health Services for the Department of Public Health, has led the way in the attempt to make its health and mental health personnel aware not only of the homophobia that exists among them but also the realities of the lives and needs of lesbians and gay men. In late 1979 and early 1980 the department's mental health division contracted with the National Sex Forum for a series of eight two-day workshops on lesbian, gay male, and bisexual life-styles. Attendance at one of the workshops was mandated for 400 mental health employees. These included physicians, nurses, clinicians, some administrators, and clerical workers who came in contact with the public. The workshops covered myths and realities about lesbians, gay men, and bisexuals, and life-style issues, sexual practices, parenting, religious concerns, health problems, and specific counseling guidelines applicable to the three groups. Presenters included women and men from the sexual orientations under discussion, chosen to cover various age ranges and ethnic diversity.

Because attendance at the workshops was mandatory, some of the professionals were angry and resistant, including some who were lesbian, gay, or bisexual. However, evaluations of the workshops were generally positive. The 400 mental health workers gained new perspectives, new techniques, and firsthand information about the lives of women and men who live under a heavy burden of societal disapproval. Ms. Norman's department has followed up the National Sex Forum workshops over the years with in-service training for additional groups of health workers.

Further, the San Francisco Department of Health has demonstrated its commitment to provide competent counseling for lesbians and gay men by creating the position of Gay Sensitive Specialist and maintaining adequate numbers of lesbian and gay clinicians on staff. To become a Gay Sensitive Specialist employees are required to become familiar with the resources of the lesbian/gay communities, to read specified books, and to complete 500 hours of supervised counseling of lesbians and gays. Supervision is conducted by those clinicians who already have the requisite experience. The Department of Health also provides some funding and oversight to Operation Concern, a lesbian/gay mental health agency, and to alcoholism programs aimed at both lesbians and gay men.

COUNSELING ISSUES FOR LESBIANS

Lesbians come to counseling with varied problems that are not inherent in lesbianism but are exacerbated by the attitudes of the dominant society and are a part of the process of self-acceptance and coming out—a process that in many ways is life long.

It is often said that mental health problems of lesbians are no different than those of heterosexual women. While there is an element of truth in the statement, it avoids the acknowledgment that lesbian lives are inevitably impacted by the prejudice, oppression, and heterosexism of the larger society. Natalie Jane Woodman and Harry R. Lenna (1980) define heterosexism as "the internalized belief in the superiority of male-female relationships." Thus, while lesbians may seek counseling for job anxiety, "fear of flying," or depression—just like other women—many of their concerns arise from, or are colored by, homophobia. Further, within the lesbian culture are subgroups with differing concerns—lesbians of color, rural lesbians, students, elder lesbians, teenagers, and lesbian mothers.

The areas of concern that follow derive from our personal experience, that of other lesbian therapists and authors (Woodman & Lenna, 1980; Moses & Hawkins, 1982).

COMING OUT

Coming out of the closet is a process of resolving one's sexual identity and acknowledging the fact of being lesbian to oneself and others. It begins with self-acknowledgment and acceptance of one's sexual orientation. It continues as decisions are made to come out to other lesbians and gay men, to family and/or close nongay friends, progressing to bosses and coworkers, and, perhaps, to a more public persona as a lesbian activist.

Lesbians must come out each time they meet someone new or as their life circumstances change (e.g., a new job, moving to a new area, a parent's sudden proximity). Coming out is probably the most important, and most traumatic, event of a lesbian's life. The awareness of same-sex attraction and one's own lesbianism can occur at any age—from before puberty or as late as the seventies. Each age range raises different problems. An independent, never-married woman in her thirties will have a very different coming out process than a 15-year-old living with her parents or a woman leaving thirty years of marriage. So, too, will the process differ for women of color, rural residents, and women with children.

Coming out is a crucial process—crucial to the woman involved and also crucial to the ultimate acceptance of lesbians by the larger society. Polls consistently tell us that nongay persons who support our human and civil rights are those who know us personally as lesbians. Research and personal testimony affirm that being open and honest about one's lesbianism is mentally healthy, while staying in the closet contributes to loneliness, deception, and alienation. Mental health workers should be sensitive to this struggle, which every lesbian faces, and help their clients understand the implications of coming out on their mental health and to weigh the consequences, both short term and long term. No lesbian should be pressured to come out. Only she can decide to whom, when, and how. If and when she does decide to come out she will need a support network among friends and/or in the lesbian community. It is difficult to convey to lesbians inhibited by the desire to conform and to therapists what a freeing and rewarding personal experience it is to come out—to be true to one's self.

DEVELOPING A POSITIVE SELF-IMAGE

Although self-image/self-acceptance play an important part in the coming out process, development of a strong, positive self-image as a lesbian takes time. When a woman recognizes and identifies her lesbian feelings she is immediately placed in conflict between her sense of being and what she has learned about acceptable social and sexual behavior. We all suffer, to a greater or lesser degree, from internalized homophobia.

Newly aware lesbians need information and some way of contacting the lesbian community, but most often they have no idea where to begin. For many women the lesbian community is a source of strength and a positive influence (Jay & Young, 1979; Moses, 1978; Wolf, 1979). A lesbian community can give one a sense of belonging, a place of refuge in which to relax and share feelings and experiences with others like oneself. Such a community can also provide positive role models, a strong support system, and an extended familylike network.

For isolated women, especially those in rural areas, finding a community of lesbians is not always possible. Knowledgeable mental health professionals may be the only source for the positive information and support they need. The transition from heterosexual misfit to a positive lesbian self-image can be one of joyous self-discovery and acceptance, or it can be a lonely and painful journey through an emotional maze of self-doubt, fear, anxiety, guilt, denial, resentment, and anger.

NEED FOR ASSISTANCE IN COPING WITH A HOSTILE WORLD

The acceptance of, and knowledge about, lesbians is infinitely greater now than ever before. However, mindless antagonism toward lesbians exists everywhere. It may be less so in San Francisco than in Paducah, but it manifests in both. Verbal slurs, physical assaults (including rape), loss of jobs, rejection by parents or friends, and attacks by religious bigots are not uncommon. Even the strongest, most centered lesbian can have need of counsel to cope with such attacks. Although she knows they are totally unjustified, they impinge on her self-image.

ENHANCEMENT OF INTERPERSONAL RELATIONSHIPS

A lesbian's relationships encompass many people: lovers, roommates, friends, parents, coworkers, children. The burden of being in the closet tends to limit relationships, inhibiting closeness with those who do not know one's orientation. This includes closeness with parents and with one's own children. There are also concerns that arise within couple relationships. With a lover, for instance, how do you cope if you are out but she is still in the closet? With money and property, do you share everything or divide it into halves? If one partner makes more money than the other what division should be made? The demands of a partner's parents can also be a problem, making holidays traumatic times, especially if the parents do not accept, or do not know about, their daughter's lesbianism and/or partner. Differences in education, class, religion, race, and upbringing may also need sorting out. Lesbian couples are families and deserve access to supportive relationship and family counseling. In some ways, lesbians sorting out these issues can help non-traditional heterosexual couples who reject the marriage partnership redefine their life-style.

WOMEN'S SOCIALIZATION

Lesbians are affected by all things that affect women in general: low pay, low status, discrimination on many fronts. Many lesbians are feminists, but not all, and this can cause problems in relationships if one is and the other is not. Because women have been socialized to wait for men to make the first move, lesbians often have difficulties meeting others, asking for dates, or even asking another woman to dance. Assertiveness training can be very helpful, as can assistance in reconciling one's self-concept with feminine sex role behavior expected by most in the dominant society.

SEXUALITY ISSUES

Despite the myth that lesbians always have orgasm and that women know instinctively how to make love to another woman, some lesbians do have sexual dysfunctions and other concerns around sexuality. These include bad body image, dislike of genitals, lack of communication with partner, desire phase disorders, and the need to overcome the socialization that women are not sexual. Other concerns have to do with relationships. Should one be monogamous or not, sexually faithful, or in an open relationship? Of current concern in some lesbian communities is the issue of bisexuality and lesbians who sometimes choose to relate sexually to men. Therapists should be aware that bisexuality is a viable option, a preferred life-style, for some women and as such should be honored by the therapist.

TEENAGE LESBIANS

High schools and colleges are dominantly heterosexist, offering scant, if any, support to young lesbians. They lack role models to prove that it is possible to make it in the world. They have fears (which are very real) that parents will commit them to a mental institution or throw them out of the house. Teenage lesbians have great difficulty in meeting others in their peer group, in finding adults who will listen to them and understand their needs.

In years past lesbian organizations limited their membership to those who were 21 or over lest they be accused of contributing to the delinquency of a minor. Today, however, many are assuming a responsibility for underage lesbians and taking on an advocacy role in dealing with such institutions as the family, schools, youth groups, and agencies involved with the well-being of children and youth.

ELDER LESBIANS

Women from 50 up, especially if they are still in the closet (which the majority are), also have difficulty meeting peers. When both are in the closet they are often like ships passing in the night, never realizing they have met. Slightly older lesbian groups can now be found in many large cities, though the "slightly" begins at 30. These groups can be helpful, however, since for the most part lesbian bars and women's organizations attract a younger crowd.

In New York, Senior Action in a Gay Environment (SAGE) is the oldest and most organized group in the country working specifically with gay and lesbian senior citizens. Other gay/lesbian communities are moving to catch up with SAGE. Elder lesbians may well need supportive help with the prolonged illness or death of a partner and coping with being left alone. The surviving partner often fears becoming ill herself and ending up in a nursing home, isolated in a heterosexual environment with nothing but her memories and no one to talk to. Also, as one ages death of friends becomes more prevalent, decimating long-time friendship networks. It is not easy for lesbians who have spent a lifetime zealously guarding their privacy, for fear of being found out, to establish new relationships amongst the other women survivors. Yet, what a wonderful opportunity is lost.

DOUBLE JEOPARDY

The conservatism of rural communities, combined with small size and the lack of anonymity, makes it doubly difficult for lesbians. The slightest hint that one is a lesbian means inability to find work, disgrace to the family, and social isolation.

Black or Hispanic communities have strong family and religious ties. Studies indicate that blacks who have come out to their families have met little or no rejection (Acosta, 1979; Dyne, 1980). They are accepted as family members first. But the family will still condemn homosexuality in general. Mexican-American lesbians are likely to experience very strong negative reactions if they come out to their families, especially if they are still living in a strongly Mexican culture with its polar-opposite gender role behavior (Vasquez, 1979). The more acculturated the family is toward American values, the less problematic. Both blacks and Hispanics have a strong religious base for their intolerance of homosexuality. Third World lesbians are likely to have a prior commitment to the struggle of their people rather than to the struggles of women or gays.

On the other hand, Doris Lunden (1978) says, "The lower-class lesbian doesn't have much 'respectability' to lose. . . .Communication is more open and direct in working class homes—they tend to fight about things. So it's common, when a lesbian comes out, for her to get kicked out of the house, to be beaten, to experience heavy reactions" (p. 230).

AFFIRMATION

What lesbianism is all about is sifting through what we have been told about our *selves* as women to find out the truth about our bodies, our feelings, our relationships to other women, and to the scheme of the world in which we find ourselves. It is a search for truth and the desire to be truthful. It is an affirmation of womanhood and of love—a love that defies and triumphs and perseveres against whatever obstacles society poses.

As Batya Bauman (1978) put it, "Zionism brought me out as a Jew. The women's movement brought me out as a feminist. The Gay Liberation Movement brought me out as a Lesbian. All are self-affirming. All are life-affirming. All have made the difference between the denial of who I am and the affirmation of who I am."

IMPLICATIONS FOR MENTAL HEALTH POLICY

HOMOPHOBIA

Homophobia—the fear and hatred of homosexuals—is the mental disorder that should be listed in the APA's Diagnostic and Statistical Manual.

Mental health professionals should launch an educational campaign to make the public aware that all the heterosexual conditioning, propaganda, pressures, proselytizing, coercion, threats, and punishment do not affect the incidence of homosexuality. The public should also be apprised that homophobia can have adverse effects upon hetero-sexuals, that it divides and creates hostility between the sexes, that it sometimes inhibits heterosexual behavior and encourages homo-sexual behavior.

SEX ROLES

Mental health professionals can be helpful in clearing up the public's confusion around gender identity, sex roles, and sexual orientation. Countless papers on these issues have been presented at professional meetings and published in academic journals, but rarely has this infor-mation been passed on to parents or efforts made to change public opinion.

All mental health specialists should read Letty Cottin Pogrebin's book *Growing Up Free: Raising Your Child in the 80s.* It is a monumen-tal work that took eight years of research into the theories, studies, practices, and effects of sex role stereotyping. The book shows how traditional childrearing methods can actually be harmful to children and how nonsexist parenting can be physically and emotionally healthy for children. The book also provides a valuable model for the transla-tion of academic jargon into terms that the average parent can understand.

LESBIAN MOTHERS

Testimony of psychiatrists in the courtroom can have a significant influence in obtaining a fair hearing for the lesbian mother. Mental health professionals who have come to terms with homophobia, who have clinical experience with lesbian families, and who have kept abreast of current research on lesbians can be helpful not only in custody suits but also in educating the public and the judiciary. Any professional testifying in a lesbian mother custody case needs to be able to critique available research to seek out heterosexual bias in the interpretation of the data. Often it is necessary to weigh the dif-ferences between competing value systems—between traditional and nonsexist approaches to childrearing.

Perhaps research is needed on the overall adjustment of adult children of lesbian mothers. More important, however, is follow-up on what becomes of the children who are arbitrarily awarded to the father because he is heterosexual, even though evidence indicates the lesbian mother is the psychological parent. Also of value would be longitudinal studies of children who are rasied by nonsexist, nonhomophobic parents, whatever their gender, martial status, or sexual orientation.

COUNSELING LESBIANS

Ethics codes mandating objectivity from psychotherapists in their counseling need to be followed. Lesbians are entitled to receive sensitive and nonhomophobic treatment. Therapists who find homosexuality repugnant should refer lesbian clients to others who are more sensitive and experienced in responding to their needs and problems. Consultation with lesbian or gay sensitive colleagues is often essential.

Mental health agencies that lack staff with the required skills to counsel lesbians should seek out and hire openly lesbian/bisexual/feminist therapists who have a unique understanding of the problems faced by women in a heterosexist society. Or they can use such therapists as consultants or as resources for in-service training. Agencies should also maintain a list of, and be familiar with, alternative support services available within the lesbian and women's communities.

SEX EDUCATION

American attitudes toward sexuality are conflicted and paradoxical. We are bombarded by exploitive sexual images in advertising, movies, and the media. On the other hand, sex education is frowned upon by parents, neglected by medical schools, and avoided by mental health professionals until individuals come to them with their hang-ups. Mental health professionals know the problems, the results of sex-negative, sex-repressive attitudes. They should be in the vanguard in the promotion of sex education for adults and children, sex-positive training for all helping professionals, understanding of the spectrum of sexual expression, and respect for women's sexuality.

CONCLUSION

Mental health professionals who claim they are placing greater emphasis on primary prevention—eliminating the sources of mental health problems—need to understand that the lesbian's stress is not inherent in her life-style but rather in society's response to her. The promotion of mental health for women includes addressing the issues of homophobia, sex role stereotyping, and forced female heterosexuality.

It might be expected that feminist theoreticians and clinicians would have a stake in resolving these issues. In many of their works, however, lesbians are invisible or treated only as marginal beings. In Jean Baker Miller's (1976) book *Towards a New Psychology for Women*, for instance, lesbians are not represented at all. The denial or the fear to acknowledge lesbian existence, we believe, is central to the plight of women in patriarchal society.

REFERENCES

Acosta, E. (1979). Affinity for black heritage: Seeking lifestyle within a community. *The Blade* (Oct. 11).

Armon, V. (1960). Some personality variables in overt female homosexuality. *Journal of Projective Techniques, 24,* 292-309.

Bauman, B. (1978). If there is a group of people who can claim more oppression than Jews, it is homosexuals. In G. Vida (Ed.), *Our right to love: A lesbian resource book* (pp. 235-236). Englewood Cliffs, NJ: Prentice-Hall.

Bell, A. P., & Weinberg, M. S. (1978). *Homosexualities: A study of diversity among men and women.* New York: Simon and Schuster.

Bess, D. (1973). 2 girls' project shocks students. *San Francisco Chronicle* (May 5).

Broverman, I. K., Broverman, D. M., Clarkson, R., Rosenkrantz, P., & Vogel, S. (1970). Sex role stereotypes and clinical judgments of mental health. *Journal of Consulting and Clinical Psychology, 34* (1), 1-7.

Bryant, B. (1975). *Lesbian mothers.* Master's thesis, School of Social Work, California State University at Sacramento.

Cotton, W. L. (1975). Social and sexual relationships of lesbians. *Journal of Sex Research, 11* (2), 139-148.

Dobash, R. E., & Dobash, R. (1979). *Violence against wives.* New York: Free Press.

Dyne, L. (1980). Is D. C. becoming the gay capital of America? *The Washingtonian* (September).

Fleener, M. G. (1977) *The lesbian lifestyle.* Paper presented at annual meeting of Western Social Science Association.

Freedman, M. (1971). *Homosexuality and psychological functioning.* Belmont, CA; Brooks/Cole.

Freud, S. (1905). Three essays on the theory of sexuality. The Standard Edition of the *Complete Psychological Works of Sigmund Freud, 7.*

Ganley, A., & Harris, L. (1978). *Domestic violence: Issues in designing and implementing programs for male batterers.* Paper presented at annual meeting of American Psychological Association.

Greenberg, S. (1979). *Right from the start: A guide to nonsexist childrearing.* Boston: Houghton Mifflin.

Gundlach, R., & Reiss, B. F. (1968). Self and sexual identity in the female: A study of female homosexuals. In B. F. Reiss (Ed.), *New Directions in Mental Health.* New York: Grune & Stratton.

Harrison, B. W. (1981). Misogyny and homophobia: The unexplored connection. *Integrity Forum,* Lent issue, 7-11.

Hopkins, J. H. (1969). The lesbian personality. *British Journal of Psychiatry, 115,* 1433-1436.

Jay, K., & Young, A. (1979). *The gay report: Lesbians and gay men speak about sexual experiences and lifestyles.* New York: Summit.

Kelly, J. (1972). Sister love: An exploration of the need for homosexual experience. In M. B. Sussman (Ed.), *Non-traditional family forms in the 1970's.* Minneapolis: National Council on Family Relations.

Kinsey, A. C., Pomeroy, W. B., Martin, C. E., & Gebhard, P. H. (1953). *Sexual behavior in the human female.* Philadelphia: Saunders.

Kirkpatrick, M., Smith, K., & Roy, R. (1977). Pilot study of the psychological status of the children of lesbian mothers. In *California Women Lawyers Child Custody Project Report* (pp. 22-24).

Lehne, G. E. (1976). Homophobia among men. In D. S. David & R. Brannon (Eds.), *The forty-nine percent majority: The male sex role* (pp. 66-88). Reading, MA.: Addison-Wesley.

Levy, T. (1960). *The lesbian: As perceived by mental health workers.* Doctoral dissertation, California School of Professional Psychology.

Lunden, D. (1978). The lower-class lesbian doesn't have much respectability to lose. In G. Vida (Ed.), *Our right to love* (pp. 235-236). Englewood Cliffs, NJ: Prentice-Hall.

Mandell, J. B., Hotvedt, M. E., Green, R., & Smith, L. (1979). *The lesbian parent: Comparison of heterosexual and homosexual mothers and their children.* Paper presented at annual meeting of American Psychological Association.

Martin, D. (1979). *Psychological implications in lesbian mother custody cases.* Paper presented at annual meeting of American Psychiatric Association.

Martin, D. (1981). *Battered wives.* San Francisco: Volcano Press.

Martin, D., & Lyon, P. (1983). *Lesbian/woman.* New York: Bantam.

Mass, L. (1979). Homophobia on the couch. *The Advocate* (Oct. 4).

Miller, B., & Humphreys, L. (1980). Lifestyles and violence: Homosexual victims of assault and murder. *Qualitative Society, 3,* 169-185.

Miller, J. B. (1976). *Towards a new psychology for women.* Boston: Beacon.

Moses, A. (1978). *Identity management in lesbian women.* New York: Praeger.

Moses, A. E., & Hawkins, R. O., Jr. (1982). *Counseling lesbian women and gay men: A life-issues approach.* St. Louis: Moody.

Nestor, B. (1977). Attitude of child psychiatrists toward homosexual parenting and child custody. In *California Women Lawyers Child Custody Project Report* (pp. 17-21).

Oberstone, A. (1974). *A comparative study of psychological adjustment and aspects of lifestyle in gay and non-gay women:* Doctoral dissertation, California School of Professional Psychology.

Pagelow, M. D. (1981). *Woman battering: Victims and their experience.* Beverly Hills, CA: Sage.

Pancoast, R. D., & Weston, L. M. (1974). *Feminist psychotherapy: A method for fighting social control of women.* Position statement of Feminist Counseling Collective, Washington, DC.

Peplau, L. A ., Cochran, S., Rook, K., & Padesky, C. (1978). Loving women: Attachment and autonomy in lesbian relationships. *Journal of Social Issues, 34* (3), 7-27.

Pogrebin, L. C. (1980). *Growing up free: Raising your child in the 80's.* New York: McGraw-Hill.

Ramey, M., Stender, F., & Dunn, G. (1977). *California Women Lawyers Project Report.*

Rich, A. (1980). Compulsory heterosexuality and lesbian existence. *Signs, 5* (4), 631-660.

Rosen, D. H. (1974). *Lesbianism: A study of female homosexuality.* Springfield, IL: Charles C. Thomas.

Schaefer, S. (1976). Sexual and social problems of lesbians. *Journal of Sex Research, 12,* 50-69.

Siegelman, M. (1972). Adjustment of homosexual and heterosexual women. *British Journal of Abnormal Psychology, 120,* 477-481.

Soiffer, B. (1981). The phobia of being close to gays. *San Francisco Chronicle* (Oct. 12).

Stack, C. (1978). *All our kin: Strategies for survival in a black community.* New York: Harper & Row.

Strouse, J. (1974). Introduction. In J. Strouse (Ed.), *Women and analysis*. New York: Grossman.

Tanner, D. (1978). *Lesbian mothers: Sexual orientation and the ability to parent.* Doctoral dissertation, University of Illinois at Chicago Circle.

Thompson, N. L., McCandless, B. R., & Strickland, B. R. (1971). Personal adjustment of male and female homosexuals. *Journal of Abnormal Psychology, 78,* 237-240.

Vasquez, E. (1979). Homosexuality in the context of the Mexican-American culture. In D. Kunkel (Ed.), *Social issues in social work: Emerging concern in education and practice.* Honolulu: University of Hawaii School of Social Work.

Walker, L. E. (1979). *The battered woman.* New York: Harper & Row.

Weinberg, G. (1972). *Society and the healthy homosexual.* New York: St. Martin's.

Wolf, D. (1979). *The lesbian community.* Berkeley: Univ. of California Press.

Wolff, C. (1971). *Love between women.* New York: St. Martin's.

Woodman, N. J., & Lenna, H. R. (1980). *Counseling with gay men and women.* San Francisco: Jossey-Bass.

9

WOMEN'S MENTAL HEALTH IN TIMES OF TRANSITION

Jessie Bernard

We know that physical health varies over time; infectious diseases are succeeded by degenerative diseases as major health hazards, and nutritional diseases change from scurvy to obesity. So also, it now appears, does mental health also seem to vary over time. There are times, as in the Middle Ages, when hysterias, visions, and obsessions take on epidemic proportions and others when depression prevails. In 1621, for example, when Robert Burton wrote his *Anatomy of Melancholy*, England was suffering from such an epidemic with few, according to him, escaping it. Lawrence Stone has characterized the sixteenth and seventeenth centuries in England in ways that can only be characterized as paranoid: people, he tells us, were suspicious, cynical, distrustful. They had little generosity, faith, or charity; there was much physical and verbal violence; people were short-tempered, and unfriendly. There was much assault and battery. The basic assumption was that "no one is to be trusted since anyone and everyone—wife, servants, children, friends, neighbors, or patrons—are only kept loyal by self-interest, and may, therefore, at any moment turn out to be enemies" (1977, p. 96). Only with the eighteenth century did more social warmth and ease and comfort—more intimacy—enter the picture.

Granted, then, that the incidence and prevalence of both physical and mental health may vary over time, is this equally true for both sexes? Unfortunately we cannot answer this question unequivocally. We do know that what "history tells us" about any period of time is biased by the "prism of sex" through which it is seen. Periodization is a highly subjective process. What is viewed as the Dark Ages, for example, may not have been dark for women. In the Middle Ages, which William Graham Sumner characterized as one in which "the passions of hatred and revenge were manifested, upon occasion, to the extremity of fiendishness" (1906, p. 212), among women the symptoms took the form of hysterias that produced "manias of falsehood, deceit [fasting women], trances, and witchcraft." But, as Schulenburg looks at that scene, it was not all that dark for women. Their mental health must have been good. They played an active part in social life. "The milieu. . . . was one of a rough-and-ready, de facto equality for women. In this frontier type of existence, women were looked upon as truly indispensable assets and as partners. Their high respect and prominence rested on a practical appreciation" (1979, p. 39). They were well integrated into the social system. The eleventh and twelfth centuries saw a silent revolution in which women lost their active roles and became isolated from the mainstream. They were no longer recognized as figures of action but rather as passive, ornamental, and highly restricted. One can only infer a negative effect on their mental health. Similarly, in the seventeenth century at a time characterized by Burton as a time of great melancholy, women were actively taking part in the English Civil War. Working women, artisans, shop girls, and laborers engaged in political action for the first time in English history (Stone, 1980, p. 308). There was a temporary overthrow of a status of female subordination and deference. Women mobbed parliament demanding peace, employment, and the release of Levellers. They demanded a share in the ordering of church and commonwealth. These activities do not sound like the activities of depressed or even paranoid women.

For recent times we have more reliable data. Thus Halliday, for example, noted some time ago that "certain of the psychosomatic affections which in the 19th century had preponderated in females (e.g., peptic ulcer, exophthalmic goiter, and perhaps essential hypertension) during the twentieth century occurred increasingly in males; whereas others that had preponderated in males (e.g., diabetes) occurred increasingly in females" (1948, p. 66). So also in mental health. In the time of Freud, narcissism was considered characteristic of women; today Christopher Lasch analyzes the narcissistic personality of our time in terms of men (1978, part 2).

We know also that until recently the norms for the female personality—passivity and dependency—were those for poor mental health, as Broverman and her associates showed us a decade and a half ago (Broverman, Vogel, Broverman, Clarkson & Rosencrantz, 1970). We know also that at the present time depression is epidemiologically much commoner among women than among men; among the factors offered to explain this fact are the role structure of the female world, including its learned helplessness, and a relational deficit. Recent research shows, however, how rapidly mental health problems can change. Not too long ago widespread incidence of involutional melancholy—an almost taken-for-granted mental-health hazard for postmenopausal women—meant that their mental health was worse than that of men. Today women no longer deteriorate in middle age. Peter N. Stearns, on the basis of French data from 1800 to 1950, notes that "prolonged employment experience followed by retirement will obviously alter the aging pattern of women in the future" (1980, p. 56), no doubt favorably, as compared with the grim past. Of prime significance in looking at the mental health of that future, as well as of today, is this "prolonged employment experience," referring to what Ralph E. Smith has labelled a "subtle revolution" (1979).

It is difficult to characterize one's own era or age. So far as the female world is concerned it is a revolutionary age. The subtle revolution, no longer subtle, gained momentum during World War II when many women entered the labor force. After the war many married women remained in their jobs. The proportion of these married women in the labor force doubled in fact between 1947 and 1976, reaching 50.2 percent in 1980 and is projected to be 66.7 percent by 1990. This revolution has already had profound repercussions on both marriage (Hofferth & Moore, 1979) and motherhood (Moore & Hofferth, 1979). The factors at work to produce these changes over time are no doubt numerous and complex. But among them is the "place" women occupy in the social structure, what is required or permitted, forbidden or sanctioned. The subtle revolution has defined two distinct categories of women—on the basis of the evaluation placed on domestic and work roles—traditionalists and modernists. The litmus-test for these categories is reponse to the question with respect to women's place. Traditional women accept the traditional family role definition: Women's place is in the home. Modern women have reservations.

TRADITIONAL AND MODERN WOMEN

Almost fifteen years ago I noted that "two polar types turn up with singular consistency in the research literature on women" (1971, p. 9). Alice Rossi was calling them "pioneer" and "housewife," and using the terms "traditional" for those who fell in between. Other terms for describing the two types were "homemaking-oriented" and "career-oriented." They are found in all kinds of populations. Samuel

Klausner, on the basis of a sample of welfare and poor working women, characterized the two categories in these terms:

> A traditionalist. . . . feels obligated principally to home and family. Her household expenditure budget emphasizes internal family needs. She expects to be supported in virtue of her position as a woman and as a mother. . . . In contrast, a mother committed to a modernizing life-style sees herself as responsible for the economic provision and protection of her children. The modernizing tendency is reinforced through the discipline of job requirements and by the variety of social influences to which work exposes her. Modernizing [women's] household expenditure budgets reflect the costs of maintaining social relations outside of the home, such as expenditures for clothing and entertaining. (1972, p. 15)

But analogous distinctions between "traditional" and "modern" women have been reported also in research on college women (Bernard, 1971). In my own exploration of the female world I found them throughout the structure (1981b). I have found the two categories not only on academic campuses but also among even the wives of top-level corporate men. Gladieux has reported it in a sample of women during the archetypical female experience of pregnancy. She concludes:

> Since traditional women are likely to be ensconced in a close-knit network of relatives or friends who are parents, their pregnancy experience tends to be more enriching and satisfying than it is for their more modern counterparts. (1978, p. 292)

More relevant here is the fact that mental health differs in the two categories. Among the traditionalists the problems have to do with the passing of the traditional family—the trauma of discovering themselves to be "deviants" rather than typical. Among the modernizing, they have to do with fatigue, overload, the revamping of role relationships. In both cases policy has some impact, directly or indirectly.

Regardless of the way we characterize an age as a whole, past or present, it is always the best of times for some and the worst of times for others. For the impact of any social system falls differentially on different segments of any population: on different age groups, on the two sexes, on the several races, on differing ethnic groups, on differing occupations, and within each of these groups, on different social classes. Policy has a great deal to do with determining where the impact will fall, and who will benefit or lose by it.

MENTAL HEALTH AND THE SOCIAL CLASS STRUCTURE

There is a fairly considerable research literature dealing with social class or socioeconomic status—SES—and mental illness. Without attempting to review it here we may use as a benchmark the work of Srole and his associates reported for Manhattan in 1962. They found four "mental-health worlds" (1962, pp. 235-236) that differed in economic underpinnings, life-styles, psychological atmosphere, and ego nurturance. In the same project, Langner and Michael found greater stresses and impairment in lower than in higher status levels (1963, pp. 467-472). In a picturesque figure of speech, Srole and his associates described this status system as "an apparatus that differentially sows, reaps, sifts, and redistributes the community's crop of mental morbidity and of sound personalities" (p. 236). We "plant" or "sow" the seeds of poor mental health—greater streses—in the lower status levels and reap the consequences—greater impairment. In other levels we "plant" other seeds and harvest sound personalities.

Actually, no status level is free of stresses but they differ in relative seriousness. Also, different levels supply more resources for dealing with them. And, of course, there are always those who have better coping skills to begin with.

Although the processes may not be identical, the social class system of the female world may also be said to "sift" and "redistribute" the community's "crop of mental morbidity and of sound personalities." There is, of course, no implication in this figure of speech that there is a fixed supply of mental morbidity or of sound personalities, as though there were an iron law of good mental health as there was once posited an iron law of wages. The hope is that with continuing research we will be able to decrease the amount of mental morbidity.

MENTAL HEALTH AND THE SOCIAL CLASS STRUCTURE OF THE FEMALE WORLD

We know from a considerable corpus of research that mental health varies by class, but so far we do not have a clean picture of what the class structure of the female world is. One attempt to make a stab at it distinguishes three elites—society women, celebrities (borrowed from C. W. Mills) and intellectuals (borrowed from Schumpeter and Mannheim)—several middle levels, welfare recipients, and outcasts (Bernard, 1981b, chapter 10).

For the two lowest levels the data here presented are from two projects: the series of studies on the Work-Incentive Program—WIN—by Samuel Klausner in and around Philadelphia (1972) and the Stress and Families Project, inaugurated by Marcia Guttentag and carried through by Deborah Belle and her staff in Boston (1982). For the other social classes the data are from the great volume of research on the subject issuing from the libraries and computers and from the growing body of work on women's health. Some of the comments are not buttressed by formal research but rest on observations of the current scene not yet subjected to rigorous scientific scrutiny.

OUTCASTS

The Oxford Dictionary defines outcast as "abject, socially despised" and as "forsaken, homeless, and neglected." There is an extensive research literature on male outcasts so defined, on bums, on tramps, on skid-row habitués, and on homeless men in general. There is less on the outcasts of the female world. Include among them are "all women who have no moorings, no place—psychologically or sociologically—to go. . . . Their family ties are tenuous or vanished. . . . They may be 'warehoused' in institutions; they may be the 'bag ladies' on the streets of large cities; they may be panhandlers; they may be runaway girls; they may be in shelters of one kind or another, including jails" (Bernard, 1981b, pp. 246-247). Klausner sees them as "banished," as outside of the social stratification system entirely. Some are no doubt the archetypically passive-dependent women who, outside of the sheltering walls of a home, are quite unable to cope. Some, no doubt, are victims of Altzheimer's syndrome—senile.

To Klausner, "the development of community is the key to the solution" of the mental-health problems of outcasts (1972, p. 66). Community "rests on participation. . . . in economic, political, religious, healing, educational, family, etc., activities." Finding ways of reincorporating the outcasts into the system is a key to treatment if or when that is feasible. In the meanwhile, the growing movement to provide shelters for abused and homeless women may be a way to salvage women before they become "confirmed" outcasts.

Some outcasts actively seek isolation from family and other ties. Some seem to be fiesty, contentious, perhaps paranoid. Some are active and successful scavengers. Lacking specific research data or direct observation, discussion of the mental health problems of these women is of necessity limited. Their mental health in some cases may be more of a problem to us than to them. It is easier to label them as deviant than to look at them in a more inclusive way that encompasses differences.

WELFARE RECIPIENTS

A considerable corpus of research has accumulated on welfare recipients from the time of Malthus on. The 1960s and 1970s saw numerous government-sponsored and individual studies on "mothers in poverty" (Kriesberg, 1970) as well as congressional hearings on the subject. The rise in the number of women in the welfare population reflects what has been called a "time of transition" (Ross & Sawhill, 1975). The 1,350 interviewees (1969-1973) in the WIN study included, in addition to the social outcasts, several other categories of women, namely the incompetent, the adjusted traditionalists, the temporary traditionalists, and the modernizers. The policies of the WIN program itself tended to select the more competent women, leaving for the welfare population women more in need of therapy of some kind, the incompetent, the conflict-prone, and the dependent. They would need rehabilitation services or traditonal forms of psychotherapy whether in the form of social case work or of mental health neighborhood or sidewalk treatment centers.

For the adjusted traditionalists, policy indicated service programs: for the temporary traditionalists, work training; for the modernizer, jobs, subsidized if necessary. If employment opportunities remained open, the modernizers would rise in the social class structure on their own. Indeed, Klausner found labor force participation in some form or other at whatever level to be the appropriate way of dealing with all categories. "The benefits of labor are not limited to welfare mothers and should even be extended to middle class and other low-income women" (1972, p. ix). Comparable conclusions were drawn from the Stress and Families project (Belle, 1982).

The Stress and Families project involved a more intensive scrutiny of 43 families. Cited here are the abstracts of chapters dealing with the correlates of stress, with the impact of social links and social support, and with the relation of work to depression.

The correlates of stress. The ongoing conditions of women's lives seemed to be related to mental health. Events that interfered with them introduced stress. The lives of the women studied seemed to be especially vulnerable to violent and uncontrollable stressful events. "Of the various conditions investigated, those relating to money were by far the most powerful correlates of mental health. Even when income level is discounted, the other life conditions relating to money were significantly related to mental health" (Makosky, 1982, p. 75).

Social links and social support. Good mental health was related to task support, such as with child care, as it was also with having a confidante. Neither of these therapeutic factors was related to neighborhood involvement. In fact, such involvement was related to high stress and depression. More adults in the household may have supplied task-related support but not availability of confidantes (Belle, 1982, p. 127).

Work and depression. "Though current work status is negligibly related to psychological well-being, long-term indicators of work experience correlate strongly with various measures of mental health and stress." As in studies of two-earner or dual-career families, so also among these women there were "difficulties coordinating work and family life" (Tebbets, 1982, p. 154). Money, overload, and psychological support work, in brief—seemed to play an important part in the mental health of these women.

The importance of work showed up here as it did in the WIN study:

> The total number of jobs a woman has held in her entire work history which is the longest-term measure of work experience, correlates negatively and significantly with. . . . anxiety, depression, life stressors in the areas of mental health, money, and parenting, and life stress in the areas of health, mental health, and total life stress. . . . The longer the duration of work experience in the last three years, the lower were the reported depressive symptoms and the higher the respondents' self-esteem. (Tebbets, 1982, p. 164)

The implications for policy could hardly be clearer. Still, it seems to have been found elsewhere that the reasons for entering the labor force has much to do with its effect on women. If they enter against their wishes, it may be negative; if in line with their wishes, positive. The proportion of women who say they plan to enter the labor force at some point in their life seems to have risen, a fact shown in the statistical trends in work force participation by women.

ELITES

The mental health problems of one of the three elites do not show up in the research literature. From time to time we hear of alcoholism, strange crochets, and long-concealed family skeletons. Wills sometimes bring to light peculiar obsessions. For the most part, however, such mental health problems are well shielded from the enquiring researcher. Limited contacts on my part have shown a certain degree of depression but certainly not enough to warrant a statement here.

The mental health of celebrities, by way of contrast, is likely to become a cause celebre in some cases, whether in the form of alcoholism, drug addiction, varietism, or depression, the archtype of which was the case of Marilyn Monroe. Worth looking into is the question, How does such media coverage affect our image of women who become celebrities? And, as a corollary, their lives? It has been suggested that the emphasis on the scandals in the lives of celebrities is a way of keeping women in line. "See what can happen if you stray too far and become a star."

Women intellectuals have been researched in depth and we do know quite a bit about them. We know that they have had to confront widespread sanctions as violators of basic role prescriptions. It was alleged that intellectual activity would ipso facto produce physical decline. Or they were caricatured as second class or ersatz males. Ravenna Helson has traced the kind of constraints traditionally impos-ed on the intellectual woman, showing how recently she has become an acceptable type. Any woman who survived the intellectual slings and arrows directed against her must surely have had good mental health. Helson's review of the research literature showed that as recent-ly as 1968, Edwin C. Lewis concluded that "the girl who aims for a career is likely to be frustrated and dissatisfied with herself as a person. . . . She is less well adjusted than those who are content to become housewives. Not only is she likely to have a poor self-concept, but she also probably lacks a close relationship with her family" (Helson, 1972, p. 36). Indeed, Lewis felt that the career was itself a compensation for personal dissatisfaction, an outlet for frustration. Helson, reviewing newer research findings, concluded that even the older case against the mental health of intellectual women was never as strong as alleged. She found that the older research was selectively received: studies that found intellectual women suffering mental health difficulties were played up, those that found them in fine fettle, ignored. The more recent studies find them "serious, competent, com-mitted, and individualistic" (1968, p. 40). For the second half of the eighties the picture will have to be looked at again.

Two mental health items deserve attention here, one positive and one negative, namely, eustress and burnout. Several years ago (1968) I wrote a paper on eustress, a concept that Dr. Hans Selye himself told me he found useful. It is the pleasurable, even sought-after, stress that accompanies challenge, the joy and excitement that over-coming obstacles makes one feel, the pleasure that mastery generates, the successful battle to the top. For some women the feminist move-ment of the 1970s generated a considerable amount of such eustress. Feminism was an elixir for them. It was indeed exhilarating. For some, symptoms of distress were replaced by eustress. They were rejuvenated. For them the feminist movement may not have been what the doctor ordered, but it should have been. It released a great burst of energy and vitality. It taught many women to direct their aggression outward rather than inward against their own bodies, as some women have done, especially when childbearing is over.

But for some other women the stress became distress. Climbing a hill that got steeper and steeper as they got higher and higher up generated more stress than they were willing or able to deal with. They became tired. There was a good deal of talk about burnout, a situation in which the returns from effort seemed less and less reward-ing. It has been suggested that the upturn in the marriage rate in the late seventies and the large number of women deciding in their mid- to late thirties to have a child may in some cases be ways of dealing with burnout. They had worked so hard to move mountains and now were finding the results of all their efforts only meager. They have had to bear too many slings and arrows of outrageous fortune. They have had to bear the brunt of male hostility. They have served as the target of surviving prejudices and discriminatory practices. They have had it. Still others have become disillusioned with one another. The sisterhood support they have counted on is withdrawn. Some of the successful women have proved to be as sexist as men. Fortunately feminist therapy is one form of treatment that is being developed to deal with these mental health hazards.

THE MIDDLE CLASSES

One common overall factor in the mental health of middle-class women has to do with the relative value they place on "women's two roles." The mental health problems differ between the tradi-tionalists and the modernizers. Among the traditionalists they have to do with the passing of traditional marriage and family and most especially with the "tipping point" in the whole female world structure. Among the modernizing, they have to do with fatigue, overload, and the revamping of gender role relationships.

TRADITIONALISTS: CRISIS AND TIPPING POINT

Among traditionalists the dizzying changes now taking place in our society are profoundly threatening. The crisis in marriage and family that occurred in the 1970s (Bernard, 1981b) could only be terrifying to traditionalists of whichever sex. There was, first of all, the almost spectacular disaffection with marriage and parenthood that occurred. This can be seen in the remarkable drop in the first marriage, the remarriage, and the fertility rates and the even more remarkable rise in the divorce rate. This disaffection was shown also in attitudes toward marriage as revealed in surveys. Between 1957 and 1976, the proportion of men and women, but especially of single women, who had positive attitudes toward marriage and parenthood declined and the proportion who felt they were all burdens and restrictions increased. The proportion of young women who said they planned to have no children doubled to almost 10 percent. The discovery and insistence on female orgasm were becoming almost an issue. This antimarriage and antiparenthood character of the 1970s seems to be passing; in the late 1970s the marriage rate turned up and the divorce rate moderated greatly and may even have begun a decline in some areas. But the end of the crisis did not mean that there was a return to the past. The decade of crisis could not help but have left a residue of threat.

Important as the crisis may have been there was another event with even more telling implications and one that was not likely to reverse itself. In 1980 the proportion of married women in the labor force reached the "tipping point," the point at which fewer than half were not employed outside the home. Being employed became, in effect, a normative life-style for married women as well as for married men. Whereas until that time married women who were not in the labor force constituted the expected norm, now for the first time they became nonconformists, a minority.

The advent of such a tipping point is like a great geological shift: A whole sociological structure had tipped and its center of gravity shifted. The concomitants were relevant for the mental health of women on both sides of the fulcrum.

Women who had remained out of the labor force from choice and had expected kudos for conforming to the traditional pattern now became defensive. They were going against the tide. For some time they had been complaining that they were looked down upon, made to feel inferior. But so long as they were in the majority there had been the support of numbers. Whereas once the kudos went to her and sanctions went against women "who worked," these traditional women came to feel shortchanged. They had been doing what had been prescribed for women and expecting the rewards. Now they found themselves denigrated. Many of them exemplified the Broverman stereotype and to this extent their mental health was not good, at least not good enough to brave the outside world.

The mental health stresses became confounded when the feminist movement began to clarify the costs traditional women had been paying for their dependency status and when the attitude toward career women had begun to change in a favorable direction. The changing attitude toward divorce did not help, nor the increasing visibility of the "displaced housewife." It was frightening for many to be told that they were only a heartbeat away from penury themselves. Further, at the time attitudes toward career women were changing in a favorable direction, attitudes toward homemaking seemed less favorable.

There has been some movement in recent years to reassure these women, to show appreciation for their services to husband and children and, through them, to the community at large, to make it clear that there was nothing denigrating about the role of homemaker. To the extent that these reassurances succeed it may be possible to protect the traditional women against depression, although for some time they will be among those who buy most of the Valium pills.

MODERNISTS: OVERLOAD AND ROLE CHANGE

One of the most nearly universal concomitants of labor force participation by married women has to do with the sheer fatigue resulting from overload. It has been found throughout the industrialized West, in socialist as well as in capitalist systems, in developing as well as in developed countries. In our society it has been found particularly serious among mothers of small children in low-paying jobs, with or without a man in the household. The challenge of child care in a society that depends on the contribution of employed women is one of the most serious at the present time. In the absence of such available help, help from support groups is among the best treatment modalities. At the higher levels there is also reported guilt generated by a conflict between family and career obligations of successful women.

A second kind of situation with mental health ramifications for the modernists has to do with the difficulties associated with gender role changes. Role sharing would seem to be a logical and feasible remedy for dealing with overload, both spouses sharing household and parental responsibilities. Early in the 1970s, about a decade ago, there was considerably more complaisance with respect to the feasibility of such role sharing. We are beginning now to understand more about the subtleties involved than we knew then. For it is becoming increasingly clear how closely gender identity itself is tied up with work roles, not only with the work itself but also with the site of the work (Bernard, 1981). It is not at all simple to restructure roles. In Washington, D.C.—admittedly far from typical—one therapist reports that attempting to work out a reasonable and feasible allocation of family responsibilities is a major source of stress. The special nature of these problems, I add parenthetically, is reflected in the special kind of therapy dual-career marriages call for, as in two-job marriages. In the world of the hard hat, the fellow workers of one man attacked him as a scab when he admitted to helping his wife around the house. The problems associated with egalitarian relationships may become stressful even with the best of intentions on both sides. The partners are treading on unmapped territory.

But modernizing women are moving with the tide and their problems are among those being given a considerable amount of attention. Now that we are defining the nature of the stresses that weigh on employed wives and mothers, we are in the process of learning how to relieve them. Now that we are discovering and analyzing the hazards that plague role relationships in two-earner or dual-career marriages, we may even be able to develop policies to avoid those hazards.

THE MID-1980S

The discussion here began with a glance at a long historical sweep tracing, however superficially, some of the ups and downs in the mental health situation of women over time. That kind of perspective is hard to get when one is engulfed in a long rise or swell oneself. Short-term changes may be more salient but judging them may be less accurate. Right now, in the mid-1980s, we are witnessing an effort by traditionalists to change the direction of policy with respect to families. There is also an effort to transfer all family issues to state and local jurisdictions. And even there, government responsibility with respect to families should be minimal. The needs of families are not denied but past policies for dealing with them have been misguided. They should be met by the private sector. Only shreds of family concerns—antiabortion legislation, for example—should remain with the federal government. Beyond a safety net for the "truly needed," government responsibility should be minimal. Foundations, industry, social service agencies, churches, voluntary groups, should bear most of the burden. That such a change in policy would have some impact on the mental health of women may be taken for granted but it would be futile at this point to speculate on its precise nature.

Nor is it any less futile to speculate whether this traditionalist movement is a long-term wave. The long-term forces—demographic, educational, technological, scientific—do not point in that direction.

In the meanwhile, among the upbeat aspects of the current mental health situation of women today is the growing discipline of feminist therapy. Jean Baker Miller in a landmark book (1976) on the psychology of women expounds the new point of view that emphasizes the strengths of women rather than their alleged weaknesses. Women are no longer to judge themselves by male standards. Qualities in themselves that have been condemned by men are not to be seen as inferior. They may even be strengths. In her own practice she has found "many women [who] now seek to explore their own needs and to evaluate themselves in their own terms. . . . [T]his may seem simple; it was not always so. In the past women tended to begin by asking what was wrong with them that they could not fit into men's needs and plans. This difference bespeaks a tremendous change. It is a kind of change that therapy cannot make. It precedes therapy, but its impact on therapy is enormous" (p. 135). These women are getting a handle on the mental health disabilities that have been inculcated in them by standards emphasizing poor rather than good mental health (Broverman et al, 1972). And there seems to be a growing feminist therapy tailored to deal precisely with the stresses engendered in women in these fast-changing times (Sturdivant, 1980). It is geared to building support systems among women, to encouraging recognition of their own values, of the validity of their own experience, of the importance of developing the standards of their own world rather than accepting unthinkingly those of the traditional male world. Of creating in women the knowledge and understanding that will make it possible for them to contribute in the formulation of policy.

The next decade, like any other, will be the best of times for some women, the worst of times for others, the best—as compared with the past—for more women than the worst. After the crisis in traditional marriage of the 1970s we may be well on our way to working through a form of marriage and family suitable for this day and age. We are at least beginning to confront the stress-producing results of overload, and a host of efforts are at least on the drawing board for dealing with them, including flexible work hours and adequate child care. We are researching ways to deal with the trauma of gender role restructuring to make egalitarian relationships more feasible. Now that we are able to pinpoint with rough accuracy the most serious stress points—and some are admittedly extremely serious—we are at least recognizing them and trying to find answers.

REFERENCES

Belle, D. (1982). *Lives in stress: Women and depression.* Beverly Hills, CA: Sage.

Bernard, J. (1968). The eudaemonists. In S. Klausner (Ed.), *Why men take chances.* Garden City, NY: Doubleday.

Bernard, J. (1971). *Women and the public interest.* Chicago: Aldine.

Bernard, J. (1981a). The good provider role: Its rise and fall. *American Psychologist, 36* (January).

Bernard, J. (1981b). *The female world.* New York: Free Press.

Broverman, I., Vogel, S., Broverman, D., Clarkson, F., & Rosencrantz, P. (1972). Sex role stereotypes: A current appraisal. *Journal of Social Issues, 28,* 59-78.

Gladieux, J. D. (1978). Pregnancy, the transition to parenthood: Satisfaction with the pregnancy experience as a function of sex role conceptions, marital relationships, and social network. In W. B. Miller & L. F. Newman (Eds.), *The first child and family formation.* Chapel Hill: North Carolina Population Center.

Halliday, J. L. (1948). *Psychosocial medicine.* New York: W. W. Norton.

Helson, R. (1972). The changing image of the career woman. *Journal of Social Issues, 28,* 33-46.

Hofferth, S. L., & Moore, K. (1979). Women's employment and marriage. In R. E. Smith (Ed.), *The subtle revolution.* Washington, DC: The Urban Institute.

Klausner, S. Z. (1972). *The work incentive program: Making adults economically independent.* Philadelphia: University of Pennsylvania.

Kriesberg, L. (1970). *Mothers in poverty: A study of fatherless families.* Chicago: Aldine.

Langner, T. S., & Michael, S. T. (1963). *Mental health in the metropolis* (vol 2). New York: McGraw-Hill.

Lasch, C. (1978). *The culture of narcissism.* New York: W. W. Norton.

Lewis, E. C. (1968). *Developing woman's potential.* Ames: Iowa State University Press.

Makosky, V. P. (1982). Sources of stress: Events or conditions? In D. Belle (Ed.), *Lives in stress: Women and depression.* Beverly Hills, CA: Sage.

Miller, J. B. (1976). *Toward a new psychology of women.* Boston: Beacon Press.

Moore, K. A. & Hofferth, S. L. (1979). Women and their children. In R. E. Smith (Ed.), *The subtle revolution,* Washington, DC: The Urban Institute.

Ross, H. L. & Sawhill, I. V. (1975). *Time of transition.* Washington, DC: The Urban Institute.

Schulenburg, J. T. (1979). Clio's daughters: Myopic modes of perception. In J. A. Sherman & E. T. Beck (Eds.), *The prism of sex.* Madison: University of Wisconsin Press.

Smith, R. E. (Ed.) (1979). *The subtle revolution.* Washington, DC: The Urban Institute.

Srole, L., Langner, T. S., Michael, S. T., Opler, M. K. & Rennie, T. (1962). *Mental health in the metropolis* (vol. 1). New York: McGraw-Hill.

Stearns, P. N. (1980). Old women: Some historical observations. *Journal of Family History, 5*(Winter), 44-57.

Stone, L. (1980). *Family, sex, and marriage in England 1500-1800.* New York: Harper & Row.

Sturdivant, S. (1980). *Therapy with women: A feminist philosophy of treatment.* New York: Springer.

Summer, W. G. (1906). *Folkways.* Boston: Ginn.

Tebbets, R. (1982). Work: Its meaning in women's lives. In D. Belle (Eds.), *Lives in stress: Women and depression.* Beverly Hills, CA: Sage.

10

VIOLENCE AGAINST WOMEN: IMPLICATIONS FOR MENTAL HEALTH POLICY

Lenore E. Walker

Concern with women's safety from men's physical, sexual, and psychological violence has been an important factor in promoting change in mental health policy in this country. In the late 1960s women began to speak out in groups against the retraumatization of rape victims by an insensitive or even sexist mental health and legal system. By the mid 1970s the horrors of battered women were being exposed and failure of the mental health system among other institutions to provide services to the victim/survivors and their children prompted the development of a whole new alternative institution, the safehouse or battered women's shelter (CAABW, 1980). The concept of marital rape, or forced sexual activity by one's own husband soon after became documented and then laws were passed in a number of states declaring such behavior a criminal act (Russell, 1982).

The psychologist's role in identifying a cluster of symptoms in victims of violence, subcategories of Post Traumatic Stress Disorder called rape trauma syndrome and battered woman syndrome, which appeared in the 1981 revision of the Diagnostic and Statistical Manual (DSM-III), made codifying of psychological injuries from assaults more precise. While everyone was still reeling from the estimated numbers of potential women victims, new figures were introduced indicating that incest and sexual molestation and assault of children was far more prevalent then ever before suspected (Finkelhor, 1979); again, mostly men committing the behavior towards girls and sometimes boys. To those of us involved in the research and delivery of services during these past 10 years, it began to seem like almost everyone was affected in some way by the psychological impact of violent behavior. How, then, could the mythology that existed before 1970 have developed and been allowed to dominate our helping professions?

HISTORICAL BACKGROUND

Feminist psychologists typically go back to Freud's influence on the profession for evidence that explains whatever is present day sex bias in a particular issue. It is interesting that Freud originally noted the frequency with which incest was reported by his women clients. In fact, his paper on the etiology of hysteria in 1896 reads as though it could have been written by one of today's feminist psychologists (Freud, 1896). He changed his original thinking about male seduction of female children, according to Masson (1984) because of the unacceptability of such ideas with his other male colleagues. Thus, Freud explained his patients reports of early sexual trauma as fantasies, fulfilling their wishes to be intimate with their fathers. From these theories came the concept of masochism, which is even more destructive to the understanding of women.

Women, Freud later believed, had an unconscious need to be punished for some sexual sin, either committed or desired as a child or an adult. The whole notion of retribution for sin was not new with Freudian theory, of course, and can be traced throughout religious teachings. The heavy impact of Jewish Kabbalah or mysticism can be found in Freud's theories, especially the notion that a person must do something positive to get rid of guilt feelings or is doomed to bear them again in each successive lifetime. Even today, with refined definitions of masochism (Shainess, 1979) victims of violence are still thought to have set up their victimization in some way to atone for their past mistakes. Those victims who are repeatedly harmed, are still thought by many psychoanalysts to psychologically need the abuse (Blum, 1982).

Perhaps the myth of masochism was necessary for people to accept the unfair laws and unjust treatment of women at the hands of some men. Dating even earlier than the Hammurabi code, handed down in ancient Babylon, women were held responsible and punished if men physically harmed or sexually defiled them. Martin (1976) documents much of the early religious and legal exhortations teaching women how to be better wives so as to avoid the discipline men must apply, should they not live up to whatever standards society had for women.

Dobash and Dobash (1981) document the influence patriarchal religion had on encouraging wife beating as does Davidson (1979) and others. The legal system, growing out of common law, perpetuated the view that women (and children) were merely men's possessions by demanding that men take legal responsibility for their families and thus permitted them to discipline wives and children at will. As social policy changed, more restrictions were placed on what kinds of discipline men could use. The last to be abolished only about 50 years ago in this country, was the "rule of thumb" that decreed that a man could beat his wife with a stick as long as it was no thicker than the man's thumb (Martin, 1976).

Although new laws against sexual or physical assault have been in effect for many years, enforcement has been slow and not equal across the country. Given the individual state's rights to set and enforce criminal behavior standards, such unevenness is to be expected. Yet, no matter what the laws, men who commit violent acts against women, especially their wives, are less likely to be punished then women who commit violent acts against men, even if in self-defense (Bochnak, 1981).

Psychological learning theory would suggest that behavior tends to be repeated if it is reinforced. Thus, it seems obvious that men who commit violent acts are accomplishing their goals or they would stop this behavior. Immediate punitive consequences would cause decrease in the offensive behavior; but no one seems to be able to offer such immediate punishment except the police. In fact, a recent study conducted for the National Police Executive Forum has demonstrated that an immediate arrest policy is the most effective technique to reduce the frequency and severity of the violence. Changing police policy, however, from a mediation or laissez-faire attitude toward treating domestic disturbances as a serious crime in progress, and instituting an arrest policy, has been so difficult that some groups have had to file class action suits to get their communities to begin to think about change (see, for example, New York city and Oakland, California). The recent election of a new mayor in Denver, Colorado, has dramatically altered the atmosphere of deadlocked community negotiations to one of cooperation in gaining better protection for battered women. Psychologists have been members of the community coalition, providing their expertise to the negotiation team.

One of the most useful ways to begin to affect public policy by changing public attitudes about this or any problem is to conduct research and widely publicize the results through the media or other ways to reach individuals. Such data now have been collected, analyzed, and published (Finkelhor, Gelles, Hotaling, & Straus, 1983). These data are helpful in telling the public how badly harmed individuals are when assaulted and explain why battered women do not have the free will to terminate the relationship. Redefining rape as a crime of violence rather than passion has also been important to change public attitudes towards sexual assault victims. So too, for sexually and physically abused children. Recent television programs on these issues have used qualified psychologist consultants to assure accuracy of their presentation. Eliminating violence and inequality between men and women are both important goals if we are to eliminate all forms of women battering in our society. Yet societal change takes a long time, maybe generations to effect. Implementation of smaller facets of public policy can make an immediate difference consistent with desired long-term policy changes.

Estimates of the number of victims of violence vary, ranging from one out of four women will be sexually assaulted as an adult, to one out of two women will be beaten by a man who loves her. Recent estimates of girl child sexual molestation victims are as least as high as those for adults. These victims will probably all suffer psychological effects that range from mild anxiety and depression, guilt feelings, heightened sense of suspiciousness, lack of trust in people, and dysfunctional relationships to serious phobias and crippling fears, paranoia, fear of going crazy, rage and anger, sexual dyfunction, and feelings of helplessness and powerlessness that generalize to a lack of motivation to go on with life. Suicides, loss of jobs, disrupted marriages, homicides, and disturbed parenting of children are some of the outcomes. Witnessing or experiencing family violence is known to affect the next generation, perpetuating the use of coercive force to get one's own way.

Given the mental health system's previous failure to provide adequate services to women victims of violence, there is great skepticism in the grassroots women's community that it can do so now that the syndromes have been identified. On the other hand, shelter and rape crisis center workers know that there are women who need the skills of a competent, trained clinician in order to heal from the trauma. Thus, mental health policy has been affected in various ways. First, policymakers have learned more about the psychological effects of violence victims; rape trauma and battered women syndromes have been identified and classified under the post traumatic stress disorders; and laws have been changed to reflect society's current intolerance of the violence.

Second, treatment modalities have been identified and studied, although widespread implementation in the mental health delivery system is yet to come (Walker, 1981, 1984a). The fear that clinicalization of victims of violence will once again result in blaming the victim rather than the perpetrator often causes women's groups to distrust mental health professionals. Sometimes this distrust creates a healthy tension that separates those clinicians more likely to be helpful to survivors of violence from those who still have much to learn about their own issues. Unless a therapist's own sexist assumptions and fears of vulnerability are personally confronted, she or he will have difficulty in being of assistance in these cases (Walker, 1981).

Third, mental health professionals have been applying the new knowledge to the legal system, minimizing further emotional trauma, educating those directly involved, sensitizing the media, and expanding the law to become more responsive to the needs of women. It is this interaction between psychology and the law that has provided the major policy changes that benefit all of us.

ASSESSMENT AND THERAPEUTIC STRATEGIES

Information obtained directly from victim/survivor's of violence indicate that initially the most therapeutic response from mental health workers is to spend time listening to their stories. Initial interviews are best when they are not very structured, allowing the woman to explain what has happened to her in her own way. Often that means beginning with a rambling narrative that eventually becomes less confused as the woman becomes more trusting. Questions or comments that suggest or emphasize the woman's possible complicity in her own abuse are countertherapeutic at this time. Learning to take better care of herself comes much later in treatment. Women who are still in danger of further violence need to help the therapist assess the danger level, especially the risk of someone dying. Browne's (1983) research indicates that the most significant difference between battered women who kill their abusers and those who don't is the level of the man's violence. An escape plan, detailing exact steps to protect herself, children, pets, and personal possessions helps reduce therapist anxiety and the client's denial of potential danger. Recognizing escalating violent behavior and teaching women to identify their own three-phase battering cycle helps women move toward safely terminating a bettering relationship. The most likely time for a homicide, suicide, or more serious emotional disturbance to occur is at the point of separation. Thus, a close professional relationship with the community safehouse task force can protect clients who need to be safe once they decide to leave home.

Techniques for crisis intervention in short- and long-term psychotherapy have been appearing in the literature since the mid-1970s. One review of strategies for working with battered women and their families can be found in Walker (1984a). Sexual assault victim assessment strategies have been developed by Burgess and Holmstrom (1978) and Kirkpatrick, Veronen, and Resick (1979). Bouhoutsos, in Chapter 11 of this volume, discusses those victims sexually exploited by other professionals. The lasting impact of childhood sexual assault on its victims has also been documented (Bass & Thornton, 1983; Butler, 1978; Finkelhor, 1979). Model programs have been designed and implemented all over the country. The Center for Women Policy Studies in Washington, D.C., keeps a current list.

PSYCHOLOGICAL ASSESSMENT FOR LEGAL CASES

Documenting psychological damage from victimization has opened the way for other societal institutions to become responsive to victims. President Reagan's Task Force on Victims of Crime (1983) analyzed testimony from victims and professionals given across the country and found that not only have we not been responsive to violence victims, but in some cases, our interventions have had a negative effect. Women and children who have been sexually assaulted are one such example. The trauma of the police investigation, medical examination, and courtroom experience revictimize women and children, and cause further harm. Victim-witness advocates who usually work for prosecutor's offices can minimize the mental health trauma caused by the legal proceedings as can good psychological intervention. It was recommended that domestic violence be further studied, and currently an Attorney General's Task Force on Domestic Violence is taking testimony all over the country. Testimony has been sought from mental health providers and recommendations for major policy changes can be anticipated. The next step will be to persuade the president, Congress, and the judiciary to implement them.

CHILD SEXUAL ASSAULT

We have learned that children who are sexually assaulted can be greatly affected by the need for their testimony in court. Adult incest and stranger assault victims tell of memories of their long-lasting psychological scars from such an experience. Development of a profile of child sexual assault psychological symptoms helped create a standard procedure for its assessment that includes videotaped play interviews with anatomically correct dolls. Such an assessment is less emotionally devastating to the victims than to have them repeat their story to all the officials who need to hear what happened. The Harbor-view Medical Center in Seattle is a prototype of its kind (Berliner, 1983).

Many states have introduced new legislation that permits substitution of the videotapes for children under the age of 10, instead of making them appear in court. The mental health professional must be able to give an opinion that the child is incompetent to testify or will be irreparably harmed but, that the child's account of the incident is reliable. The professional then testifies as to what the child said, the emotional reactions, and reliability of the account. The defendant has the right to cross-examine the psychologist, not the child, which both puts a tremendous burden on the professional and takes away some of the accused's right under our laws. The court must balance the alleged offender's rights against the victim's rights not to be further harmed. Higher courts will be asked to rule on the constitutionality of the use of these procedures in the criminal courts (State v. Thiret, Colorado, 1984). Meanwhile, in the less punitive and more treatment oriented juvenile courts, these proceedings allow dependency and neglect cases to be more easily resolved with a minimum of additional emotional harm from the system designed to protect the victims. At Walker & Associates, we are developing videotape procedures that meet the psychology profession's assessment standards as well as stand the scrutiny of the legal system.

CIVIL LITIGATION

In cases where the damage has already been done, documentation of psychological injuries may be used to pursue a civil lawsuit. In our tort laws, financial compensation may be awarded to the victim for injuries sustained by another person. Many victims frustrated by the slow process and minimal punishment meted out by the criminal justice system have chosen to file civil actions against their assailants or against others for malpractice or negligence in allowing conditions that facilitated the assault. Although these cases can take up to several years to be heard, out of court settlements and large financial awards by jurors and judges who have heard expert witness testimony as to the extent of the psychological damages make them a particularly attractive addition to the victim's healing process. Many hotels and major corporations are instituting procedures to demonstrate good faith attention to women's safety following large financial awards to women who have been harmed, in part, by their negligence. This has been somewhat successful in battered women cases and much more successful in rape cases. Attorney General offices have been using similar procedures in revocation of licensure hearings as Bouhoutsos describes in the next chapter.

ADMISSIBILITY STANDARDS

In order to get expert witness testimony admitted, it must meet the standards set by the rules of evidence. Most states adopt the Federal Rules of Evidence standard that calls for a three-part test: (1) The information experts will testify to is beyond the general knowledge of the average juror; (2) the qualifications of the experts meets their own profession's standards; and (3) the methodology used is based on the state of knowledge in the field that is sufficiently developed so as to allow the formation of a reasonable opinion. In criminal cases, even if an expert's opinion is found to meet all three tests, if it is judged to be more prejudicial (harmful to the defendant) than probative (assisting in finding the truth), the evidence can be kept out of the proceedings. So, the same opinion offered by a psychologist in a civil case or administrative hearing, can be barred from that defendant's criminal trial.

Evidence of rape trauma syndrome has not been admitted in several states because it was judged too prejudicial (see in re State v. Saldana. 324 N.W. 2d 227, 1982), while it has been admitted in others (see in re State v. Marks. 647 P.2nd 1292, 1982). It has been the reason for not admitting battered women syndrome testimony in only one case (Thomas v. State, Ohio, 1978). In the other cases where admissability of an expert has been challenged, the predominant reason has been questioning the sufficiency of the scientific knowledge base and methodology upon which the expert's opinion is formed. A more extensive discussion can be found in Walker (1984b).

The American Psychological Association (APA) has assisted individual members by submitting an Amicus Curiae Brief in two cases appealing the trial court's opinion that there is insufficient data upon which a psychologist can offer an opinion about why they were justified in killing their batterers. (Kinsports, Bersoff & Ennis, 1983). In these cases, battered women killed their abusers after years of abuse. Both claimed they were terrified of further imminent bodily harm or death, and so killed in self-defense. They argue that jury needs the testimony of an expert to understand their state of mind. (see in re Hawthorne v. State, Florida, and Kelley v. State, New Jersey, where the New Jersey Supreme Court agrees). The APA's friend of the court argument reviews the relevant psychological literature, legal opinions, and comments to demonstrate that the state of the knowledge in their field is indeed well enough developed so as to support an expert's opinion. A discussion of how much testimony was presented at one woman's trial can be found in Sandiford and Burgess (1984).

IMPACT ON WOMEN'S MENTAL HEALTH POLICY

The psychological and legal developments outlined above are representative of a newer kind of policy formulation. The law has been a harbinger of sexism against women, especially those who are victims of violence (Bochnak, 1981). Until the admissability of expert witness testimony for battered women who kill in self-defense, it was typical for such women to plead guilty to a murder charge and spend at least 10 years in prison. Today, acquittal or perhaps at most a manslaughter conviction with probation is a more likely outcome. Women who kill their husbands are more likely to be charged with first degree murder while men who kill their wives more likely receive a manslaughter charge (Brown, 1983).

A recent homicide case illustrates the sexist biases. Richard and Debra Janke both had been physically abused, and Debra had been sexually abused, by their father. Maria Janke, their mother also had been abused throughout her marriage. Sixteen-year-old Richard shot and killed their father as he returned home, while Debra waited inside the house near other guns. He was convicted of manslaughter and sentenced to five years in prison; she was convicted of a higher-level crime, conspiracy to commit murder, and sentenced to seven years in prison. In neither trial was expert testimony permitted, and it can only be surmised that the jurors determined levels of guilt and judges imposed sentences based on outdated sex-biased information. Certainly no one would suggest homicide is a preferable solution to ending violence against women; but society's institutions must become more responsive to the pain and horror victims experience. Changing the legal system and psychological system makes an important contribution to women's mental health.

REFERENCES

American Psychiatric Association (1981). *Diagnostic and statistical manual, third edition (DSM-III).* Washington, DC: Author.

Bass, E., & Thornton, L. (1983). *I never told anyone: Writings by women survivors of child sexual abuse.* New York: Harper & Row.

Berliner, L. (1983). Impact of sexual assault and therapeutic intervention, in *Sexual assault: representing the victim*. Seattle: Northwest Women's Law Center.

Blum, H. P. (1982). Psychoanalytic reflections on the "beaten wife syndrome," in Kirkpatrick, M. (Ed.), *Women's sexual experiences: Explorations of the dark continent* (pp. 263-267). New York: Plenum Press.

Bochnak, E. (1981). *Women's self defense cases: Theory and practice.* Charlottesville, VA: The Michie Company Law Publishers.

Browne, A. (1983). *When battered women kill.* Doctoral dissertation for the Union of Experimenting Colleges and Universities.

Burgess, A. W., & Holstrom, L. L. (1978). Recovery from rape and prior life stress. *Research in Nursing and Health, 1*(4), 165-174.

Butler, S. (1978). *Conspiracy of silence.* San Francisco: Glide.

Colorado Association for Aid for Battered Women (CAABW) (1980). *A monograph on services to battered women.* DAHS Publication No. OHDS79-05708.Washington, DC: Government Printing Office.

Davidson, T. (1979). *Conjugal crime: Understanding and changing the wife-beating pattern.* New York: Hawthorne.

Dobash, R., & Dobash, R. (1981). *Violence against wives.* New York: Macmillian.

Finkelhor, D. (1979). *Sexually victimized children.* New York: Free Press.

Finkelhor, D., Gelles, R., Hotaling, G., & Straus, M. (1983). *The dark sides of families.* Beverly Hills, CA: Sage.

Freud, S. (1896/1959). The aetiology of hysteria. In Jones, E. (Ed.), *The Collected papers of Sigmund Freud* (vol. 1, pp. 183-219). New York: Basic Books.

Kinports, K., Bersoff, D. N., & Ennis, B. J. (1983), *Brief of Amicus Curiae American Psychological Association in Support of Appellant.* Washington, DC: APA.

Kirkpatrick, D. G., Veronen, L., & Resick, P. A. (1979). Assessment of the aftermath of rape: Changing patterns of fear. *Journal of Behavorial Assessment, 1*(2), 133-148.

Martin, D. (1976). *Battered wives.* San Francisco: Glide.

Masson, J. M. (1984). *The assault on truth: Freud's supression of the seduction theory.* New York: Farrar, Straus & Giroux.

President's Task Force on Victims of Crime (1983). *Final report,* Washington, DC: U.S. Government Printing Office.

Russell, D. (1982). *Rape in marriage.* New York: Macmillian.

Sandiford, K., & Burgess, A. (1984). *Shattered night.* New York: Warner Books.

Shainess, N. (1979). Vulnerability to masochism: Masochism as a process. *American Journal of Psychotherapy, 33*(2), 174-189.

Walker, L. E. (1979). *The battered woman.* New York: Harper & Row.

Walker, L. E. (1981). Battered women: Sex roles and clinical issues. *Professional Psychology, 12*(1), 81-91.

Walker, L. E. (1984a). *The battered woman syndrome.* New York: Springer.

Walker, L. E. (1984b). Battered women, psychology and public policy. *American Psychologist* (October).

11

SEXUAL INTIMACY BETWEEN PSYCHOTHERAPISTS AND CLIENTS: POLICY IMPLICATIONS FOR THE FUTURE

Jacqueline C. Bouhoutsos

The problem of sexual intimacy between healers and their patients may be traced to antiquity, and its prohibition to the Hippocratic oath, which cautioned physicians to "abstain from lasciviousness with women or men, free or slaves." Whether this fiat was based on moral principles of the time or on observed damage to the participants is not clear.

In modern times, the healing professions nominally continued the proscription against patient-therapist sex by including oblique references to such activity under provisions concerning client welfare, negligence, or community standards in ethics codes and licensing laws. Violations of the prohibition did occur, however, even among such well-known figures in the history of psychotherapy as Ferenczi and Jung. Their sexual activities with patients were viewed by their colleagues in a mildly reproving but hardly outraged manner and there was no disciplinary action taken.

During the 1960s, proliferation of growth groups that emphasized increased physical and emotional intimacy appeared to extend the boundaries of patient-therapist sexuality. There were even a few psychotherapists who openly advocated sexual intimacy between therapist and patient, purportedly to improve sexual identity and functioning (McCartney, 1966; Shephard, 1971).

Data about the frequency of such sexual activities were largely unavailable. When research was suggested to obtain such data, one proponent was threatened with expulsion from a professional organization (Butler, 1977); in another instance where research was allowed, the results were suppressed (Forer, 1968). The patients involved in almost all of the reported incidents with therapists were women; the therapists and the researchers were men. Publications by women on the topic of sexual intimacy between patients and therapists are conspicuously absent from the literature of those years.

It was not until the 1970s that serious attention was given to the problem. Perhaps this was due to the increase in the number of women entering the field of psychology. In 1972, the percentage of women who received doctorates in psychology was 26.7 percent; this rose to 42.3 percent in 1981. Approximately one-half of the students enrolled full time in psychology doctoral programs at this time are women. "Unless there are factors that differentially and adversely affect earning of the doctorate by women. . .a continued increase in the percentage of women doctorate holders is to be expected" (Russo, Olmedo, Stapp, & Fulcher, 1981).

In addition to the increase of women in the mental health fields, further impetus to research in the therapist-patient sex area was the growth of consumerism and the unwillingness of the public to accept unquestioningly whatever was offered by professionals. The Nader report began a series of explorations of various schools of therapy and their effectiveness and introduced the concept of "shopping for a therapist" through more than one initial interview. In the early 1970s, a number of civil suits filed against psychotherapists for including sex as part of their therapy were decided in favor of women plaintiffs, raising the issue of patient-therapist sex to the public consciousness. The growth of the women's movement was also a factor. As women became more active politically, they became increasingly aware of the social policy issues involved in sexual acting out against women, whether this involved spousal battering, rape, incest, or psychotherapeutic abuse.

Women mental health professionals began to become more active on local and national levels, forming infrastructures to provide support networks. Many women psychologists had themselves experienced sexual harrassment in their training; this is not surprising, since one out of our four female graduate students will have had sexual relations with a supervisor or teacher before obtaining her degree (Pope, Levenson, & Schover, 1979).

An increasing number of female therapists in private practice were consulted by clients who reported intimacy with a previous therapist, and revealed the negative consequences of such relationships. In the 1970s female therapists became a visible and angry subgroup of professionals concerned about patient-therapist sex. More often than men they suggested punishments for offending therapists and expressed anger toward those therapists (Holroyd & Bouhoutsos, 1984). It became apparent that research was needed not only for academic interest, but to provide information about the frequency and effects of patient-therapist sexual involvement on which to base social policy changes.

RESEARCH

The first studies on therapist-client sexual involvement were directed toward the question of frequency: How many therapists of what gender, ages, and so forth were involved sexually with patients? Roughly 6 percent admitted sexual contact: 5.5 percent of male and .5 percent of female therapists in a study of Los Angeles County physicians (Kardener, Fuller & Mensh, 1973), a subsequent national study of psychologists (Holroyd & Brodsky, 1977), and a recent California study of the effects of such intimacy on patients (Bouhoutsos, Holroyd, Lerman, Forer & Greenberg, 1983). The apparent consistency of these figures has not diminished speculation (*Los Angeles Times, Parade,* August 23, 1983) that the real incidence is substantively higher, since self-report tends to encourage underreporting. Also, these figures pertain only to therapists, not their clients.

Of therapists who act out sexually, 75 percent to 80 percent do so with more than one client (Butler, 1975; Holroyd & Brodsky, 1977). In one instance, a therapist was reported to have been involved with more than 100 clients (Siegel, 1983). Attempts to estimate the number of "victims of therapists" in the United States have led to diverse speculations from one out of three clients (*Los Angeles Times,* August 23, 1983) to hundreds of thousands of clients. A more realistic estimate might be 60,000, using a figure of 20,000 male psychologists in the service delivery system, an equal number of psychiatrists, about twice that number of master's level counselors (based on the California figure of licensed counselors compared with the number of licensed psychologists), and approximately 30,000 social workers (based on an estimate from the National Association of Social Workers of the number of social workers in private practice). If only one client were involved with each therapist; 6 percent of the resultant 200,000 providers would yield 12,000 clients sexually involved with therapists; assuming an average of five clients (to provide for the multiple incidence data), we have an approximation of 60,000. There are many possible sources of error in this estimate. Victims of persons who are not licensed have been omitted. Therapists who serve in institutions are not listed as private providers and are therefore not included. However, 14 percent of the sexual acting out occurred in institutions (Bouhoutsos et al., 1983). Only the core disciplines and counselors have been included, but many other types of individuals in the human services have sexual involvements with clients, such as psychiatric technicians, nurses, para-professionals, religious workers, and the like. All of these factors may cause underestimation of the number of "victims." On the other hand, such predominantly female occupations as social work, counseling, and nursing might lower the estimate. Social workers, and marriage and family counselors have not as yet been studied for incidence of sexual activity with clients. Such research is now in progress (Pope & Bouhoutsos, in preparation; Gechtman, Pope, & Bouhoutsos, in preparation). Should the percentage prove to be considerably lower in predominantly female professions, a diminution of the sexual intimacy problem may come about serendipitously as women enter the mental health professions.

A second group of studies (Belote, 1974; Butler, 1975; D'Addario, 1977; Stone, 1982; Bouhoutsos, 1983) examined the types of patients and therapists who became sexually involved with one another, and the effects of such involvements.

The female clients were approximately 12 to 16 years younger than their therapists; many, but by no means all, were sexually dysfunctional and nonoragasmic. The studies described them as lonely, searching, unhappy, looking for acceptance and friendship. Belote (1974) found them to be vulnerable and high in traditional feminism, which she described as being other-directed, having poor self-regard and low self-actualization with little acceptance of their own aggressive impulses. Often they were not sexually attracted to the therapist, but had a need for acceptance and love and a desire for "cuddling" rather than sex (Forer, 1969). In most instances they abdicated their right of choice and submitted to the therapist because of his status, authority, and the aura of the profession. Many remained in treatment because they trusted the therapist or were afraid to question the therapist lest he stop seeing them. Some of the more disturbed women were diagnosed as borderline or psychotic, seeking a lifesaving attachment. Frequently depressed, dependent, delusional, and even frankly psychotic, they were vulnerable to exploitation. Female institutionalized patients of this kind are often seen as ideal targets for sexual acting out by staff. They are unlikely to turn against therapists, since they are seen as the only solution to an insoluble life situation. Even if they do complain about the treatment, they are often not believed since they are obviously disturbed. Many, but by no means all, have had a history of eroticized relationships with father, brothers, other family members, and with other professionals. These women are easily talked into sexual activity under the guise of therapy, especially when a psychiatrist prescribes medication or hypnosis to assist the seduction. There are several instances of public record where psychiatrists have literally held patients hostage by prescribing and withholding drugs to keep a patient obedient and providing the desired sexual favors. When such women become involved sexually with their therapists, they sustain substantively more damage than less initially disturbed patients (Feldman-Summers, 1984). This is an important finding that contradicts the common public misconception that sexual involvement with disturbed persons does not matter since they were mentally ill anyway.

Who are the sexually involved therapists? The literature shows a mean age of 43.5, with 5 to 30 years of private practice experience. About 90 percent of the therapists reported feeling vulnerable, needy, or lonely when the sexual contact occurred (Butler & Zelen, 1977). They were separated, divorced, or unhappily married. About 95 percent reported fear or guilt; 55 percent were frightened of intimacy. "These aging men, some in a depressive and needy period, somehow let themselves be convinced by their patients' fantasies that they might recapture their youth" (Dahlberg, 1971). Other researchers have postulated an analytic causality: an infantile sadistic tendency based on unsolved relationships with the mother, which are then replayed with patients when the patients refuse to mother them indefinitely (Smith, 1981). Most studies agree that power needs motivate the therapists, a desire to play the guru, to dictate the course of clients' lives, or to collect followers and adherents.

Mostly, the therapists were limited in their sexual activity (Keith-Spiegel, 1979). Sometimes, the sexual relationship consisted totally of the client performing fellatio on the therapist, without attempts to reach an orgasm of her own. In all of these studies, damage accrued to the clients. Terminations were frequently traumatic; the original dysfunctions were not improved, and the complications of the new relationships were added. The women became angry over the change in role and experienced hurt, loneliness, and feelings of abandonment.

All of these studies of clients and therapists dealt with small numbers. In the early 1980s, it became apparent that a large scale research study on the effects of sexual intimacy between clients and therapists was necessary to test the generalizability of the findings in individual cases. The inaccessibility of subjects proved to be problematic. Clients were not available directly, because of the confidential nature of the therapeutic relationship, and experimental research was unfeasible, despite Riskin's (1979) naive suggestion that it should be done (a suggestion published in a reputable law journal!). The only feasible approach appeared to be an indirect one, utilizing therapists' information rather than clients'. A California State Psychological Association Task Force sent questionnaires to all of the licensed psychologists in the state (4385), asking about patients who had reported being intimate with a previous therapist. The study was thus limited by errors of memory and second hand reporting, subjective inferences of causality on the part of the respondents, and a truncated sample that included only those patients returning to therapy after sexual intimacy. Nonetheless, the research was useful in that it examined reports on 559 patients who had been sexually involved with their therapists.

In 90 percent of the cases reported, patients were harmed (Bouhoutsos et al., 1983). The damage ranged from an inability to trust men and hesitation about entering therapy again, to major depressions, hospitalization, and even suicide. The client's personality was seen to have been affected in 34 percent of the cases. This included increased depression, loss of motivation, impaired social adjustment, significant emotional disturbance, suicidal feelings or behavior, and increased drug or alcohol use. Of the 559 cases reported upon, 11 percent were hospitalized. Among the 26 percent for whom sexual, marital, or intimate relationships worsened, mistrust of the opposite sex increased for 14 percent, marriage and/or family were negatively affected for 9 percent and sexual relationships were impaired for 7 percent. Almost half (48 percent) had problems recommencing therapy. Clients were suspicious and mistrusted therapists, and were hesitant in returning for treatment, despite the lack of solution to the original problems. The more intense the sexual involvement with the therapist had been, the greater the difficulty the clients had in returning to therapy. Of the previous therapists reported to have engaged in sexual intimacies, 96 percent were male, 4 percent were female. Of the reported sexual relationships, 92 percent occurred between female patients and male therapists. Other research, however, has revealed that male therapists also act out with male patients in far greater number than female therapists with female patients. In the California study, 58 percent of those male patients reported by subsequent therapists as sexually involved with their therapists had male therapists. It is not clear whether this acting out by male therapists is a regional phenomenon or whether it exists nationwide. Additional research is clearly needed.

ACTION

Because sexual involvements with therapists have been shown to be so harmful to clients, it is particularly important that women in the mental health arena recognize the seriousness of the problem and assist in bringing about changes in public policy that will facilitate prevention and/or containment of this phenomenon. Sexual intimacy between therapists and patients has been described as "the quintessence of sex-biased therapeutic practice" (Holroyd, 1983).

Approximately 13 percent of allegations of professional misconduct in malpractice suits handled by the APA insurance trust (Wright, 1981) and 18 percent of the American Psychological Association ethics complaints in 1982 (Hall & Hare-Mustin, 1983) involved sexual offenses. Nonetheless, suits and complaints are rarely filed. Action is taken in about 4 percent of the cases where sexual intimacy occurs between patient and therapists, and only half of these are carried to completion (Bouhoutsos et al., 1983). Obviously, offending therapists have little to fear from legal or ethics actions. Why are actions so rarely filed?

Many patients who have been harmed feel powerless. They have been told about, and have themselves experienced, the protectionism maintained by professional associations that have functioned traditionally as guilds, and that have sought to protect members, regardless of their transgressions. Fortunately, this trend has been reversed somewhat in the last few years, with the increasing responsivity of the mental health professions to the expanding literature on the harm done to patients and the involvement of women professionals in action programs. However, the aura of protectionism remains.

Another deterrent to reporting is the fear of bureaucracy and its complexity. Most clients are unsophisticated in dealing with professional organization or state government systems, and the ponderousness of the processes and the lack of responsivity discourage efforts to file complaints. Even the commonly accepted written complaint forms are sufficiently impersonal and forbidding to negatively impact the distressed and powerless client.

Frequently, clients are ashamed or guilty about their role in therapist-patient sex and are unwilling to make public their confessions of having been duped and used. Or they have guilt feelings about being seductive and assume their complicity in what resulted, not recognizing that the responsibility for the course of therapy rests entirely with the therapist. Some are embarrassed that they sought therapy in the first place and are unwilling to admit this in a public forum. Many are angry with the mental health professions and are reluctant to trust other professionals to carry on the process of investigation or punishment of colleagues.

Some have unresolved transference feelings that remain, despite the damage done to them, and they hesitate to cause the offending therapists pain. They need to protect the therapist, to look after him, despite the harm he has caused them. These feelings frequently complicate the complaint process and the ambivalence often results in a withdrawal of charges, even after filing. Many therapists choose clients for sexual relationships whom they evaluate as low risk for disclosure, especially confused, vulnerable women who have had a history of being battered, or victims of incest.

Perhaps the most powerful deterrant to reporting is the fear of the consequences of disclosure. In many instances this fear is realistic, since information obtained in the context of the therapy relationship can be twisted and used against them. Disclosure often removes the therapist-client confidentiality privilege and it is frightening to know that the therapist is legally free to use any "secrets," even if they are not directly harmful. But some instances of direct harm have occurred. Husbands have divorced their client-wives after learning about their involvement with therapists. Children have been taken away in custody battles, with the husband using the therapist-patient sexual relationship as grounds.

Even when clients have chosen to disclose details in the legal system, many have found that it is impossible to take action because the sexual intimacy occurred many years before and there is frequently a statute of limitations. Clients in such relationships often are involved for many years before the denouement, and often further years are necessary before the clients have worked through the experiences to arrive at a place in their lives where they can take the step to complain against the therapist who damaged them. As in cases involving medical responsibility for birth injury to a child, a reasonable time for filing after discovery of the injury should be provided in the law. The American Psychological Association has had a five-year limitation for filing, but a recent increase in the number of "old" cases being filed plus a growing sensitivity to the issues involved has convinced the committee to reconsider the ruling. Administrative law regulating licensing frequently does not have statutes of limitations. However, financial considerations often militate against undertaking cases that are more difficult to prove. In older cases there are fewer witnesses, memory is frequently called into question, and judges are often loathe to impose penalties on therapists without additional later charges having been filed.

The reluctance on the part of the clients to come forward and file complaints is matched by the resistance of the systems charged with the investigation and resolution of such complaints. Most frequent reasons given for inaction is lack of funding, whether by government agencies or professional associations. Liability to suit is also a concern. Allocation of resources to a protracted trial can drain coffers and divert assets, and this spector haunts every enforcement agency or ethics committee. Client-therapist sex is often weighed against "serious crimes" such as murder, robbery, rape, and so on, by which society is overwhelmed, and law enforcement agencies are loathe to spend time on a category of offenses where the victims are perceived as having cooperated in their victimization. This view is not unlike the way in which rape was formerly perceived. As rape prosecutions become more successful, attorneys general are more likely to go forward on professional sexual intimacy cases.

Another deterrent to action on complaints is the fear of "false positives," that innocent men might be designated as rapists by angry women wanting vengeance. This fear is buttressed and complicated by the fact that sexual activity between therapist and client, like rape, is an offense that is difficult to prove, since there are usually only two people present, the therapist and the client. The therapist, usually older, is in a position of authority, with colleagues to testify to the therapist's good character. The client is usually young, insecure, and dependent. Attorneys are understandably not fond of aligning themselves with poor risks and thereby risking the loss of cases, so they are hesitant to take on such clients. In small communities, there are frequently no attorneys available to provide the client with a "day in court."

Despite the reluctance on the part of clients to report and on the part of systems to respond, there has been a recent dramatic rise in the number of sexual intimacy cases handled by ethics committees, state psychology boards, civil and criminal courts. Growing public sensitivity to the problem has led to a greater willingness to seek redress on the one hand, and limitation or punishment of the sexually acting out therapist on the other. The choice of arena for action by the consumer is still bewildering. A quick review of the possibilities, their advantages and disadvantages is in order.

PROFESSIONAL ASSOCIATION ETHICS COMMITTEES

A complaint may be filed with local, state, or national professional organization ethics committees if the psychotherapist is a member of that organization. Frequently, local organizations do not have the finances or the expertise to deal with cases of sexual intimacy. The state or national association is usually more appropriate, but the national associations meet only rarely and the process is slow.

State associations usually meet regularly and can be responsive to a complaint. However, if the psychotherapist is not a member of that professional organization, the association has no jurisdiction. Since association membership is not obligatory, and only about half of the persons practicing a profession belong to professional associations, loss of membership is frequently seen as a mild penalty.

If the therapist admits the sexual relationship occurred, often no appearance is necessary by the complainant, and the matter is dealt with "in camera." Frequently, the complainant is not informed what action was taken, and until very recently, not told that there was any action at all. This has added to the aura of protectionism and has discouraged reporting.

The ethics committee decides on the best way to rehabilitate its errant members. The choices are limited in most cases to supervision, therapy, or a mix of the two. In some instances, a list of approved senior psychologists is presented to the offending therapist, who may choose among the proffered names. Confidentiality is waived for the purpose of reporting to the ethics committee, which may require quarterly written assessments of progress. When the established time for supervision/therapy has passed, the committee reviews the reports and makes a decision whether to continue the treatment/supervision on the basis of the reports. In most instances, the decision is made that rehabilitation has taken place and no further action is taken. Records are kept on these types of cases in the majority of instances, so that if the difficulty recurs, appropriate weighting can be given to the seriousness of the evidence. Despite these precautions, and a process that sounds satisfactory in written description, many difficulties are entailed.

The primary problem is that with so few offenses reported, it is highly unlikely that two or more clients of one therapist would report, or that another instance involving the same therapist would come to the attention of an ethics committee. Also, there is no way of monitoring the therapist after the end of the imposed supervision/therapy, so if the offense does recur, it is unlikely to be discovered. Since, as mentioned above, 75 to 80 percent of the therapists act out with more than one client, the assumption must be made that repetition is likely but undiscoverable. The targeting of those therapists who will act out repeatedly is akin to the prognostication of dangerousness, and there is little statistical evidence to show that mental health professionals are able to predict successfully (Megargee, 1980).

If a therapist denies sexual involvement with a client, the situation is even more complicated. It is unusual for ethics committees to conduct investigations other than writing letters. Committee members rarely give time to personal interviews with either complainant or respondent, let alone with witnesses, and professional associations do not have the finances available to hire investigators. Recent refusal by malpractice insurance carriers to pay damages in sexual intimacy cases has caused many therapists to deny their guilt, not only in civil cases, but in ethics cases. Previously, it was not unusual for a therapist to admit involvement with a client, especially when only one patient complained. The therapist would claim that he "fell in love," and throw himself on the mercy of his colleagues, usually receiving a suspension of membership, with reinstatement contingent upon a stipulated number of months of supervision and/or therapy. With the present possibility of civil suit and lack of insurance coverage if the charge is proven, it is likely that there will be increased denials, with resultant mandatory formal hearings. Such hearings are time consuming and can utilize the lion's share of a professional association budget. Objections to such expenditures are frequently raised by members, who claim that ethics actions are not only costly, but if brought to public attention, put the profession in a poor light.

Ethics committees are aware that due process must be provided for the respondent-therapists, and usually it is necessary for associations to retain attorneys to advise them on methods of protecting their members. Generally, these attorneys insist on courtroom procedure, with a member of the ethics committee taking the role of prosecutor against the defendant's attorney. Opposing an attorney on the attorney's turf, the courtroom, is a difficult feat. Small wonder that ethics committees are not eager to handle sexual intimacy cases. Recent insistence by the American Psychological Association Ethics

Committee that hearings be run by the committee, with attorneys merely present to serve as consultants, has made their formal hearings more palatable. But the limited repertoire of solutions, the lack of funding, the legal complexities involved in the protection of due process, the possibilities of suit, the disinterest of the membership, the human tendency to deny or repress unpleasantness combine to make resolution of the problem of sexual intimacy between therapists and clients through professional associations relatively unsuccessful.

Licensing boards. Protection of the public is mandated in most states through a code regulating the professions. If a psychotherapist is licensed by the state, the state also has the power of removing or suspending that license if that therapist is a danger to the welfare and safety of the public. If the offending therapist is removed from practice and cannot further damage members of the public, is this not the solution to the problem?

Licensure for mental health professionals other than psychiatrists (who are licensed as physicians) is a recent phenomenon, commensurate with the growth of the various mental health professions. Psychologists are now licensed in all 50 states, social work in about 31 as of this writing. Fewer states recognize by licensure the more nebulous designation of marriage and family counselors. Throughout the history of state licensure of the professions, from its 1639 inception in Virginia, boards made up of members of the professions have administered the licensure laws (Council of State Governments, 1980). These boards have traditionally received and investigated consumer complaints, conducted hearings and applied disciplinary measures. However, there is a whole range of decision-making authority among the various states, from complete autonomy (26 states) to mere advisory function (2 states). In about half of the states, there are some limitations placed on professionals' controls over their own licensees, usually through review by a central agency. This agency may limit professionals' functions through control of budgets, personnel, or other administrative functions. Over the past 20 years there has been a trend toward such centralization.

How does the structure of the board affect the licensure and disciplinary process in reference to sexual intimacy between clients and therapists? In all states a complaint is necessary to start the disciplinary process. A complaint may be filed by the individual involved sexually with the therapist, by a professional association, or by any member of the public. The complaint is filed with the board that issues the license: medical board if a psychiatrist is involved; psychology board or a supraordinate board if certain professions have been combined for administrative purposes (in California, psychiatry and psychology are under the Board of Medical Quality Assurance, while marriage and family counselors, licensed clinical social workers and licensed educational psychologists are under the Board of Behavioral Science Examiners).

In most states, the office of the attorney general has responsibility for determining if the case is sufficiently strong to file; in other states, the licensing board itself may make that determination. In contrast to professional assocation ethics committees, the deputy attorneys general or licensing boards may utilize investigators, many of whom have been trained in law enforcement functions. These investigators interview complainants and respondants, and when no witnesses are available, do undercover work to test the therapists' behavior with female patients. If the decision is made that the case is not sufficient for court presentation, the complaint is tabled. If prosecution does go forward, it may take from one to five years or even longer to prepare the case and move it through crowded court calendars.

What is the relationship between licensing boards and professional organizations? There is a wide diversity of relationships, and these affect the handling of the cases of sexual intimacy. For example, in states where the professional association leaders sit on licensing boards in judgement of their peers, there is no duplication of function between ethics committees and licensing board. Where the licensing functions are separate, and the board is made up of predominantly public members, distrust of the professional association may exist, with the view that professional associations are guild oriented and reluctant to discipline their membership, even when guilty. In such cases, states frequently prefer to do their own investigations and disciplinary actions and duplication may result. One state board executive has described the optimal relationship between the board and the professional association as "healthy tension" (Levy, 1981) that maintains the focus on the welfare of the public. This does not address the question of duplication, however. Whatever the model, cooperation is important. A resistant and hostile board and an unwilling legal support system impedes progress in dealing with the problem of client/therapist sexual relations. An involved professional organization that is cooperative with the licensing board can be helpful in providing consultation and training for the investigators and the attorneys general. Sensitivity to the vulnerabilities of complainants and an understanding of the problem of sexual intimacy between clients and therapists on the part of both groups can help make the legal process less traumatic.

Another area where cooperation is necessary between professional organization and licensing board is the penalty phase. When a therapist is found guilty of sexual misconduct with a patient and the license is suspended or revoked, most state codes contain a provision for reinstatement. Usually, the licensee may reapply after a period of time, usually a year, when proof of rehabilitation is required. Such proof usually consists of testimony by supervisors and/or therapists that the offender has completed the prescribed rehabilitative process. The supervisors/psychotherapists may be required to appear personally at a hearing for restoration of license, and to testify as to the efficacy of their treatment of the offender. In most instances, they indicate that they have been successful and that the individual will not act out again. A recent study has shown that consultants to therapists who become sexually involved with patients tend not to see them as negatively as those who have worked with the patients involved (Holroyd & Bouhoutsos, 1984). We also know that 75 to 80 percent of therapists who act out do so with more than one person. What we do *not* know is if that percentage still obtains after treatment/supervision, nor if the judgment of those professionals who supervise/treat is accurate. Findings from other areas of sexual offenses show very low "cure" rates (Shah, 1980) so we must recognize the high risk. Research is needed in this area. If supervision and therapy are the only interventions utilized, if relicensure is almost routine, then the public is not being protected against those therapists who will act out again. The difficulties of doing research in this area are immediately apparent. The percentages of psychotherapists found guilty and placed in treatment is miniscule in comparison to the number who become sexually involved with patients. Even in those instances where they are apprehended, most of the information about their propensity for such behavior is privileged, unless the case was handled in open court. Since prior history is crucial to estimate future behavior, this is indeed a public policy dilemma.

Ethics committees and licensing boards face a similar dilemma: the protection of the public versus the right of the individual to earn a living. When experts testify that the therapist is no longer a danger, it is likely that they will be believed if there is no evidence to the contrary. And as of this writing, there is little evidence available.

Several interim measures are possible: (1) A requirement by the licensing board that there be an independent evaluation of the treatment record and the prior history of the individual requesting relicensure, with subsequent report to the board on the advisability of relicensure. (2) The actual placement of the burden of proof on the applicant for relicensure to show why the applicant should be reinstated rather than on the board to show why they should not reinstate. (3) Education of the public about the inadvisability of allowing acting-out therapists to continue practice unsupervised and without accountability. (4) Recognition by insurance companies that they must share responsibility since they pay for treatment that includes sexual intimacy with therapists in 78 percent of such cases (Bouhoutsos et al., 1983), and therefore they should support research to assist in diagnosing potential abusers and/or recidivists. Insurance companies pay to have the damage in the initial therapy corrected through subsequent therapy, raising premiums and/or cutting mental health coverage for the public to control costs.

Civil and criminal courts. Since the early 1970s several successful cases have been filed against therapists alleging damage as a result of sexually intimate relations, or against the institutions employing them. The first, a New York suit against a popular author-psychiatrist, was the subject of a book (Freeman & Roy, 1976), and later, a motion picture for television. In 1979, a 26-year-old woman was granted 4.5 million dollars in a jury trial in which she sued her psychiatrist. She later settled for 2.5 million to avoid a long appeals process, and has spent much of the monies to fund self-help support groups for women victims of therapists. In the same year, another psychiatrist settled for $200,000, when he was found guilty of having intercourse with a patient under threat of cutting off her prescription drugs and hospitalizing her. He also counselled the plaintiff how to succesfully commit suicide after she unsuccessfully attempted it. Such cases are heard in open court, with press coverage and full disclosure of all details in the lives of both parties to the suit. This process can be stressful and debilitating to a client who has already been damaged in the relationship with the therapist. But it can also provide her with impetus to heal once the facts are no longer her secret burden.

A recent and somewhat troubling development in civil suits has been the out of court settlement, which, while it reduces the stress on the client, provides a loophole for the offending therapists to continue the same behavior with other patients. Some states limit the amount of money that can be paid without automatic notification of the licensing board. In California $30,000 is the most that can be paid to buy the silence of the client. Frequently, women who have been sexually involved with a therapist, who are not working, and who have been divorced by their husbands as a result of the affair with the therapist, are willing to settle out of court. In such instances, the client agrees not to reveal the details of the incident or the settlement nor to file a complaint with a professional association ethics committee or licensing board. The court may be a party to the settlement, with stipulation that abridgement of the agreement will result in contempt of court charges. Fortunately, this particular type of agreement is now being considered by the courts in California, and the current unofficial opinion of several government attorneys is that such contempt charges are illegal. The case is still pending on appeal. The need for action in other states against such out of court settlements is clear.

Attorneys working at all levels of government are charged with filing charges against psychotherapists who are a threat to the safety or welfare of public. In an instance of sexual intimacy with a client, the laws of the state determine the nature of the charges and the severity of the sentence. It has been possible to charge a psychotherapist with sexual abuse, call expert witnesses, and show that such sexual behavior has been a threat to the client's safety or welfare. Proving that the effects of sexual intimacy between therapist and client are harmful has been difficult until the recent publication of research data supporting such findings (Bouhoutsos et al., 1983). The enactment of legislation that states simply that sexual intimacy between therapist and client is illegal obviates the need for experts and requires only the determination of guilt. Some 15 states have enacted such legislation, which simplifies the process. Under Minnesota Criminal Code (#609.231, 1982), such sexual activity is punishable by a maximum fine of $1000, and/or imprisonment of one year. In Arizona, a recent criminal court action against an osteopathic psychiatrist for sexual abuse of eight or nine women resulted in a conviction on two counts, each count carrying a sentence of two-and-one-half years, to be served consecutively. Because of the severity of such sentences, proof of the sexual act is crucial, and there is careful scrutiny of the complainants and witnesses. Frequently, there are attempts to discredit the witnesses through discussion of previous sexual history, mental instability, mental hospitalizations, and so forth.

A bill recently introduced in the California Senate would have made sexual intimacy between therapist and patients a felony, and would have defined it as rape. Resistance came not from the professions, as might be expected, but from the public. Objection was raised that the element of force was absent, and that the definition of rape should not be broadened to include sexual intimacy with clients, which was viewed as having "voluntary" elements on the part of those clients. Proponents argued that clients involved in transference with therapists do not have the ability to make decisions to leave treatment to avoid sexual intimacy, and that the betrayal of trust constitutes rape. Others compared sexual intimacy between clients and therapists to incest, since the therapist acts *in loco parentis*. The bill was amended to drop the rape designation and to include provisions similar to a 1982 Minnesota "Vulnerable Adults" act. This law contains a controversial provision that mandates the reporting of sexual intimacy between therapist and patient by the subsequent therapist. This second therapist is thus placed in an ethical bind. Ethics codes, and frequently state business and professions codes, prohibit betrayal of confidences; this law would require the reporting of the offending therapist, whether or not the patient gives permission. The psychology board of Minnesota has chosen to prioritize confidentiality below that of sexual abuse (Minnesota Board of Psychology, 1983). Arguments within the mental health professions center on the erosion of confidentiality that has already taken place because of legal child abuse mandatory report requirements, and in some states, the necessity of notifying the authorities when there is danger to the client or others.

A requirement to report a previous therapist over the objections of a client might severely damage the relationship, especially when the previous therapeutic relationship was negative and the established trust was impugned. There are those who claim that it is therapeutic for the damaged client to confront the previous therapist and/or take action to report such behavior. But what about the client's right *not* to do so, however therapeutic we might think it is for her? There are some interesting constitutional issues involved here.

An alternative to mandatory reporting by the subsequent therapist is suggested by A. Stone (1983), who proposed the use of a consultant to allow the present therapist to continue the relationship without discussing the legal or ethical steps that are mandated. The consultant meets with the client around the legal issues and around advocacy, and may also notify the offending therapist that consultation has taken place, or issue a warning about recurrence. Such consultation appears unwieldy and time consuming. It would necessitate either volunteer services or undue financial drain on clients, and would create a nerve-wracking and threatening obligation for the consultant in situations where the possible penalties can be so severe.

Another concern about the Vulnerable Adults Act is the definition of psychotherapy clients as "vulnerable." Since 92 percent of the clients involved in sexual intimacy with therapists are women (Bouhoutsos et al., 1983), this designation may add to the depiction of women as weaker, vulnerable, and needing protection, thus perpetuating a stereotype. Women would also sustain the most damage from the mandatory reporting requirement, since they are already suffering an erosion of trust through their betrayal by a previous therapist. Perhaps the betrayal of confidentiality of a known individual should also outweigh the possibility of harm to an unknown member of the public, who might refuse the advances of a therapist anyway (Koocher, 1983). But the most salient objection is the possible harm to the individual client who would have to deal with the results of mandatory reporting. Many of these women are fragile, and cannot withstand confrontation by the previous therapist, questioning by investigators, and the rigors of a trial. Some discretionary power is necessary for subsequent therapists. They are in the best position to assess the strength of their clients and to judge whether the mandatory reporting process might endanger their emotional or mental health. Clinical judgement should determine the choice. This represents a less than satisfactory solution, but mandatory reporting, with exceptions for clients judged at risk would at least impress upon mental health professionals the negative sequellae of sexual acting out with clients.

PREVENTION

Preferable to containment or rehabilitation is prevention. Current public attention brought to the problem has been helpful in obtaining legislative and legal cooperation. It has also served to alert potential or present clients of psychotherapists about the illegal and unethical nature of sexual activity with clients on the part of therapists. Only 50 percent of those clients involved in such relationships are aware of these facts (Bouhoutsos et al., 1983). Patients' rights personnel in California have been given in-service training by the Task Force to assist them in recognizing the signs of such abuse. Instruction booklets to patients have been amended to inform patients that sexual abuse by caretakers or fellow patients is illegal and unethical and should be reported. Distribution of Ethics Codes and Standards for Providers of mental health services by therapists in private practice might also serve to alert consumers as to what is legal and ethical and what possibilities of redress are available. Usually, the only time the public is given a copy of the ethics code of a profession is *after* a complaint is filed. Informing consumers involves minimal effort and little expenditure.

A frequently advanced hypothesis for client-therapists sexual involvement is poor training of the therapist. An examination of the standard texts for the teaching of psychotherapy reveals that no mention is made of sexual arousal on the part of the neophyte therapist, nor are instructions given on how to deal with it should it occur. This deficiency may be a result of the lack of research data and of our reluctance to look into this taboo area. However, such research is now underway (Keith-Spiegel & Pope, 1984). The extensive sexual involvements between faculty and students in mental health services (Pope, Levenson & Schover, 1979) speak to the necessity for both preventive and remedial intervention in educational institutions. Modeling of this type cannot help but effect future professional behavior. Reluctance on the part of universities to deal with the problem suggests that the possibility of modifying such behavior through university or professional school structures is somewhat limited. Nonetheless, this is an area of continuing concern to those professionals desirous of impacting patient-therapist sexual behavior.

With better modeling in mental health training programs, agencies sensitized to selection and in-service training of personnel, an educated public aware of the negative effects of sexual intimacy between clients and therapists, and legal systems responsive to complaints, many of the current problems of containment and prevention could be ameliorated. Rehabilitation of those therapists who have already been so involved, or assistance to those who are sufficiently disturbed to act out in the future continues to be problematic. Programs for impaired mental health professionals, begun in medicine, now have been established in psychology and social work. The goal is to provide assistance to those professionals who are experiencing difficulties in their own lives, which could lead them to act out with clients. Continuing education of mental health professionals, with periodic relicensure has been suggested. The current open admission by the mental health professions that the problem of sexual intimacy between psychotherapists and clients exists is a positive development. Prevention of the problem requires policy changes in many areas of the mental health system. Women in mental health can be instrumental in achieving such changes.

REFERENCES

American Psychological Association. (1975). Report of the task force on sex bias and sex-role stereotyping in psychotherapeutic practice. *American Psychologist, 30,* 1169-1175.

Belote, B. (1974).*Sexual intimacy between female clients and male psychotherapists: Male sabotage.* Doctoral dissertation, California School of Professional Psychology, Los Angeles.

Bouhoutsos, J., Holroyd, J., Lerman, H., Forer, B., & Greenberg, M. (1983). Sexual intimacy between psychotherapists and patients. *Professional Psychology: Research and Practice, 14,*(2), 185-196.

Butler, S. E. (1975). *Sexual contact between therapists and their patients.* Dissertation, California School of Professional Psychology, Los Angeles.

Butler, S., & Zelen, S. (1977). Sexual intimacies between psychotherapists and their patients. *Psychotherapy: Theory, Research and Practice, 139,* 143-144.

Council of State Government. (1980). *Occupational licensing: Centralizing state licensure functions,* (pp. 1-29). Council of State Governments, Iron Work Pike, Lexington, KY.

D'Addario, L. (1977). *Sexual relationship between female clients and male therapists.* Dissertation, California School of Professional Psychology, San Diego.

Dahlerg, C. C. (1977). Sexual contact between patient and therapist. *Contemporary Psychoanalysis, 6,* 107-124.

Edelwich, J. & Brodsky, A. (1982). *Sexual dilemmas for the helping professional* (pp. 1-232). New York: Brunner/Mazel.

Feldman-Summers, J. & Jones, G. (1984). *Psychological impacts of sexual contact between therapists or other health care practitioners and their clients.* Manuscript submitted for publication.

Forer, B. (1968). Personal communication.

Forer, B. (1969). The taboo against touching in psychotherapy. *Psychotherapy: Theory, Research and Practice, 6*(4), 229-231.

Freeman, L., & Roy, J. (1976). *Betrayal.* New York: Stein & Day.

Gechtman, L., Pope, K., & Bouhoutsos, J. *Sexual intimacy between social workers and clients.* Manuscript in preparation.

Hall, J., & Hare-Mustin, R. T. (1983). Sanctions and the diversity of ethical complaints against psychologists. *American Psychologist, 38,*(6), 714-729.

Holroyd, J. (1983). Erotic contact as an instance of sex-biased therapy. In Murray, J. & Abrahamson, P. (Eds.), *Handbook of bias in psychotherapy.*

Holroyd, J. & Bouhoutsos, J. (1984). *Sources of bias in reporting effects of sexual contact with patients.* Manuscript submitted for publication.

Holroyd, J. C., & Brodsky, A. M. (1977). Psychologists' attitudes and practices regarding erotic and nonerotic contact with patients. *American Psychologist, 32,* 843-849.

Kardener, S., Fuller, M., & Mensh, I. (1973). A survey of physicians' attitudes and practices regarding erotic and nonerotic contact with patients. *American Journal of Psychiatry, 130,* 1077-1081.

Keith-Spiegel (1979). *Sex with clients: Ten reasons why it is a very stupid thing to do.* Paper presented at the convention of the American Psychological Association, New York, September.

Keith-Spiegel, K., & Pope, K. (1984). Manuscript in preparation.

Koocher, J. (1983). Personal communication.

Levy, H. (1981). Personal communication.

McCartney, J. (1966). Overt transference. *Journal of Sex Research, 2,* 227-237.

Megargee, E. (1980). Methodological problems in the prediction of violence. In Hay, Roberts, Solway, (Eds.), *Violence and the Violent Individual,* (pp. 179-191). New York: S. P. Medical & Scientific Books.

Minnesota. (1980). *Laws of Minnesota for 1980.* Chap. 542-HF No. 1942. 626.557, 712-718.

Minnesota (1982). Criminal Code 609.231.

Pope, K. S., & Bouhoutsos, J. (1984). *Sexual intimacy between marriage and family therapists and clients.* Manuscript in preparation.

Pope, K. S., Levenson, H. & Schover, L. R. (1979). Sexual intimacy in psychology training: Results and implications of a national survey. *American Psychologist. 34,* 682-689.

Riskin, L. (1979). Sexual relations between psychotherapists and their patients: Toward research or restraint. *California Law Review, 67,* 1000-1027.

Russo, N. Oledo, E., Stapp, J. & Fulcher, R. (1981). Women and minorities in psychology. *American Psychologist, 36*(11), 1315-1163.

Shah, S. A. (1980). Dangerousness: Conceptual, prediction and public policy issues. In Hays, R. & Solway (Eds.), *Violence and the violent individual* (pp. 151-178). New York: S. P. Medical & Scientific Books.

Shepard, M. (1971). *The love treatment: Sexual intimacy between patients and psychotherapists.* New York: Wyden.

Siegel, S. (1983). Personal communication.

Smith, S. (1981). *Analytic explorations of therapists involved with patients.* Paper delivered at California State Psychological Association, San Diego, February.

Stone, A. (1983). Commentary. *American Journal of Psychiatry, 140*(2).

Stone, A. (1976). The legal implications of sexual activity between psychiatrist and patient. *American Journal of Psychiatry, 133,* 1138-1141.

Stone, L. G. (1980). *A study of the relationships among anxious attachment ego functioning, and female patients' vulnerability to sexual involvement with their male psychotherapists.* Unpublished doctoral dissertation. California School of Professional Psychology, Los Angeles.

Stone, M. H. (1976). Boundary violations between therapist and patient. *Psychiatric Annals, 6*(12), 670-682.

Wright, R. W. (1981). Psychologists and professional liability (malpractice) insurance: A retrospective review. *American Psychologist, 36,* 1485-1493.

12

WOMEN AND WORK:
IMPLICATIONS FOR MENTAL HEALTH

Esther Sales
Irene Hanson Frieze

The dramatic increase in women's labor force participation has been one of the most noted social trends in recent decades. This change from the traditional pattern is most pronounced in the increasing number of women continuing their employment after childbirth (Masnick & Bane, 1980). More women are choosing to retain their jobs after becoming mothers, or are reentering the labor force while their children are still young. Women are also employed outside the home for longer periods of their lives because they are marrying later, having fewer children, and experiencing divorce and widowhood for longer periods of their adult lives (Mott, 1982; O'Rand & Henretta, 1982). In general, these social trends can be seen as reducing women's involvement in family roles, while enhancing their occupational involvement. By the late 1970s, women spent an average of 22.9 years in the labor force (Pifer, 1979).

In view of these shifting patterns, it becomes increasingly important to understand the impact of paid employment on women's lives. Some writers have suggested that women's employment during the early years of childrearing may increase stress by adding to their role demands (Bernard, 1974; Hoffman & Nye, 1974). If this is true, current social trends could result in more mental health problems and breakdown for women in the future. On the other hand, if work is a central contributor to adult adjustment, participation in the labor force may be health-enhancing for women.

This issue also has crucial implications for the planning of mental health services. Women have long been heavy users of such services (Guttentag, Salasin & Bell, 1980; Veroff, Kulka, & Douvan, 1981). In part, this may be attributed to their greater help-seeking tendencies, but it also reflects the greater psychological distress they report on a variety of measures (Dohrenwend & Dohrenwend, 1976; Goldman

& David, 1980; Gove & Tudor, 1973; Pearlin,1975; Rice & Cugliani, 1980; Veroff et al., 1981). If labor force participation affects a woman's mental health, we would expect to see changes in the demands for mental health services due to increasing female employment.

Over the last decade, a number of investigators have examined the relationship between employment and women's well-being. In general, no evidence has been found of any negative associations between employment and women's physical or mental health. Furthermore, women have shown no increase in either physical or mental health symptomatology in recent years, despite their increasing work involvement (Kessler & McCrae, 1981; Rice & Cugliani, 1980). Thus, women's increasing labor force involvement probably will not lead to greater physical or mental health problems for them in the future.

Many studies, in fact, report a modest *positive* association between work and both physical and mental health indicators (Baruch, Barnett, & Rivers, 1983; Brown, Bhrolchain, & Harris, 1975; Gove & Geerken, 1977; Wheeler, Lee, & Lee, 1983). However, other investigators have found no direct relationship between employment and well-being (Iglehart, 1978; Pearlin, 1975; Veroff et al., 1981; Woods & Hulka, 1979). These discrepant findings suggest that the impact of work must be examined in relation to other factors in a woman's life. Fortunately, recent research has increased our understanding of some of the central factors affecting the impact of employment, including a woman's personal need priorities, her family status and stage in life, and her social class background.

CENTRAL FACTORS AFFECTING
THE IMPACT OF EMPLOYMENT

PERSONAL FACTORS IN THE MEANING OF WORK FOR WOMEN

Personality differences among women affect their occupational involvement in many ways. Based on their different needs and motivations, women make many choices regarding their adult lives. Some women, for example, choose to acquire more education, prepare for high status occupations, delay marriage and childrearing, and maintain their labor market involvement through early parenthood and more continuously throughout their lifespans. Others do not.

Nieva and Gutek (1981) have outlined a model of career choice for women that differs somewhat from the typical pattern for men.

To start, girls, like boys, make initial decisions about job goals. These decisions are based on societal stereotypes about the types of occupations appropriate for females or males (Eccles & Hoffman, in press). Role models and media influences are also important. Frieze, Bailey, Mamula, and Moss (1983) have suggested that girls first narrow their range of possible occupational choices on the basis of such social factors and then make more specific choices by matching their own motives and values to their perceptions of the demands of specific jobs. Another choice point occurs for a woman at some point after she has made her initial choice of a job. She will have to decide whether she will actually continue to work in this field throughout her life, or work only until she marries or has children.

How do empirical data support this model? Looking first at the factors that detemine initial career choice, there is evidence that both extrinsic and intrinsic motives are important in occupational selection. In many cases females choose occupations much as males do. Astin (1978) reports that both female and male college students are concerned with selecting a field in which there are many job openings. However, there are some differences found between men and women in job choices. For example, a large survey study found that adolescent females saw helping others as relatively more important, while males rated having a high income, leadership, and leisure time as more important (Tittle, 1981). Similar data have been reported for college students (Norris, Katz, & Chapman, 1978). For both sexes, then, such extrinsic factors as income, security, and status are the most important aspects of job choice.

Another way of understanding the possible reasons for job selection is to identify the types of motives that jobs may satisfy (Herzberg, Mausner & Snyderman, 1959). Motivation researchers have suggested that such needs can be classified into three basic groups; the desire (1) for affiliation, (2) for achievement, and (3) for power (Atkinson, 1964). Affiliation is defined as a need to be with someone else and to enjoy mutual friendship. Achievement motivation involves wanting to perform well or to do better than others. Power is the desire to have an impact on others or make an impression on them. Power motivation can be expressed in either of two ways: (1) personal power motivation, which is directed toward building reputation or glory for oneself, or (2) social power motivation, which is expressed by using one's talents to help others, and in so doing to have an impact on their lives (McClelland & Steele, 1972). Thus, job satisfaction can come either from the intrinsic aspects of the work itself that may satisfy one or more of these basic motives, from extrinsic working conditions, or from the change in self-image resulting from the job's status (Rabinowitz & Hall, 1977). A major motivational need met by jobs is the need to achieve and experience "success." For men, success has traditionally been seen as synonomous with career attainment. Because of women's lesser career involvement, it had been falsely assumed that they did not experience achievement needs (Frieze, Parsons, Johnson, Ruble, & Zellman, 1978). Socialization of girls in our society has typically placed less emphasis on competitive achievement and on having a good (i.e., successful and money-making) job. Some research has even suggested that women may fear societal rejection, which may be associated with high career attainment (Condry & Dyer, 1976; Horner, 1972; Tressemer, 1976). Others have argued that women have always had achievement needs; however, because of social pressure and the internalization of socialized values, women have expressed their achievement motives through being good homemakers or through other "feminine" activities (Stein & Bailey, 1973). We also know now that although some women fear success, so do many men (Tressemer, 1976). Until recently, however, women's achievement concerns have often been diverted away from career success.

As job opportunities increase and societal attitudes toward women's employment become more accepting, we can assume that women will increasingly find that paid employment satisfies their achievement needs. However, some women's achievement needs may still differ from the traditional competitive form, being expressed instead through vicarious achievement, relational achievement, or deriving intrinsic satisfactions from the task (Lipman-Blumen & Leavitt, 1976). Parsons and Goff (1980) have also suggested that many women want jobs that satisfy both affiliative and achievement needs.

Motivational differences between women and men may be a major factor in the types of jobs each sex commonly chooses. Female-dominated jobs such as nursing, teaching, social work, librarianship, or secretarial work appear to be selected by those women who place high importance on affiliative or helping needs (Angrist & Almquist, 1975). Such jobs are often low paying and allow little opportunity for promotion or for the expression of personal power or achievement needs (as traditionally defined). However, they may permit the expression of affiliative or social power needs (Oppenheimer, 1975). Since many of these "female" fields involve giving advice or helping others, these jobs provide a mechanism for women to satisfy social power needs (Winter, 1973). In addiiton, doing these jobs well may generate feelings of mastery that allow for the satisfaction of certain types of achievement motivation. Finally, female fields often offer flexible or nontraditional work schedules that permit women to better juggle work and family responsibilities.

The reasons for selecting male-dominated jobs are similar for both sexes. O'Farrell (1982) reports that women in traditionally male blue-collar jobs appear to be motivated by money as well as by interest in the work, challenge, skill, and security. Similarly, Greenfeld, Greiner, and Wood (1980) found that women in male occupations indicated a greater tendency than other women to define success as recognition from others, being an authority, and having a high salary. Such definitions of success have more typically been associated with men (Parsons & Goff, 1980). In addition, Greenfeld et al. (1980) report that women in male-dominated fields also find satisfaction of expressive affiliative needs. Thus it appears that, for some women, choosing to work in a traditionally male field may allow for the satisfaction of achievement, affiliation, and power needs, as well as extrinsic needs such as money.

As mentioned earlier, Nieva and Gutek suggest that once they married, and especially after the birth of children, women could choose to be full-time homemakers. Like other female occupations, this job is most likely to satisfy the affiliative, nurturant, or social power needs of women with traditional values and personalities (Greenglass & Devins, 1982; Hoffman & Fidell, 1979). Being a full-time homemaker can be a satisfying choice for some mothers. Baruch et al. (1983) found that married full-time homemakers with children expressed more pleasure with their lives than did any other group of women. And Veroff et al. (1981) found that homemakers had fewer worries and more life satisfaction than other women.

For most women, however, the homemaker role is insufficient for need satisfaction. Baruch et al. (1983) suggest that women who have a high need for mastery will not find this need satisfied in their own homes. And Pearlin (1975) found that women who were disenchanted with homemaking were quite high in depression. More recently, the dissatisfied homemakers in Verbrugge's (1982) study showed the highest symptoms of physical and mental problems and drug use of all women in her sample. Thus, homemakers who find this role unsatisfying are at high risk of negative mental health consequences.

All this suggests that a key element in the mental health of a woman may be found in her ability to *choose* roles that best mesh with her personal needs (Filer, 1983; Kessler & McCrae, 1981). Possibly because many women have chosen to take jobs outside the home, they are more likely to emphasize that they are working because of the intrinsic interest they have in their jobs, while men are more concerned with high pay and economic stability (Astin, 1978; Burke, 1966; Goldber & Shiflett, 1981; Turner, 1964). And employed women generally like their jobs more than men do (Verbrugge, 1982). Overall, the ability of women to choose work that satisfies their personal needs may add to its meaning. If employment is freely selected by women, one would expect the work role to satisfy personal needs. If, in contrast, employment is sought out of economic necessity, or if a woman has few job options, her work may not satisfy as many needs. Most occupations provide some opportunities for social exchange that may satisfy affiliative motives and the need to do things well. They also provide a source of income that may give the woman enhanced power within the family (Gillespie, 1971). Employment may also provide a basis for enhanced self-esteem that can serve as a buffer when a woman experiences difficult life events (Brown et al., 1975).

FAMILY CIRCUMSTANCES

While a woman's personal motives provide a base for her job choices, her life status is a crucial element in her reaction to employment. Childless, unmarried women are able to be highly involved in their jobs and show clear mental health benefits from employment. Generally, married women who work outside the home are in better psychological health than are married homemakers (Birnbaum, 1975; Gove & Geerken, 1977; Verbrugge, 1982). However, both Pearlin (1975) and Radloff (1975) found that the positive relationship between work and health holds only when women's family and work roles are well-integrated and when their marriages are satisfying. In general, work appears to be associated with positive health for married women as long as they are in good marriages.

For most women, employment and childbearing are closely inter-twined (Gould & Henretta, 1982). For traditional women, this has meant that employment decisions are adjusted according to childrearing demands. In contrast, highly career-oriented women's decisions about timing and numbers of children were likely to be influenced by the demands of their jobs. Although recent evidence suggests that the direct association between fertility and work patterns is diminishing (because more women maintain their work involvement after childbirth and more couples espouse a two-child norm regardless of the wife's work aspiration (Mott, 1982) the pervasive impact of children on women's lives remains.

In general, mental health problems seem most acute among mothers of preschool children (Brown et al., 1975; Gove & Geerken, 1977; Pearlin, 1975; Radloff, 1975). Chapter 7 in this volume documents the particular difficulties of low-income mothers, where rates of depression can exceed 40 percent for women with preschool children who are heads of households (Belle, 1980; Brown et al., 1975). It is clear that early motherhood is a vulnerable period in women's lives.

Since the early childrearing period is particularly difficult for women, we need to pay close attention to the impact of work during this stage. Currently, the majority of women still choose to remain home with their preschool children. However, it is this group of women who are now increasing their labor force participation in record numbers, and may be most vulnerable to mental health problems generated by employment. At present, the data relating work during early motherhood to mental health remain equivocal. Some have found that employed mothers are in somewhat better mental health than those not employed (Brown et al., 1975; Wheeler et al., 1983). The Brown et al. study (1975) is particularly relevant in finding lower depression for employed working class mothers of preschool children, compared to homemaker mothers. Since this group of women generally has very high stress, the beneficial effects of employment are especially noteworthy. However, other researchers have found no differences in the well-being of employed mothers and homemakers (Barnett, 1982; Woods & Hulka, 1979).

Combining outside employment with motherhood may be beneficial because it allows women to satisfy diverse needs. Radloff (1975), for example, states that employed mothers may show less depression because they have dual sources of satisfaction. Her arguments are supported by Stewart and Salt's (1981) finding that employed mothers showed fewer symptoms of stress than their nonemployed counterparts. They suggest that the ability to obtain rewards in one role acts as a buffer to the problems and frustrations of other roles. Baruch et al. (1983) used a similar interpretation of their finding that women with the most roles had the highest overall scores on indicators of mental health. Brown et al. (1975) argue that employment can create a psychological buffer for women who have problems in other areas of their lives. And Gove and Geerken (1977) suggest that outside work diminishes the loneliness and burdens felt by mothers, thereby insulating them from emotional difficulties.

The direct effect of work on women in the early years of parenting is complicated by other factors that affect women's mental health during this period. In fact, Woods & Hulka (1979) suggest that family pressures are much more important than employment in determining the health of mothers. When family stresses are high—because women have more young children, more problematic living conditions, less social support from husbands, or because other circumstances exist that demand additional coping resources—a high potential exists for psychological breakdown (Belle, 1980; Brown et al., 1975; Warren, 1976).

In view of the psychological demands of childrearing, it is not surprising that women's psychological distress seems to decrease as they (and their children) get older. Despite the popular belief that women are vulnerable to depression after their children leave home or during menopause, women generally show decreased symptoms once their children are grown (Campbell, Converse, & Rodgers, 1976). Consistently, mothers report higher life satisfaction in the postparental period (Campbell et al., 1976; Gove & Geerken, 1977; Pearlin, 1975; Radloff, 1975; Veroff et al., 1981; Wheeler et al., 1983). Once the demands of childrearing diminish, the impact of work on women in the later years of their lives is more uniformly positive. At midlife, employed women have fewer psychological problems than those who remain home-centered (Lowenthal, Thurnher & Chiriboga, 1975), are happier (Rose, 1965), have higher self-esteem (Birnhaum, 1975), and fewer marital conflicts (Dizzard, 1968). And in old age, work-centered mothers report higher life satisfaction and activity than more traditional home-centered women (Maas & Kuypers, 1974).

SOCIAL CLASS

In addition to a woman's personal needs and her family circumstances, the socioeconomic status in which she was raised and in which she currently lives creates another set of conditions affecting her response to employment. As we have seen in Chapter 7 (Belle's chapter), social class exerts a powerful influence on women's lives in many ways. Therefore, it should not be surprising that it also has strong impact on a woman's work experiences. A woman's class background influences her educational training, the timing and form of her marriage and parenting roles, the type of available work options, the reasons for working, and the availability of domestic and child care help. Until recently, most research has focused on the employment experiences of educated middle-class women, a group more accessible (and perhaps of greater interest) to academic researchers. For highly educated women, work has clear mental health benefits (Birnbaum, 1975; Campbell et al., 1976; Ginzberg, 1966; Hoffman & Nye, 1974; Wheeler et al., 1983). Educated, employed women have more life satisfaction, higher self-esteem, and fewer mental health symptoms than nonworking educated women. These findings are not surprising, since these women would be most motivated toward careers. Furthermore, highly educated women often structure their lives in ways that facilitate employment. They spend more years obtaining skills that can lead to more challenging and better paying jobs, delay marriage and childbearing, and have fewer children. They are also more likely to have companionate marriages with husbands who are supportive of their occupational roles. And, because of their greater economic security, they can afford to drop out of the labor force when their role demands become too high, or pay for more child care and domestic help (Hoffman & Nye, 1974; Mott, 1982).

For working-class women, employment involves fewer benefits and greater costs. Their jobs are less desirable and less lucrative, and at the same time they perform more tasks in the home. Despite these adverse conditons, the limited data available suggest the same positive relationship between employment and mental health. That is, working-class women who are employed show mental health patterns that echo, albeit with diminished intensity, those found in middle-class women. Specifically, they report less symptomatology and lower use of mental health services than their nonworking counterparts (Belle, 1980; Brown et al., 1975; Wheeler et al., 1983). We can conclude, therefore, that employed women are in better mental health than those who remain in their homes, regardless of social class background.

LIMITATIONS OF CURRENT RESEARCH

The above discussion of research findings regarding work and mental health should be viewed as somewhat speculative. While it is based on empirical knowledge, it is, nevertheless, limited by three crucial problems in interpretation.

The first problem involves the variety of measures currently used as indicators of physical and mental health. Some investigators (such as Kessler & McCrae, 1981; Verbrugge, 1982, 1983; Waldron, Herold, Dunn, & Staum, 1982; Woods & Hulka, 1979) focus on women's physical or psychological symptoms, or their actual use of medications and health care sevices. Other investigators (such as Baruch et al., 1983; Wheeler et al., 1983), using a definition of mental health that goes beyond the absence of health symptoms or service use, measure positive indicators of well-being. Such measures can focus on the pleasures and satisfactions reported by women, or they can examine other indicators of good adult adjustment, such as feelings of self-esteem or competence. Any of these measures can be based on women's self-reports, on medical records, or on the assessments of professionals.

While it is useful to use a variety of indicators to measure a concept as complex as mental health, problems arise when one observes differences in the findings from various studies. Such inconsistencies could be due to differences in the measures of mental health employed. For this presentation we have drawn on both physical and mental health data, in the belief that many physical symptoms result from psychological factors. But it is possible that women's employment may have differential impact on varied aspects of physical or mental health. For example, Verbrugge (1983) suggests that employed women may delay their initial seeking of health care services, but may have more in-hospital or at-home days (possibly because of this delay). Furthermore, Baruch et al. (1983) found that employment related to women's feelings of mastery, but not to her postive feelings about life. It is possible that employment may be positively related to some aspects of well-being, be unrelated to others, and be negatively related to still other measures. Thus, employed women may feel better about their competence and self-worth, but may be no happier or healthier than other women, and may also have greater stress because of additonal role demands.

A second problem relates to the influence on employment of other factors in a women's life. Early studies of the impact of work did not consider variations due to age, economic status, or childrearing stage. Recent studies have used more sophisticated strategies to isolate the contribution of employment, but few studies control for all relevant factors simultaneously. For example, we cannot conclude that the mental health advantage of educated working women derives from their jobs or from other positive life circumstances such as smaller family size, more income that can be used to hire child care and domestic help, or more supportive husbands. As another example, the finding that married nonemployed women show more health symptoms that those with jobs may be due to the older average age of married homemakers. Thus, before we conclude that work is beneficial for certain groups of women, we must control for other variables (such as age or economic status) that may be the actual source of these benefits.

This discussion now brings us to the third, and perhaps most crucial, interpretive dilemma. Women who seek and maintain employment are significantly healthier than their nonworking counterparts (Verbrugge, 1982; Waldron et al., 1982). However, even the best evidence of a positive relationship between employment and mental health does not necessarily mean that employment has led to these mental health benefits. Women select themselves into the labor force. It may be that such women, when compared with homemakers, are in better physical or mental health prior to their employment. That is, women who are physically stronger, better adjusted, and have greater abilities, self-confidence, and coping skill may enter the labor market in greater numbers than their homemaker counterparts. In fact, Waldron et al.'s longitudinal study (1982) found that, while healthier women chose employment, working had no further benefits for their health. Thus, finding that women who work during early motherhood are in good health does not permit us to conclude that *all* women with young children would benefit from employment. In fact, such advice may be quite harmful for women already feeling overextended by role demands, who may be in circumstances that make employment more difficult (a recalcitrant or easily angered husband, less child care support, and the like), or whose needs are well satisfied by being full-time homemakers.

Waldron et al.'s findings notwithstanding, not all of the findings reported here can be seen as stemming from self-selection effects. For example, the increased labor force participation of women in recent years has not attenuated the general relationship between health and employment (Kessler & McCrae, 1981; Rice & Cugliani, 1980). Even if one views the early entrants into work roles as an elite that were unusually blessed with physical stamina and strong psychological motivation, the majority of women now in the labor force can no longer be seen as unusual specimens of health. Furthermore, while earlier female employees may have more commonly elected to seek employment because of unusual capacities or motivation, factors such as economic need, divorce, widowhood, or social pressure have led many other women to enter the labor force. These circumstances may be assumed to be largely independent of prior psychological health. Yet the entry of these women into the labor force has not diminished the mental or physical health profile of employed women. This again suggests that their jobs may be contributing to women's well-being.

IMPLICATIONS FOR MENTAL HEALTH POLICY

Thus far, the accumulating evidence regarding the mental health consequences of work for women is reassuring. Many positive relationships and few negative effects have been found. It is very clear that work is an additional source of satisfaction and self-esteem for most women. Such differences in mental health seem especially likely to reveal themselves in the later years of life (Bart, 1976).

Therefore, we can encourage women to seek and maintain employment without fear for their well-being. Our concerns about role overload notwithstanding, most women seem to thrive in high-demand situations. Rather than be concerned about either the physical or mental health of working women, we probably should focus our attention on creating work situations that more fully draw on their capacities and skills. This would mean reducing the variety of structural barriers to women's employment that now exist (Zellman, 1976). The current work situation often segregates women in low-skill, low-income jobs that lack any potential for significant advancement. Child care and other family responsibilities must be accommodated to the demands of their jobs. In view of all these problems, it is rather remarkable that women are increasingly choosing to work outside the home, and it is even more noteworthy that they seem to enjoy their work more than men do (Verbrugge, 1982).

The social policy implications of the above analysis seem clear. Changes in the formal policies of work settings, including more equitable hiring practices for desirable jobs, reduced pay differentials and greater possibilities for on-the-job training and promotions would increase the attractiveness of employment for women. Employers also need to recognize that work roles interface with other roles in their employees' lives. Many companies have come to accept, as sound business practice, the premise that they should help employees with personal problems affecting job performance. While family demands may not be considered directly relevant to work performance, they cannot be totally ignored by the employer. Already we are seeing protests by dual-worker couples against indiscriminate job transfers. We also find more employers accommodating to their workers' status as new parents by offering parental leaves. More structural supports by employers, such as flexible work schedules or work site child care services during early parenthood, would probably overcome the main deterrent to women's employment. In addition, governmental policies could encourage child care use through tax benefits, subsidizing of programs, and quality standards.

Women also need more realistic preparation for the demands of the marketplace. This would include more early experiences for girls with independence, competition, and teamwork in home, school, and community (Moss & Frieze, 1984). These experiences would facilitate women's entrance into the labor force on a coequal basis with men.

These proposals are neither innovative nor dramatic. In fact, they are recommendations that we might encounter in any analysis of women and work. The central contribution of this discussion lies in the recognition that employment is significantly related to the mental health of women. Therefore, policies that enhance the conditions of female employment would also enhance the mental health of women. Such health gains could be manifested most tangibly in fewer days of illness, lower health care needs, reduced medication cost, and an overall reduction in women's use of all health care services. Since women have been such heavy users of these services, the economic impact of diminished utilization could be consequential.

VULNERABLE GROUPS OF WOMEN

There is another, less obvious implication of our current understanding of mental health correlates for women. Consistently, one finds that women living under conditons of cultural, economic, or interpersonal deprivation are at major risk of both physical and mental breakdown. For example, Wheeler et al. (1983) found that 65 percent of nonwhite, nonmarried, nonemployed women were psychologically distressed. Similarly, Verbrugge (1983) found that women with the fewest roles, that is, lacking work, husband, and children, had the worst health profile. Such roles all involve restrictions in social contacts. Since women have appeared to need and benefit from interpersonal supports more than men, such conditions of isolation may be especially detrimental to them. In fact, their heavy use of health care services may be viewed partly as a way of seeking more personal contact. Unfortunately these isolated women often lack visibility outside of treatment settings, making them very easy to overlook. However, they may be the women most in need of preventive mental health services.

Other researchers have concluded that people who have lost previously held roles through divorce, widowhood, or unemployment are at great health risk (Veroff et al., 1981). These reduced role statuses are often nonvoluntary, and may be problematic because such role reductions make people aware of their own helplessness and lack of choices (Belle, 1980; Brown et al., 1975; Radloff, 1975). Such women must grapple with their subjective feelings of having been placed in these roles involuntarily, as well as with the objective difficulties of their lives. These circumstances can lead to feelings of helplessness that commonly are associated with depressive symptoms (Bart, 1976; Brown et al., 1975; Kerman & Weissman, 1980; Radloff, 1975, 1980). If such is the case, we may expect to see less depression in women of the future as they increase their labor force participation. Such women should feel more control over their lives. While we have no direct evidence that encouraging these women to seek jobs would help reduce their problems, we do know that women in these vulnerable categories who are employed currently frequently show better mental health.

Despite the general evidence for the positive relationship between role involvement and mental health, there may be a point at which more activity ceases to be health-enhancing. Woods and Hulka (1979) found that women with more roles had more symptoms of distress than did women with fewer roles. And Veroff et al. (1981) suggested that heavily overloaded women, such as single or divorced working mothers, may be highly distressed. Thus, when a woman holds too many demanding roles simultaneously, her physical and mental health may suffer. Based on these patterns, at least one writer (Verbrugge, 1983) suggests that the relationship between role demands and mental health may be curvilinear. If so, a woman may do better psychologically by reducing some of her other role involvements while her children are young. However, the increasing numbers of divorced mothers who are heads of households, receiving little or no child support from their ex-husbands, may find this suggestion impossible to follow. Society may need to focus more attention on the needs of this overstressed, and often highly vulnerable, group of women.

We also should be monitoring the consequences for men and children of women's changing roles. If women's health gains are achieved at the expense of their children or husbands, we need to consider policies for maintaining the mental health of other family members. Thus far, however, there is little evidence that women's employment impacts negatively on other family members (e.g., Hoffman, 1979).

FUTURE DIRECTIONS

In conclusion, we can view the future involvement of women in the labor force with cautious optimism. It is likely that women will need fewer mental health services, and will particularly be less likely to suffer from depressive symptoms. Their self-esteem and sense of mastery may increase. The gains of employment are likely to increase even more as women grow older. The women who may most need mental health services may be those *not* in the work arena, especially those who are isolated or homebound because of young children or limited social roles.

When we consider the mental health needs of women in the future, we may need to help them deal more with issues that are work related. That is, they may need more help in young adulthood to clarify their occupational goals, help in the middle years to resolve dilemmas of multiple roles, and help in the later years in planning for retirement. In many ways, these problems are closer to those traditionally experienced by men. However, women's greater tendency to seek help from others for problems may bring them into treatment in greater numbers. Thus, the mental health system may need to think of innovative services to support the normal problems of adult women as they integrate employment roles into their other roles over their life span.

REFERENCES

Angrist, S., & Almquist, E. M. (1975). *Careers and contingencies.* New York: Dunellen.

Astin, H. S. (1978). Patterns of women's occupations. In Sherman, J., & F. Denmark (Eds.), *Psychology of women: Future directions of research.* (pp. 258-283). New York: Psychological Dimensions.

Atkinson, J. W. (1964). *An introduction to motivation.* Princeton: Van Nostrand.

Barnett, R. (1982). Multiple roles and well-being: A study of mothers of preschool age children. *Psychology of Women Quarterly, 7*(2), 175-178.

Bart, P. (1976). Depression in middle-aged women. In S. Cox (Ed.), *Female psychology: The emerging self.* Chicago: Science Research Associates.

Baruch, G., Barnett, R., & Rivers, C. (1983). *Lifeprints: New patterns of love and work for today's women.* New York: McGraw-Hill.

Belle, D. (1980). Mothers and their children: A study of low-income families. In C. Heckman (Ed.), *The evolving female: Women in psychosocial context.* New York: Human Sciences Press.

Bernard, J. (1975). *Women, wives and mothers: Values and options.* Chicago: Aldine.

Birnbaum, J. A. (1975). Life patterns and self-esteem in gifted family oriented and career committed women. In M.. T. Mednick, S. S. Tangri, & L. W. Hoffman (Eds.), *Women and achievement: Social and motivational analyses.* Washington, DC: Hemisphere.

Brown, W. B., Bhrolchain, M., & Harris, T. (1975). Social class and psychiatric disturbance among women in an urban population. *Sociology, 9*(2), 225-254.

Burke, R. J. (1966). Differences in perception of desired job characteristics of the same sex and the opposite sex. *Journal of Genetic Psychology, 109,* 37-46.

Campbell, A., Converse, P., & Rodgers, W. (1976). *The quality of American life: Perceptions, evaluations and satisfactions.* New York: Russell Sage Foundation.

Condrey, J., & Dyer, S. (1976). Fear of success: Attribution of cause to the victim. *Journal of Social Issues, 32,* 63-83.

Dizzard, J. (1968). *Social change in the family.* Chicago: Community Family Study Center, University of Chicago.

Dohrenwend, B., & Dohrenwend, B. (1976). Sex differences and psychiatric disorders. *American Journal of Sociology, 81*(6), 1447-1454.

Eccles, J. S., & Hoffman, L. W. (in press). Sex roles, socialization, and occupational behavior. In H. W. Stevenson & A. E. Siegel (Eds.), *Research in child development and social policy* (vol. 1). Chicago: University of Chicago Press.

Filer, R. K. (1983). Sexual differences in earnings: The role of individual personalities and tastes. *Journal of Human Resources, 18,* 82-99.

Frieze, I. H., Bailey, S., Mamula, P., & Moss, M. (1983). *Life scripts and life planning: The role of career scripts in college women's career choices.* Paper presented at the annual meeting of the Society for Experimental Social Psychology, Pittsburgh.

Frieze, I. H., Parsons, J. E., Johnson, P. B., Ruble, D. N., & Zellman, G. (1978). *Women and sex roles: A social psychological perspective.* New York: W. W. Norton.

Gillespie, D. L. (1971). Who has the power? The marital struggle. *Journal of Marriage and the Family* (August), 445-458.

Ginzberg, E. (1966). *Lifestyles of educated women.* New York: Columbia University Press.

Goldberg, A. S., & Shiflett, S. (1981). Goals of male and female college students: Do traditional sex differences still exist? *Sex Roles, 7,* 1213-1222.

Goldman, N., & David, R. (1980). Community surveys: Sex differences in mental illness. In M. Guttentag, S. Salasin, & D. Belle (Eds.), *The mental health of women,* (pp. 31-55). New York: Academic Press.

Gove, W., & Geerken, M. (1977). The effect of children and employment on the mental health of married men and women. *Social Forces, 56*(1), 66-76.

Gove, W. R., & Tudor, J. F. (1973). Adult sex roles and mental illness. *American Journal of Sociology, 98,* 812-835.

Greenfeld, S., Greiner, L., & Wood, M. M. (1980). The "feminine mystique" in male-dominated jobs: A comparison of attitudes and background factors of women in male-dominated jobs. *Journal of Vocational Behavior, 17,* 291-309.

Greenglass, E. R., & Devins, R. (1982). Factors related to marriage and career plans in unmarried women. *Sex Roles, 8,* 57-71.

Guttentag, M., Salasin, S., & Belle, D. (Eds.). (1980). *The mental health of women.* New York: Academic Press.

Herzberg, F., Mausner, B., & Snyderman, B. (1959). *The motivation to work.* New York: John Wiley.

Hoffman, D. M., & Fidell, L. S. (1979). Characteristics of androgynous, undifferentiated, masculine, and feminine middle-class women. *Sex Roles, 6,* 765-781.

Hoffman, L. W. (1979). Maternal employment: 1979. *American Psychologist, 34,*859-865.

Hoffman, L. R., & Nye, F. I. (1974). *Working mothers: An evaluative review of the consequences for wife, husband and child.* San Francisco: Jossey-Bass.

Horner, M. S. (1972). Toward an understanding of achievement-related conflicts in women. *Journal of Social Issues, 28,* 157-175.

Iglehart, A. (1978). *Married women and work.* Lexington, MA: D. C. Heath.

Kessler, R., & McRae, J. (1981). Trends in the relationship between sex and psychological distress: 1957-1976. *American Sociological Review, 46* (August), 443-452.

Klerman, G., & Weissman, M. (1980). Depression among women: Their nature and causes. In M. Guttentag et al. (Eds.), *The mental health of women,* (pp. 57-109). New York: Academic Press.

Lipman-Bluman, J., & Leavitt, H. J. (1976). Vicarious and direct achievement patterns in adulthood. *The Counseling Psychologist, 6,* 26-31.

Lowenthal, M., Thurnher, M., Chiriboga, D., & associates (1975). *Four stages of life: A comparative study of women and men facing transitions.* San Francisco: Jossey-Bass.

Maas, H. S., & Kuypers, J. A. (1974). *From thirty to seventy: A forty-year longitudinal study of changing life styles and personal development.* San Francisco: Jossey-Bass.

Masnick, G., & Bane, M. J. (1980). *The nation's families: 1960-1990.* Cambridge, MA: Joint Center for Urban Studies of MIT and Harvard University.

McClelland, D. C., & Steele, R. S. (1972). *Motivation workshops.* New York: Genreal Learning Press.

Moss, M., & Frieze, I. H. (1984). *College students' perceptions of career success strategies for male and female occupations.* Unpublished manuscript, Department of Psychology, University of Pittsburgh.

Mott, F. L. (Ed.). (1982). *The employment revolution: Young american women in the 1970's.* Cambridge: MIT Press.

Nieva, V. F., & Gutek, B. A. (1981). *Women and work: A psychological perspective.* New York: Praeger.

Norris, L., Katz, M. R., & Chapman, W. (1978). *Sex differences in the career decision-making process.* Final Report NIE-G-77-0002. Princeton, NJ: Educaton Testing Service.

O'Farrell, B. (1982). Women and nontraditonal bluecollar jobs in the 1980's: An overview. In P. A. Wallace (Ed.), *Women in the workplace.* (pp. 135-165). Boston: Auburn House.

Oppenheimer, V. K. (1975). The sex-labeling of jobs. Chapter in M.T.S. Mednick, S. S. Tangri, & L. W. Hoffman (Eds.), *Women and achievement: Social and motivational analyses.* (pp. 307-325). Washington, DC: Hemisphere.

O'Rand, A., & Henretta, J. (1982) Women at middle age: Development transitions. In F. Berardo (Ed.), *Middle and late life transitions. Annals, 464,* 57-64.

Parsons, J. E., & Goff, S. B. (1980). Achievement motivation and values: An alternate perspective. In L. J. Fyans (Ed.), *Achievement motivation: Recent trends in theory and research.* (pp. 349-373). New York: Plenum.

Pearlin, L. (1975). Sex roles and depression. In N. Datan & L. Ginsberg (Eds.), *Life-span developmental psychology: Normative life crises.* (pp. 191-207). New York: Academic Press.

Pifer, A. (1979). Women working: Toward a new society. In K. W. Feinstein (Ed.), *Working women and families.* (pp. 13-34). Beverly Hills, CA: Sage.

Rabinowitz, S., & Hall, D. T. (1977). Organizational research on job involvement. *Psychological Bulletin, 84,* 254-288.

Radloff, L. (1975). Sex differences in depression: The effects of occupation and mental status. *Sex Roles, 1*(3), 249-265.

Radloff, L. (1980). Risk factors for depression: What do we learn from them? In M. Guttentag et al. (Eds.), *The mental health of women.* (pp. 93-109). New York: Academic Press.

Rice, D., & Cugliani, A. (1980). Health status of american women. *Women and Health, 5*(1), 5-22.

Rose, A. (1965). Factors asociated with the life satisfaction of middle-class, middle-aged persons. In C. B. Vedder (Ed.), *Problems of the middle-aged.* Springfield, IL: Charles C. Thomas.

Stein, A. H., & Bailey, M. M. (1973). The socialization of achievement motivation in females. *Psychological Bulletin, 80,* 345-366.

Stewart, A., & Salt, P. (1981). Life stress, life-styles, depression and illness in adult women. *Journal of Personality and Social Psychology, 40*(6), 1063-1069.

Tittle, C. K. (1981). *Careers and family: Sex roles and adolescent life plans.* Beverly Hills, CA: Sage.

Tressemer, D. (1976). The cumulative record on research of fear of success. *Sex Roles, 2,* 2;17-236.

Turner, R. H. (1964). Some aspects of women's ambition. *American Journal of Sociology, 70,* 271-285.

Verbrugge, L. (1982). Work satisfaction and physical health. *Journal of Community Health, 7*(4), 262-282.

Verbrugge, L. (1983). Multiple roles and physical health of women and men. *Journal of Health and Social Behavior, 24* (March), 16-30.

Veroff, J., Douvan, E., & Kulka, A. (1981). *The inner American: A self-portrait from 1957-1976.* New York: Basic Books.

Waldron, I., Herold, J., Dunn, D., & Staum, R. (1982). Reciprocal effects of health and labor force participation among women: Evidence from two longitudinal studies. *Journal of Occupational Medicine, 24,* 126-132.

Warren, R. (1976). Stress, primary support and women's employment status. In D. McGuigan (Ed.), *New research on women and sex roles,* (pp. 146-159). Ann Arbor: University of Michigan, Center for Continuing Education of Women.

Wheeler, A., Lee, E. S., & Loe, H. (1983). Employment, sense of well-being, and use of professional services among women. *American Journal of Public Health, 73*(8), 908-911.

Winter, D. G. (1973). *The power motive.* New York: Free Press.

Woods, N. F., & Hulka, B. S. (1979). Symptom reports and illness behavior among employed women and homemakers. *Journal of Community Health, 5*(1), 36-45.

Zellman, G. (1976). The role of structural factors in limiting women's institutional participation. *Journal of Social Issues, 32*(3).

13

NEW SEX THERAPIES: POLICY AND PRACTICE

Lorna P. Cammaert

Shifts in societal values and norms concerning sexuality have been dramatic in this century. The nineteenth-centry ideology viewed sexuality as perverse and in need of repression. Therapy centered on controlling sexual expressiveness in all areas for all people (Leiblum & Pervin, 1980). Movement toward more modern views about sexuality was instigated by three men in different countries. The first was Henry Havelock Ellis in England who emphasized that sex was a natural human instinct and that women had sexual feelings. The second was Sigmund Freud in Austria who felt sex was central to every aspect of human development. His theories about female sexuality have been very influential, particularly his outdated view that women have two different kinds of orgasms: the clitoral, related to infantile sexuality, and the vaginal, related to mature sexuality. The third man was Alfred Kinsey in the United States who systemically surveyed sexual practices of Americans culminating in two classic works: *Sexual Behavior in the Human Male,* (Kinsey, Pomeroy, & Martin, 1948) and *Sexual Behavior in the Human Female* (Kinsey, Pomeroy, Martin, & Gebhard, 1953). His studies revealed data that challenged the current myths: Women were capable of rapid sexual arousal, 62 percent of women surveyed masturbated at some time of their life, 84 percent had relied primarily on labial and clitoral stimulation in masturbation, and 25 percent had engaged in extramarital sex.

Until the 1960s, sex therapy primarily focused on psychoanalytic dynamics, which involved treating the underlying neurotic causes of sexual dysfunction and resolving unconscious conflicts arising from the patient's past experiences. With the publication of *Human Sexual Response* (Masters & Johnson, 1966) and *Human Sexual Inadequacy* (Masters & Johnson, 1970), major steps were made in the physiological study of sexual response and in the development of a method for brief treatment of sexual dysfunctions. William Masters and Virginia Johnson reemphasized that sexuality was a natural human response and was a source of pleasure for both partners. Sexual dysfunctions, they contended, were primarily caused by psychological, not physical reasons, and could be overcome rapidly through reeducation rather than through intensive and lengthy psychotherapy.

Although psychologists utilizing behavior modification theory and techniques had tackled some sexual problems prior to the publication of the works of Masters and Johnson, for example, aversion therapy (Feldman, 1966), systematic desensitization to treat "chronic frigidity" (Lazarus, 1963), masturbation techniques with anorgasmic women (Hastings, 1963), and the importance of individual cognitions and beliefs about sexual behaviors (Ellis, 1958, 1975), many now turned to the application of behavior modification techniques for treatment of sexual dysfunctions. This popular modality utilizes five basic techniques: anxiety-reduction techniques, directed masturbation, orgasmic reconditioning, imagery techniques, and explicit homework assignments. Initial assessment of the problem and design of a treatment program are essential in the behavioral approach (Jehu, 1979). The treatment itself is educative through provision of information, modification of attitudes, and management of sexual assignments. An integral part of behavior modification is evaluation of the effectiveness of the technique used, which has led to the majority of research on sex therapy and the evolvement of more sophisticated concepts and techniques.

These advances in knowledge and therapy have encouraged women and men to slough off repression of their sexuality and to express themselves in active sexual behavior. As Leiblum and Pervin (1980) succinctly state:

> Current expectations enjoin women to be well versed in their sexual preferences, lubricate promptly, enjoy a variety of sexual acts, experience a minimum of one orgasm at some point during a sexual encounter (and preferably more), and take active delight in pleasuring their partner. (pp. 19-20)

More recently, the G spot (Belzer, 1981; Weisberg, 1981) and its specific orgasm and ejaculation have been added to the performance expectations for women. The increased liberation of sexuality appears to have produced a concomitant expectation of responsibility and performance that may cause anxiety and sexual dysfunction.

FEMALE SEXUAL DYSFUNCTION: DEFINITION
AND FREQUENCY

In clinical settings, the concerns expressed by women about their sexual functioning generally fall into four areas: (1) general sexual dysfunction (Kaplan, 1974), (2) orgastic dysfunction (Kaplan, 1974), (3) vaginismus (Kaplan, 1974), and (4) dysparunia, or painful intercourse (Jehu, 1979).

General sexual dysfunction. General sexual dysfunction has also been labelled frigidity (Kaplan, 1974), female sexual unresponsiveness (Kaplan, 1974), vasocongestive dysfunction (Jehu, 1979), and low sexual desire (Schover & LoPiccolo, 1982). These terms

> refer to conditions which are characterized by an inhibition of the general arousal aspect of the sexual response. On a psychological level, there is a lack of erotic feelings; on a physiological, such a patient suffers from an impairment of the vasocongestive component of the sexual response. (Kaplan, 1974, p. 324)

Kaplan provided an invaluable service to women in relabelling the old term "frigidity," which she felt failed to convey the fact that there are two components to the sexual response: arousal and orgasm, which can be impaired separately. Also, she felt it was an "inaccurate and pejorative" term (Kaplan, 1974, p. 339) as women who suffer from sexual inhibition or unresponsiveness are not necessarily cold and hostile but are often still warm and responsive.

The frequency of inadequate arousal is scantily documented in the literature. Bancroft and Coles (1976) reported that 63 of 102 women seen at a sexual problems clinic had "general unresponsiveness" as their principal sexual dysfunction. Levine and Yost (1976), when studying 59 black women, found 7 who exhibited "excitement-phase dysfunctions." Frank Anderson, and Rubenstein (1978) in analyzing data from a sample of 100, predominately white, nonclinical couples found 35 percent of the women complained of "disinterest" in sex and 28 percent experienced being "turned off" by sex. In reviewing data collected from 1974-1981, Schover and LoPiccolo (1982) note increases in the prevalence of desire phase problems. The seeming increase in this area may be an artifact of increased sophistication in assessment and treatment or be due to increased expectations. Whatever the reason, dysfunctions in this area are clinically held to be more difficult to treat and have a poorer prognosis (Schover & LoPiccolo, 1982) than other sexual dysfunctions.

Orgastic dysfunction. Orgastic dysfunction is the most common sexual complaint presented by women. It refers to the impairment of the orgasm phase in the female response cycle. Primary orgastic dysfunction, anorgasmic, or preorgasmic are terms used to describe a women who has never experienced an orgasm. If the woman has been able to reach orgasm but over a period of time has no longer been able to do so, it is labelled secondary or situational orgastic dysfunction.

Research by several authors indicates the high frequency of this concern. Most recently, Wiesmeier and Forsythe (1982) reported that the most common sexual concern expressed by 1034 female college students involved orgasmic difficulties (74 percent). Kinsey et al. (1953) reported that 11-25 percent of the married women surveyed had never reached orgasm during coitus. Figures for married women who have never experienced orgasm during coitus as reported by other researchers are lower: 8 percent (Terman, 1951), 5 percent (Fisher, 1973), and 8 percent (Butler, 1976). In a computer search through *Psychological Abstracts,* 113 articles were cited as referring to orgastic dysfunctions. Self-help books outlining effective treatment strategies for orgastic dysfunction, especially for preorgasmic women, are available (e.g., Barbach, *For Yourself,* 1975; Heiman, LoPiccolo, & LoPiccolo, *Becoming Orgasmic,* 1976).

Vaginismus. The third common area of sexual dysfunction for women is vaginismus. This refers to a spastic contraction of the vaginal entrance causing the vagina to "shut tight" involuntarily whenever entry is attempted. Intromission is prevented or if possible is accomplished with great difficulty and pain. Frequency of vaginismus is difficult to ascertain from the literature but Masters and Johnson (1970) found 29 percent of the women seeking their treatment fit this category. Bancroft and Coles (1976) reported that 11 of 102 clients (11 percent) seeking help at their clinic suffered from vaginismus.

Painful intercourse. Painful intercourse or dysparunia may involve burning, itching, or aching sensations that occur during or after intercourse and may be associated with other sexual dysfunctions as the pain logically leads a woman to be disinterested in sex and may generalize to vaginismus. The incidence of dysparunia appears to vary greatly in normal women from 7 percent (Purtell, Robins, & Cohen, 1951) to 15 percent (Winokur, Guze, & Pfeiffer, 1959), to 59 percent (Wiesmeier & Forsythe, 1982) and is mentioned as "common" by Wabrek and Wabrek (1975).

FEMALE SEXUAL DYSFUNCTION: TREATMENT AND EFFECTIVENESS

Modern treatment for these sexual dysfunctions is usually conducted in a directive manner or by using techniques developed by psychologists using behavior modification theory. For complete descriptions of typical treatment strategies, see Kaplan (1974), Leiblum and Pervin (1980), and Jehu (1979). These techniques quickly became popular due to the rapid effectiveness and high success rates of the treatment as experienced by clinicians.

General sexual dysfunction. General sexual dysfunction is a term so encompassing that research must define it more specifically. Thus early research is difficult to interpret due to the definitions of the problem, and because criteria for improvement and/or cure are seldom clearly delineated. Kaplan (1974) states experience at the Cornell clinic indicates that prognosis for change in general sexual dysfunction is highly dependent on the relationship the woman has with her partner. In defining "cure" she states:

> The usual outcome of treatment is that the woman now enjoys sex and is orgastic in heterosexual situations. Such patients often become orgastic on coitus as a result of treatment, but this reponse is by no means universal. (Kaplan, 1974, p. 440)

Leiblum and Ersner-Hershfield (1977) question whether orgasm through coitus alone is a reasonable goal of sexual therapy.

Writing in 1979, Jehu stated there was no information available on outcome of behavioral approaches to the treatment of inadequate interest, with the exception of some uncontrolled case reports. Schover and LoPiccolo (1982) have reanalyzed archival data from the Sex Therapy Center at Stoney Brook that indicates positive outcome statistics on "marital adjustment, overall sexual satisfaction, the frequency of intercourse and masturbation, and patterns of initiation of sexual activity" (p. 179), but they add that the posttreatment picture "represents respectable gains so that there is an absence of distress, but does not suggest striking enhancement of intimacy or pleasure above the common run" (p. 196). Thus this area of sexual dysfunction remains one that perhaps need reconceptualization and much more research.

Orgastic dysfunction. Orgastic dysfunction has been treated with four major models: systematic desensitization, sensate focus, directed masturbation, and hypnosis with each methodology being empirically supported (Anderson, 1983). Effectiveness of the treatment appears high particularly when directed masturbation is used. For instance, in treating primary orgastic dysfunction, Masters and Johnson (1970) report 82 percent of 193 women treated for this problem with a sensate focus approach reached orgasm. Barbach (1974), utilizing a five-week masturbatory training program for 83 women in group treatment, indicated 91.6 percent of the subjects were experiencing orgasm consistently through masturbation. She added that the transfer of this capability to partner-related activities within eight months after the group ended occurred for women who were in satisfactory emotional relationships. The goal of the group treatment was orgasm with a partner, rather than orgasm during intercourse (Barbach & Ayres, 1976). In her book, Barbach (1975) mentions that although the majority of the 600 women who have participated in her preorgasmic programs were involved in heterosexual relationships, some of the women were currently in same-sex relationships or in no relationship at all. The techniques were effective regardless of the type of relationship involved but the issue raises questions about definition of the goal and criteria for success, which are amply covered by Kuriansky and Sharpe (1981). Although variation in outcome criteria and assessment methods makes it difficult to make direct comparisons across studies, the high rate of effectiveness in all studies lends support to the techniques used (Barbach & Ayres, 1976; Kuriansky & Sharpe, 1981).

The studies cited above did not include a no-treatment control group or attempt to determine whether individual, couple, or group treatments were most effective. Nemetz, Craig, and Reith (1978) randomly assigned 16 women to either individual or group treatment consisting of relaxation training and viewing videotaped vignettes depicting graduated sexual behaviors over a period of five sessions. Six other women were assessed but not treated. The results indicated significant decreases in anxiety and significant increases in behavioral and attitudinal measures for both treatment groups, but a trend was observed for greater improvement by those in the group treatment.

Concern has been expressed that a lack of partner involvement when women seek treatment individually and in all-female groups may be undesirable (Payn & Wakefield, 1982). However, when Ersner-Hersfield and Kogel (1979) assessed the effects of couples versus women-only group treatments with 23 couples assigned to four treatment modalities, the couples groups were not superior on measures that assessed couple activities and frequency of orgasm. Analysis of the data on the women in women-only groups revealed significant improvements in both self sexuality and couple sexuality. Without participating in the groups, the men with whom the women were involved showed significant improvements on the majority of couple activity measures.

Most of the studies have involved relatively young women, but Schneidman and McGuire (1976) utilized a group treatment with sensate focus and directed masturbation with 10 women below and 10 women above 35 years of age. At termination of the treatment, 70 percent of the young and 40 percent of the older women were orgasmic with self-stimulation. These figures increased at the six-month follow-up to 80 percent and 60 percent for younger and older women, respectively. None of the younger women and only one of the older women were coitally orgasmic. The authors concluded group treatment may be less successful for older women necessitating individual treatment, but since a high rate has not been shown for this alternative, the 60 percent success rate of the group treatment in this study should not be disregarded.

Secondary orgasmic dysfunction appears to respond less well to treatment, although Masters and Johnson (1970) report success with 75.2 percent of the 149 women who sought treatment for secondary orgastic dysfunction. Two aspects appear to impinge on this dysfunction: low sexual desire and marital discord, which may mitigate against effectiveness of sex therapy for the specific dysfunction in isolation from marital therapy or more extensive personal therapy. This is supported by Barbach and Flaherty (1980), who reported on an all-women group treatment program for those not experiencing orgasms with their partner. Two-thirds of the women were successful, but the program was most effective for women in casual relationships or those of less than 1.5 years duration. In relationships that were committed and over three years duration, the outcomes were mixed.

Individual and group formats have been used in treatment of secondary orgastic dysfunction. The only study found in the literature that compared the two treatments was done by Golden, Price, Heinrich, and Lobitz (1978) where men who were prematurely ejaculating and their female partners who were inorgasmic during intercourse were treated as a couple or in couple groups for 12 weekly sessions. Although the group format initially showed a slight tendency toward more rapid progress, by the two-month follow-up there was significant improvement for couples in both treatment formats.

The need for extended foreplay and intromission had been hypothesized to be beneficial to woman's orgastic response but in a retrospective review of data from 619 women who sought treatment for sexual dysfunction, Huey, Kline-Graber, and Graber (1981) did not find support for this. They found that 44 percent of the anorgasmic women estimated foreplay lasted 10 minutes or less, while 56 percent estimated it lasted more than 10 minutes. These figures are almost identical to those reported by Kinsey et al. (1953) for a normal sample of American women. In a study of approximately 1000 nonclinical Dutch women, de Bruijn (1982) also concluded that the amount and length of foreplay did not relate directly to orgasm during coitus. These findings may indicate that the typical sensate focus pleasuring concept in sex therapy may not be essential to women reaching orgasm in coitus but relates more to other aspects of sexuality and caring that women value more. In de Bruijn's sample, 75 percent of the women stated flatly that "the experience of orgasm contributes little or nothing to their sexual satisfaction. Within their personal frame of reference, other things are usually more important" (de Bruijn, 1982, p. 160).

Vaginismus. Vaginismus has been primarily treated with vaginal dilation, systematic desensitization, and hypnosis. High success rates are noted. Masters and Johnson (1970) treated 29 women who after treatment were all able to engage in intercourse over a five-year follow-up period. Fuchs et al. (1973), utilizing two different treatment methods, reported 66 percent and 91 percent of their patients were successful.

Some authors contend that more lengthy treatment of vaginismus utilizing sex therapy, psychotherapy, and marital therapy is required because it is not merely a physical dysfunction but may be more akin to phobic anxiety (Davidson & Yftach, 1976; Duddle, 1977; Kaplan, 1974; O'Sullivan, 1979), especially when causes may lie in previous experiences such as rape or incest (Lesnik-Oberstein, 1982; McGuire & Wagner, 1978). It should be noted that vaginismus has been treated surgically. Kaplan (1974) notes that although surgical procedures are anatomically successful, "they often give rise to adverse emotional reactions and sexual problems of sufficient severity to contraindicate their use" (p. 442). The literature review also revealed one study (Mikhail, 1976) where four women complaining of vaginismus were given doses of diazepam (Valium) after which the patients reported having succesful intercourse and two of the four reported being orgasmic for the first time. Treatment by surgery and drugs seems contraindicated since the process of recognizing and learning the sexual response is taken out of the woman's control, making her a passive recipient and thus perpetuating negative sexual stereotypes.

Painful intercourse. Little research appears to be available on treatment effectiveness of dysparunia with only a few uncontrolled cases reported (Jehu, 1979).

CONCEPTUALIZATION AND POLICY ISSUES

RECONCEPTUALIZATION OF FEMALE SEXUALITY

Much progress has been made since the nineteenth century when female sexuality was repressed, denied, and believed to be nonexistent. Today, women are encouraged to express themselves sexually, and sex therapy must be commended for recognizing that the scope of sexuality goes far beyond the young to those who are old, sick, and institutionalized (Leiblum & Pervin, 1980). However, women and men are often still caught in stereotypic attitudes and behaviors that maintain men should be dominant and women passive in heteroexual relationships. In discussing power and sexuality, Lips (1981) describes the male sexual role as "initiator, leader, expert, and teacher" (p.112), in contrast with the female sexual role of "follower and gatekeeper" (p. 112). This traditional role division is reinforced in the media but particularly finds expression in pornography, which holds up male dominance and female submission as ideal, erotic, and desirable.

Pornography may be defined as "erotica that debases—erotica in which the theme is sexual degradation of another person" (Lips, 1981, p. 120). Several studies (Malamuth & Check, 1979; Malamuth, Haber, & Feshbach, 1980; Malamuth, Reisin, & Spinner, 1979) indicate the close relationship between violent pornography and attitudes toward women. In answering a questionnaire, 50 percent of male undergraduates in one study (Malamuth, Haber & Feshbach, 1980) and 69 percent in another (Malamuth & Check, 1979) thought that they might rape a woman if they could be assured of no legal consequences. This proclivity to rape was associated with acceptance of the belief that women enjoy rape (Malamuth & Check, 1979). This coupled with the finding that the incidence of sexual violence has escalated between 1973 and 1977 in the soft-core erotica of *Playboy* and *Penthouse* (Malamuth & Spinner, 1980) indicates the traditional ideas of a passive female recipient enjoying violent sex are alive and well. Some feminists contend that rape is a crime of power, not sex, and that this is an efficient means of controlling women (Brownmiller, 1975; Clark & Lewis, 1977). There appear to be strong forces at work to maintain a passive image of female sexuality and a male dominance that may involve power and violence.

Yet the media and sex therapy encourage women to be more active in giving pleasure, initiating sexual activity, and experimenting with new sexual behaviors. The dilemma for women increases when authors contend that men are sexually ambivalent about such activity on the part of women (Komarovsky, 1976) and that this may result in increased impotence for men (Ginsberg, Frosch, & Shapiro, 1972). This leads to two major questions for women and for sex therapy: (1) What is female sexuality? and (2) What is normative sexual behavior for women?

Traditional socialization and current media, including pornography, portray one image of female sexuality that is severely limited and that does not appear to fit women's own image of their sexuality (Hite, 1976; de Bruijn, 1982). However, the sexual diversity of women is just beginning to emerge in the professional literature (Hoon & Hoon, 1978; Loewenstein, 1978). It is being recognized that female sexuality encompasses much more than heterosexual intercourse. Masturbation and orgasm with a partner of the opposite or same sex are now recognized as valid expressions of sexuality that are ends in themselves and not just steps along the way to the old ultimate goal of orgasm in intercourse. Female reproductive functions involving pregnancy, childbearing, and breast-feeding are now included in discussions of female sexuality. Professionals are exploring the effects on women's feelings of sexuality of various functions such as menstruation, menopause, and the premenstrual syndrome, or as a result of diseases such as breast cancer and the consequent surgery, and other surgical interventions, for example, hysterectomies. The emphasis is on the women's self-reports rather than the professionals' description of how she should feel. Thus we are on the brink of discovering much more about the breadth, depth, and diversity of female sexuality from women rather than the conceptualizations laid on women by men through socialization, fantasy, or theory.

A feminist critique of sex therapy by Seidler-Feller (in press) suggests that female sexual dysfunction may be a reflection of sexual politics. Thus sexual dysfunction may be a woman's only possible expression of the following: (1) a general status protest against the sexual ritual of subordination; (2) unacknowledged power conflicts intended to preserve or alter power relations; (3) self-ownership or a right to privacy; (4) conflict around the necessity of role adjustment and possible loss of power incurred through changes related to the female reproductive cycle; or (5) a dispute or strike over working conditions preceded by fatigue and role overload. Viewing sexual dysfunction from this perspective would necessitate a complete reconceptualization of female sexuality and of where the problems or dysfunctions lie, with the subsequent treatment being quite different from that which is currently being used.

It must be noted that the image of female sexuality that emerges from the literature is severely limited or biased not only conceptually but also in terms of the women who are surveyed or treated. The vast majority of studies involve white, middle-class, well-educated, and married women (Baisdea & Baisdea, 1979). Only one study in the literature utilized black women (Levine & Yost, 1976), one study compared treatment effects for women at two age levels (Schneidman & McGuire, 1976), one suggested sexual enhancement for elderly couples (Rowland & Haynes, 1978), and one involved lower-class couples (Heiman & LoPiccolo, 1983). Although some articles appear on treatment of homosexual couples, very few articles were found in the review of literature about sexual dysfunctions of lesbian women singly or as couples. This large omission has been noted and criticized by Sharratt and Bern (in press). It is clear that in reconceptualizing female sexuality, this glaring limitation must be expanded so that experiences of all women are included in the new conceptualization. Thus much more research is required on the sexuality of women who are poor, who have less than college education, who choose to be single, who choose to be celibate, who choose to have same-sex relationships, and who are of color.

RECONCEPTUALIZATION OF SEXUAL SATISFACTION

Sex therapy for women has focussed primarily on genital functioning with an emphasis on orgasm. The underlying assumption has been that by learning to masturbate to orgasm, women can then be taught to generalize this response to orgasm through intercourse. This is exemplified by the Orgasm Hierarchy Scale developed by Kuriansky, Sharpe, and O'Connor (1982), where orgasm through intercourse is rated higher than orgasm by self-stimulation or orgasm with a partner present.

Several writers, all female, have begun questioning this attitude (Brunley, 1979; Leiblum & Ersner-Hershfield, 1977). Barbach's (1974) effective treatment for female orgasmic problems through self-directed masturbation has led the way for women to explore, become aware of, respect, and like their own anatomy. Some women have discovered that masturbation is "not just a second-rate outlet, but [is] a first-rate way to cherish and love one's own body" (Coyner, 1976, p. 222). Thus women's experience in learning that sex is not something done to her but rather is something she controls and feels for herself leads to increased pleasure and possibly more self-determination of that pleasure.

Articles on secondary orgasmic dysfunction (Barbach & Flaherty, 1980), on sexual versus marital communication (e.g., Chesney, Blakeney, Chan, & Cole, 1981; Everaerd & Dekker, 1981), and on the role of orgasm in sexual enjoyment (Waterman & Chiauzzi, 1982) emphasize that relationship factors play an important role in an individual's assessment of sexual satisfaction and that orgasm may not necessarily be correlated with sexual enjoyment. In fact, Waterman and Chiauzzi (1982) found that for most activities, for both men and women in their sample of 42 couples, pleasure ratings were significantly higher when the activity occurred without orgasm. Thus the goal orientation of orgasm may be detrimental to sexual pleasure. In the study of normal women by de Bruijn (1982), the majority of women (58 percent) experienced orgasm more often outside coitus and 75 percent felt that orgasm was not an important factor contributing to their sexual satisfaction.

These writings from various viewpoints combine to bring into question the emphasis on orgasm and its centrality to women's sexual satisfaction and to sex therapy. Sexual satisfaction for women must be reconceptualized to fit their experiences from their perspectives. The whole idea of sexual satisfaction must be added to simply being sexually functional (Jayne, 1981), and sexual therapists along with marital therapists have to expand their perspective to include societal, political, and economic determinants of sexual functioning and satisfaction. In the opinion of Laws (1975), there is "evidence for neglect, not exploration of this area in research" (p. 105); and yet sexual functioning and satisfaction appear to be linked to happy, healthy, functioning women who value sexuality both within and outside marriage (Baruch, Barnett, & Rivers, 1983). This could lead to a complete reconceptualization of female and male sexual dysfunctions. The focus could change from the genital functioning related to orgasmic dysfunction, vaginismus, painful intercourse, and impotence to much more emphasis on sex role definition, examination of beliefs about sexuality, negotiations in relationships, and responsibility for one's own sexuality. This would have the added benefit of removing sexuality from only the heterosexual realm and normalizing sexual pleasure with same-sex partners.

This deemphasis on orgasm for sexual satisfaction may serve another purpose, too, in finally disarming the psychoanalytic viewpoint that judges which female orgasms are mature or immature. The research of Masters and Johnson (1970) resolved for most professionals the question of the duality of orgasm hypothesized by Freud, with the female orgasm clearly linked physiologically to both clitoral stimulation and vaginal contractions. In spite of the research evidence, some writers still cling to the concept of two types of orgasm, regarding the vaginal superior to the clitoral because it is a mark of greater maturity (Hogan, 1975) and the Freudian concepts of penis envy and female masochism. Writing in 1977, Eissler concluded that ''a. masochism is still necessary for a psychoanalysis of femininity, b. motherhood is destiny for women, and c. the daughters of the present generation of feminists will revert to the traditional role of women in society'' (p. 79). For a person with such beliefs to be providing therapy for orgasmic dysfunctions appears to be contrary to the APA Guidelines on Therapy for Women (American Psychological Association, 1978) and against the APA ethical code, which prohibits functioning in an area outside the psychologists' knowledge.

Reconceptualization of sexual satisfaction with its concomitant deemphasis on orgasm, will encourage women and researchers to look beyond genital function to encompass many other aspects of women's lives. For example, depression is often cited as a possible underlying cause of low sexual desire (Kaplan, 1974; LoPiccolo, 1980; Munjack & Staples, 1976). Depression is the most common diagnostic label used in conjunction with all women who present themselves for treatment (Fidell, 1980). Yet, only one study (Mathew & Weinman, 1982) has investigated the incidence of sexual dysfunctions in depressed patients. The lack in the professional literature of systematic evidence linking depression, sexual functioning, and self-esteem, especially for women, is unexpected and appalling. It is imperative that research be conducted on this possible interaction.

A related issue is the effect of drugs on women's sexual responsiveness and sexual desire. Some research has been conducted into the validity of woman's concerns that contraceptive drugs cause loss of interest (Adams, Gold, & Burt, 1978; Royal College of General Practitioners, 1974; Trimmer, 1978), but definitive answers have not been found. Effects of other drugs, for example, sedatives, tranquillizers, antihypertensives, and narcotics, on female responsiveness appear to have been underresearched (Jehu, 1979), although some studies have been conducted on the effects of drugs on men especially in relationship to erectile and impotence dysfunctions. Since tranquillizers and antidepressants are so frequently prescribed for women presenting a variety of physical complaints to physicians (Fidell, 1980), the relationship between drugs and sexual functioning appears to be a logical and imperative area of research that remains to be done.

SEXISM IN SEX THERAPY

Sexual therapy is provided by people from a multitude of disciplines: general practitioners, gynecologists, nurses, psychiatrists, psychologists, social workers, and sociologists. Some of those practicing in the area may or may not have appropriate background, training, and supervised experience to offer themselves as sexual therapists, especially for women. There is a danger that besides inappropriate treatment, stereotypes and outdated ideas of women's sexual function will be reinforced in therapy. Because of the interdisciplinary nature of sex therapy and with the major reconceptualization of what constitutes appropriate sex therapy, credentialing of sex therapists is an important policy issue. Until a solution and official recognition of some type is available, it is essential that the consumer be knowledgeable and conscientious in choosing a sex therapist. A consumer wanting sex therapy must shop carefully, asking concrete questions about the therapist's qualifications, experience, attitudes toward women, and fees. Available consumer guides to choosing a therapist (e.g., Federation of Organizations for Professional Women, *Women and Psychotherapy,* 1982) are undoubtedly useful in deciding on a sex therapist.

Sexual therapy, particularly that with a basis in behavior modification theory, operates with an underlying assumption that egalitarianism in treatment and for a couple is desirable (Gurman, 1978). In treatment this is most often communicated implicitly through assignment of homework tasks on an equal basis, and respecting input from both partners about assessment and decision-making. This implicitness appears to overlook important issues about the sex role socialization of the individuals, the degree to which the individuals perceive their relationship to be equal (Margolin, Fernandez, Talovic, & Onorato, 1983), and the power issues that are involved (Lips, 1981). A therapist who ignores these dynamics may be perceived by the clients as naive, insensitive, and possibly incompetent. Even worse, the client may not be sophisticated enough to perceive this in therapists and may be damaged by the therapy.

This naiveté on the part of therapists appears to extend to the co-therapy relationship so often stressed due to the Masters and Johnson model, although not proven in terms of research (Jehu, 1979; Kaplan, 1974; Zilbergeld, 1980). Based on anecdotal reports in the literature often by couples providing therapy, Jehu (1979) reports that possible threats to a positive co-therapy relationship arise from problems between the therapists such as

> clashes in values,. . .differences in their therapeutic styles,. . .discrepancy in their levels of experience,. . .professional stereotypes, role expectations, status differences,. . .discrepancies in the gender role expectations of each therapist in relation to the other, or transfer of conflicts from the personal relationship between them in the therapeutic situation. (p. 199)

In 1975, Rice and Rice discussed status and sex role issues in co-therapy for marriage counseling. One issue germane to sexual therapy that Rice and Rice raise is differential status of the two therapists. Often the co-therapy team in sexual therapy is a married couple representing two disciplines, with the male in the higher status occupation, for example, psychiatrist and social worker. Many implicit and explicit aspects about the co-therapy couple may impact on the clients: whose office is used, the professional labels that are used, such as Dr., who does most of the talking, to whom is the fee or the largest fee paid, the marital attitudes and life-styles of the co-therapists, and who controls the interview. In the view of Rice and Rice (1975):

> Perceived co-therapist status differences become a critical factor in this treatment format. Few therapists (married or unmarried) seem willing to face, or are even cognizant of the status role model they present to patients in its egalitarian or nonegalitarian forms. (p. 146)

Although seemingly not known or dealt with by the majority of co-therapy teams, it is obvious that these issues plus that of control or power must be acknowledged, dealt with openly, and continuously as they are "usually omnipresent" (Rice & Rice, 1975, p. 146). Jehu (1979) warns that nonresolution of such issues "is likely to be stressful and unrewarding for the therapists, and quite possibly damaging to the clients" (p. 199). This warning is too mild considering the impact on clients that such naivete and bias can have, especially in such a value-laden area as sex therapy. Obviously, training and ongoing consultation for the therapists is essential to ensure that clients are provided sex-fair counseling where sex role and power issues are acknowledged and incorporated into therapy when appropriate.

CONCLUSION

What is female sexuality? Answers to this question are just beginning to emerge. Women are awakening to their own sexuality and its variety and are not willing to accept the traditional passive role in sexual intimacy. Instead, women are beginning to value their bodies, their needs, and their desires. They are searching for responsive, sensitive sexual partners. Research is beginning to recognize and value responses from women. Researchers and sex therapists are coming to see that sexual needs and desires of women are just as important as, and are not necessarily identical to, those of men. Yet there is much that is not known.

The little that is known is based on samples of predominantly white, well-educated, middle-class, heterosexual American women. Conceptualization of female sexuality must include experiences of all women: poor, of color, single, lesbian, celibate, of all ages, and from a variety of educational levels.

With a change in focus from simple sexual functioning to a much broader conceptualization of female sexual satisfaction, and from orgasm during intercourse to sexual feelings from a variety of activities, a fuller understanding of female sexuality may finally be possible. Female sexuality may be placed into perspective of women's lives and how their various roles impinge on or facilitate women's sexuality and mental health. Hard questions will have to be answered. For example: Is monogamy with a male partner mentally and sexually healthy for a woman? Is the nuclear family the best arrangement for raising mentally healthy children? For mentally healthy men and women? Is the increase in violent pornography an attempt to keep women in their traditional passive place? What effect do different sex roles have on relationships? On power? On mental health? If women adopt more assertive attitudes about their own sexuality, will men adapt and change? If so, in what ways? And how? By being more knowledgeable and comfortable with their own sexuality, will women have more power in their self-determination? In their relationship? There is every possibility that by finding answers to these and other questions, the fabric of our society may gradually change to one where more choices are available and acceptable for expressing one's sexuality and where men and women accept the responsibility of their choices.

Sex researchers and therapists have a professional responsibility to address the many existing gaps in research, practice, and theory. This requires that they first examine their own socialization and attitudes to ensure they are not perpetuating myths and stereotypes in their practice. Then they can proceed to further understand this new, ever-changing but old phenomenon: female sexuality.

REFERENCES

Adams, D. B., Gold, A. R. & Burt, A. K. (1978). Rise in female-initiated sexual activity at ovulation and its suppression by oral contraceptives. *New England Journal of Medicine, 23,* 1145-1150.

American Psychological Association Report of the Task Force on Sex Bias and Sex-Role Stereotyping in Psychotherapeautic Practice (1978). Guidelines for therapy with women. *American Psychologist, 13,* 1122-1123.

Anderson, B. L. (1983). Primary orgasmic dysfunction: Diagnostic considerations and review of treatment. *Psychological Bulletin, 93*(1), 105-136.

Baisdea, M. J. & Baisdea, J. R. (1979). A profile of women who seek counseling for sexual dysfunction. *American Journal of Family Therapy, 1*(1), 68-76.

Bancroft, J. & Coles, L. (1976). Three years' experience in a sexual problems clinic. *British Medical Journal, 1,* 1575-1577.

Barbach, L. G. (1974). Group treatment of preorgasmic women. *Journal of Sex and Marital Therapy, 1*(2), 139-145.

Barbach, L. G. (1975). *For yourself: The fulfillment of female sexuality.* Garden City, NY: Doubleday.

Barbach, L. G. & Flaherty, M. (1980). Group treatment of situationally orgasmic women. *Journal of Sex and Martial Therapy, 6*(1), 19-29.

Barbach, L. G. & Ayres, T. (1976). Group process for women with orgasmic difficulties. *Personnel and Guidance Journal, 54*(7), 389-391.

Baruch, G., Barnett, R. & Rivers, C. (1983). *Lifeprints: New patterns of love and work for today's women.* New York: McGraw-Hill.

Belzer, E. G. (1981). Orgasmic expulsions of women: A review and heuristic inquiry. *Journal of Sex Research, 17*(1), 1-12.

Brownmiller, S. (1975). *Against our will.* New York: Bantam Books.

Brunley, W. (1979). When is therapy indicated for female sexual concerns? A clinician's view. *Australian Journal of Clinical and Experimental Hypnosis, 7*(3), 231-234.

Butler, C. A. (1976). New data about female sexual response. *Journal of Sex and Marital Therapy, 2*(1), 40-46.

Chesney, A. P., Blakeney, P. E., Chan, F. A. & Cole, C. M. (1981). The impact of sex therapy on sexual behavior and marital communication. *Journal of Sex and Marital Therapy, 7*(1), 70-79.

Clark, L. & Lewis, D. (1977). *Rape: The price of coercive sexuality.* Toronto,: Women's Press.

Coyner, S. (1976). Women's liberation and sexual liberation. In S. Gordon and R. Libby (Eds.), *Sexuality: Today and tomorrow* (pp. 216-228). New York: Wadsworth.

Davidson, S. & Yftach, R. (1976). The therapy of the unconsummated marriage. *Psychotherapy: Theory, Research, and Practice, 13*(4), 418-419.

de Bruijn, G. (1982). From masturbation to orgasm with a partner: How some women bridge the gap— and why others don't. *Journal of Sex and Marital Therapy, 8*(2), 151-167.

Dekker, J. & Everaerd, W. (1983). A long-term follow-up study of couples treated for sexual dysfunctions. *Journal of Sex and Marital Therapy, 9*(2), 99-113.

Duddle, M. (1977). Etiological factors in the unconsummated marriage. *Journal of Psychosomatic Research, 21*(2), 157-160.

Ellis, A. (1958). *Sex without guilt.* New York: Lyle Stuart.

Ellis, A. (1975). The rational-emotive approach to sex therapy. *Counseling Psychologist, 5,* 14-22.

Eissler, K. R. (1977). Comments on penis envy and orgasm in women. *Psychoanalytic Study of the Child, 32,* 29-83.

Ersner-Hershfield, R. & Kogel, S. A. (1979). Group treatment of preorgasmic women: Evaluation of partner involvement and spacing of sessions. *Journal of Counseling and Clinical Psychology, 47*(4), 750-759.

Everaerd, W. & Dekker, J. (1981). A comparison of sex therapy and communication therapy: Couples complaining of orgasmic dysfunction. *Journal of Sex and Marital Therapy, 7*(4), 278-289.

Federation of Organizations for Professional Women (1982). *Women and psychotherapy.* Washington: Author.

Feldman, M. P. (1966). Aversion therapy for sexual deviations: A critical review. *Psychological Bulletin, 65,* 65-79.

Fidell, L. S. (1980). Sex role stereotypes and the American physician. *Psychology of Women Quarterly, 4*(3), 313-330.

Fisher, S. (1973). *The female orgasm: Psychology, physiology, fantasy.* London: Allen Lane.

Frank, E., Anderson, C. & Rubenstein, D. (1978). Frequency of sexual dysfunction in "normal couples." *New England Journal of Medicine, 299*(3), 111-115.

Fuchs, K., Hoch, Z., Paldi, E., Abramovici, H., Brandes, J. Timor-Tritsch, I. & Kleinhauser, M. (1973). Hypno-desensitization therapy of vaginismus. I. In vitro method. II. In vivo method. *International Journal of Clinical and Experimental Hynopsis, 21,* 144-156.

Ginsberg, G. L., Frosch, W. A. & Shapiro, T. (1972). The new impotence. *Archives of General Psychiatry, 26,* 218-220.

Golden, J., Price, S., Heinrich, A. G. & Lobitz, W. C. (1978). Group vs couple treatment of sexual dysfunctions. *Archives of Sexual Behavior, 7*(6), 593-602.

Gurman, A. S. (1978). The patient's perception of the therapeutic relationship. In A. S. Gurman & A. M. Ruzin (Eds.), *Effective psychotherapy: A handbook of research* (pp. 503-543). Oxford: Pergamon.

Hastings, D. W. (1963). *Impotence and frigidity.* London: Churchill.

Heiman, J., LoPiccolo, L. & LoPiccolo, J. (1976). *Becoming orgasmic: A sexual growth program for women.* Englewood Cliffs, N.J.: Prentice-Hall.

Heiman, J. R. & LoPiccolo, J. (1983). Clinical outcome of sex therapy: Effects of daily versus weekly treatment. *Archives of General Psychiatry, 10*(4), 443-449.

Hite, S. (1976). *The Hite report.* New York: Dell.

Hogan, R. A. (1975). Frigidity and implosive therapy. *Psychology, 12*(2), 39-45.

Hoon, E. F. & Hoon, P. W. (1978). Styles of sexual expression in women: Clinical implications of multivarate analyses. *Archives of Sexual Behavior, 7*(2), 105-116.

Huey, C. J., Kline-Graber, G. & Graber, B. (1981). Time factors and orgasmic response. *Archives of Sexual Behavior, 10*(2), 111-118.

Husted, J. R. (1975). Desensitization procedures in dealing with female sexual dysfunction. *Counseling Psychologist, 5*(1), 30-37.

Jayne, C. (1981). A two-dimensional model of female sexual response. *Journal of Sex and Marital Therapy, 7*(1), 3-30.

Jehu, D. (1979). *Sexual dysfunctions: A behavioural approach to causation, assessment, and treatment.* Bath, England: Pitman Press.

Kaplan, H. S. (1974). *The new sex therapy.* New York: Brunner/Mazel.

Kinsey, A. C., Pomeroy, W. B. & Martin, C. E. (1948). *Sexual behavior in the human male.* Philadelphia: Saunders.

Kinsey, A. C., Pomeroy, W. B., Martin, C. E. & Gebhard, P. H. (1953). *Sexual behavior in the human female*. Philadelphia: Saunders.

Komarovsky, M. (1976). *Dilemmas of masculinity: A study of college youth*, New York: Norton.

Kuriansky, J. B. & Sharpe, L. (1981). Clinical and research implication of the evaluation of women's group therapy for anorgasmia: A review. *Journal of Sexual Marital Therapy, 7*(4), 268-277.

Kuriansky, J. B., Sharpe, L. & O'Conner, D. (1982). The treatment of anorgasmia: Long-term effectiveness of a short-term behavioral group therapy. *Journal of Sexual and Marital Therapy, 8*(1), 29-43.

Laws, J. L. (1975). A feminist view of marital adjustment. In A. S. Gurman & D. G. Rice (Eds.), *Couples in conflict: New directions in marital therapy* (pp. 73-123). New York: Jason Aronson.

Lazarus, A. A. (1963). The treatment of chronic frigidity by systematic desensitization. *Journal of Nervous and Mental Disease, 136,* 272-278.

Leiblum, S. R. & Ersner-Hershfield, R. (1977). Sexual enhancement groups for dysfunctional women: An evaluation. *Journal of Sexual and Marital Therapy, 3*(2), 139-152.

Leiblum, S. R. & Pervin, L. A. (1980). *Principles and practice of sex therapy*. New York: Guilford.

Lesnik-Oberstein, M. (1982). Iatrogenic rape of a fourteen-year old girl: A note. *Child Abuse and Neglect, 6*(1), 103-104.

Levine, S. B. & Yost, M. A. (1976). Frequency of sexual dysfunction in a general gynecological clinic: An epidemological approach. *Archives of Sexual Behavior, 5,* 229-238.

Lips, H. M. (1981). *Women, men, and the psychology of power*. Englewood Cliffs, N.J.: Prentice-Hall.

Loewenstein, S. (1978). An overview of some aspects of female sexuality. *Social Casework, 59*(2), 106-115.

LoPiccolo, L. (1980). Treatment of sexual desire disorders. In S. R. Leiblum & L. A. Pervin (Eds.), *Principles and practice of sex therapy* (pp. 29-64). New York: Guilford.

LoPiccolo, J. & LoPiccolo, L. (1978). *Handbook of sex therapy*. New York: Plenum.

Malamuth, N. M. & Check, J. V. P. (1979). Penile tumescence and perceptual responses to rape as a function of victim's response. Paper presented at Canadian Psychological Association, Quebec City, June.

Malamuth, N. M., Haber, S. & Feshbach, S. (1980). Testing hypotheses regarding rape: Exposure to sexual violence, sex differences, and the "normality" of rapists. *Journal of Research in Personality, 14*(1), 121-137.

Malamuth, N. M., Reisin, I. & Spinner, B. (1979). Exposure to pornography and reactions to rape. Paper presented at the Annual Meeting of the Western Psychological Association, San Diego.

Malamuth, N. M. & Spinner, B. (1980). A longitudinal content analysis of sexual violence in the best selling erotic magazines. *Journal of Sex Research, 16*(3), 226-237.

Margolin, G., Fernandez, V., Talovic, S. & Onorato, R. (1983). Sex role considerations and behavioral marital therapy: Equal does not mean identical. *Journal of Marital and Family Therapy, 9*(2), 131-145.

Masters, W. H. & Johnson, V. E. (1970). *Human sexual inadequacy*. Boston: Little, Brown.

Masters, W. H. & Johnson, V. E. (1966). *Human sexual response*. Boston: Little, Brown.

Mathew, R. J. & Weinman, M. L. (1982). Sexual functions in depression. *Archives of Sexual Behavior, 11*(4), 323-328.

McGuire, L. S. & Wagner, N. N. (1978). Sexual dysfunction in women who were molested as children: One response pattern and suggestions for treatment. *Journal of Sex and Marital Therapy, 4*(1), 11-15.

Mikhail, A. R. (1976). Treatment of vaginismus by i. v. diazepam (Valium-super (R)) in abreaction interviews. *Acta Psychiatrica Scandinavica, 53*(5), 328-332.

Munjack, D. J. & Staples, F. R. (1976). Psychological characteristics of women with sexual inhibition (frigidity) in sex clinics. *Journal of Nervous and Mental Disease, 163*(2), 117-123.

Nemetz, G. H., Craig, K. D. & Reith, G. (1978). Treatment of female sexual dysfunction through symbolic modeling. *Journal of Consulting and Clinical Psychology, 46*(1), 62-73.

O'Sullivan, K. (1979). Observations on vaginismus in Irish women. *Archives of General Psychiatry, 36*(7), 824-826.

Payn, N. & Wakefield, J. (1982). The effect of group treatment of primary orgasmic dysfunction on the marital relationship. *Journal of Sex and Marital Therapy, 8*(2), 135-150.

Purtell, J. J., Robins, E. & Cohen, M. E. (1951). Observation of clinical aspects of hysteria. *Journal of the American Medical Association, 146,* 902-909.

Rice, J. K. & Rice, D. G. (1975). Status and sex role issues in co-therapy. In A. S. Gurman & D. C. Rice (Eds.), *Couples in conflict: New directions in marital therapy* (pp. 145-150). New York: Jason Aronson.

Rowland, K. F. & Haynes, S. N. (1978). A sexual enhancement program for elderly couples. *Journal of Sex and Marital Therapy, 4*(2), 91-113.

Royal College of General Practitioners (1974). *Oral contraceptives and health: An interim report.* London: Pitman Medical.

Schneidman, B. & McGuire, L. (1976). Group therapy for nonorgasmic women: Two age levels. *Archives of Sexual Behavior, 5*(3), 239-247.

Schover, L. R. & LoPiccolo, J. (1982). Treatment effectiveness for dysfunctions of sexual desire. *Journal of Sex and Marital Therapy, 8*(3), 179-197.

Seidler-Feller, D. (in press). A feminist critique of sex therapy. In L. Bravo Rosewater & L. Walker (Eds.), *A handbook of feminist therapy.* New York: Springer.

Sharratt, S. & Bern, L. (in press). Lesbian couples and families: A co-therapeutic approach to therapy. In L. Bravo Rosewater & L. Walker (Eds.), *A handbook of feminist therapy.* New York: Springer.

Terman, L. M. (1951). Correlates of orgasm adequacy in a group of 556 wives. *Journal of Psychology, 32,* 115-172.

Trimmer, E. (1978). Reducing the side effects of the pill. *British Journal of Sexual Medicine, 5*(33), 3.

Wabrek, A. J. & Wabrek, C. J. (1975). Dyspareunia. *Journal of Sex and Marital Therapy, 1,* 234-241.

Waterman, C. K. & Chiauzzi, E. J. (1982). The role of orgasm in male and female sexual enjoyment. *Journal of Sex Research, 18*(2), 146-159.

Wiesberg, M. (1981). A note on female ejaculation. *Journal of Sex Research, 17*(1), 90-91.

Wiesmeier, E. & Forsythe, A. B. (1982). Sexual concerns and counseling needs of "normal" women attending a student health service women's clinic. *Journal of American College Health, 30*(5), 212-215.

Winokur, G., Guze, S. B. & Pfeiffer, E. (1959). Developmental and sexual factors in women: A comparison between control, neurotic, and psychotic groups. *American Journal of Psychiatry, 115,* 1097-1100.

Zilbergeld, B. (1980). Alternatives to couples counseling for sex problems: Group and individual therapy. *Journal of Sex and Marital Therapy, 6*(1), 3-18.

14

FEMINIST THERAPY:
IMPLICATIONS FOR PRACTITIONERS

Lynne Bravo Rosewater

Feminism and psychotherapy can be viewed as polarities: feminism the radical pole and psychotherapy the traditional pole. Feminism is a forward-looking ideology calling for action and change; psychotherapy is a more conservative ideology calling for adjustment and continuity. Combining the two can have powerful results for individual women as well as impact on mental health policy as it has been.

Traditional psychotherapics have been based on the medical model that looks for underlying pathology to cure by its specialized treatment. The basic assumption, as the phrase "mental illness' attests, is that patients are sick. Behavior is defined as pathological according to the majority view of societal needs. The question arises as to who decides what is pathological behavior. Chesler (1973), whose study was one of the first to document the damage the mental health profession was causing women, asserts that women are diagnosed as crazy either for underconforming or overconforming to sex role stereotypes. The classic Broverman, Broverman, Clarkson, Rosenkrantz, and Vogel study (1970), which confirmed mental health professionals' biases against women, delineated the double bind of women. They found therapists believed a woman cannot be a healthy woman AND a healthy person at the same time. Horner's (1981) study of women's achievement motivation found the same double standard: if a woman fails she is not living up to her own standards of performance; if she succeeds she is not living up to the societal's expectation of a feminine role. Wells (1977) has dubbed this phenomenom "society's femininty game: You win by losing" (p. 228). Ten years after the Chesler, Broverman, and Horner studies, Sherman (1980) reviewed 16 studies investigating sex role stereotyping of mental health standards and concludes: "Data indicate there is sex role stereotyping in mental health standards and that sex role discrepant behaviors are judged more maladjusted" (p. 60).

Feminist therapy, on the other hand, is one of the psychotherapies based on a presumption of health. Individuals' behaviors are seen as a function of being oppressed rather than confused or sick. Women are encouraged to separate their individual problems from those common to all women because of societal's oppression. New behavior skills are taught in a therapeutic educational manner. As Gilbert (1980) states, "The basic assumption underlying feminist therapy is that ideology, social structure and behavior are intricably woven" (p. 247). The feminist therapist, then, rejects the notion of therapist as social controller (Brown, in press) and instead sees her role as effecting change by inhancing individuals' problem-solving skills and political awareness (Wycoff, 1977).

Feminist therapy aims to integrate self-exploration and action (Mander & Rush, 1977). The basis for action is a positive rather than a negative focus. A 30-year-old female client of mine, in therapy with me for six months after previous treatment with a psychiatrist, articulated the difference:

> I think one reason therapy has worked so well for me with you is that you take things from a positive approach. . . .you approach it not as, "What is wrong with you?", but, "What is right with you?", where in the past it's been "What's wrong with you?" That's very destructive; it just automatically builds in a poor self image. With you, you're approaching it as, "Well let's look at what's good about you and then we'll try to solve the problems that are getting in your way of making you feel totally good and totally right.". . .It started off on a better foot, because I didn't feel like I was hopeless; I didn't feel like there was something dramatically wrong with me. I felt more like it's just that I've got a few problems that need to be straightened out. . . . I came into this very apprehensive, because the couple of times I did experience this (therapy) before and it was just wrong. . . . It just made things worse because. . . o.k., let's rip you apart to build you back together rather than o.k., let's start from where you are now and go forward. And that ripping apart process was totally unnecessary; it just brought me down to a low way down at the bottom to a point where I was almost having a nervous breakdown, and that's not constructive at all.

DIFFERENT PERSPECTIVES OF FEMINIST AND TRADITIONAL THERAPY

In a study of 50 women therapists, Bosma (1975) found that feminists rated clients shown in videotaped vignettes as stronger and less ill than did nonfeminists. Similarily, Brodsky and Hare-Mustin (1980) found that feminist therapists rate female clients as stronger and healthier than do nonfeminists. Kahn and Theurer (in press), in an attempt to measure the effectiveness of a course on counseling women given at the University of British Columbia, found that the 17 female graduate students who had taken the course had a greater awareness of gender role issues than the control group who had not taken the course. Further, they found that students who are interested in women as a special client group already hold liberal attitudes toward women.

Thus, the way a women is viewed significantly affects decisions about the problems in her life. Rawlings and Carter (1977) showed the dramatic difference between traditional therapy and feminist therapy in the conception of the problem, treatment goals, style of treatment, treatment outcome, and implied and explicit values. While the former was aimed at helping a woman "adjust" to her environment, the latter was aimed at validating the reality of the woman client's perceptions and supporting change rather than adjustment.

Miller (1976), discusses the need for a new viewpoint in therapy; which is to view behavior symptoms in a new light,

> no longer as defenses, maneuvers or other such tactics, but as struggles to preserve or express some deeply needed aspects of personal integrity in a milieu that will not allow for their direct expression. The task of the therapist then becomes the co-operative search for an understanding of those needs and an understanding of how they have been diverted or distorted. (p. 381)

Understanding those needs means seeing the problems from the individual's or woman's point of view. Traditional psychotherapy, though dealing primarily with women, defined their problems from the generic male viewpoint resulting in further oppression of women. Criticism of such psychoanalytic thinking has been rampant in the woman's movement. Women don't envy a man's penis; they envy his power (Thompson, 1973; Mander & Rush, 1977). Freud's viewpoint is too narrow, constricted by a biological and determanistic foundation, thereby reducing psychological qualities to anatomical causes (Horney, 1967). Most importantly, male-defined psychological theories, fashioned from studies of male development, valued "male" thinking. Caring, nurturing, and other relational thinking, which are female traits, were devalued. Miller (1976) addresses the necessity of revaluing female traits, which previously have been labeled "weaknesses," such as emotionality and vulnerability. Gilligan (1982), in the same vein, expresses the positive value of female style, which she has labled a "morality of care," a concern for the impact of decision-making, which, while different from, is not inferior to, the male concept of "impartial (i.e., unfeeling) justice."

THE NEED FOR A FEMINIST THEORY OF PERSONALITY

Thus far, a feminist theory of personality has been defined more by what it is not, than a clear doctrine in its own right. Lerman (1983), however, has taken a step in this direction by formulating a set of criteria for a feminist theory of personality: It should be clinically useful, that is, practical and easily applied to working with women. It should encompass all life-styles for women and address issues relevant to women. It should include as a basic premise that internal psychological reality exists separate and apart from the social circumstances in which women live. Last, and most important, the viewpoint should be female.

We may be closer than we think to developing a feminist theory of personality. What we may in fact be doing is taking the route backward. Theory usually develops first, then is followed by applications of the theory to practice. For feminists, however, experiential practice has come first. Feminist therapy's commitment to a political and philosophical base differentiates it from other therapies. The belief is that males and females should have equal opportunity for gaining personal, political-institutional, and economic power and that interaction between persons should be egalitarian (Rawlings & Carter, 1977). Thus, Lerman's suggestion that the concept "the personal is political" is a starting point for the development of such a feminist theory of personality: "In my view a strong possibility exists that, whatever the cultural set-up, emotional ills might most easily arise in the conflict between what a society says that a woman (or man) ought to be and what is actually in the nature of that particular person to become" (in press). Lerman seems to be suggesting that women's mental health is directly related to the degree women are valued in their culture for their personal attributes as well as for their performance at the roles society's policy dictates them to do. Policy, in this case, can create mental health problems!

CHANGING THE RELATIONSHIP BETWEEN CLIENT AND THERAPIST

An egalitarian therapist-client relationship does not mean both are equal, but is based on mutual respect for each other's skills. Therapists accept that they do not know what the client's perceptions are until she discloses them. Clients accept that the therapist's skills in understanding human behavior can help define her feelings, thoughts, and actions differently, to facilitate her personal growth. To actually behave in this manner radically changes the concept of therapy. Such therapy is not aimed at adjustment, as defined by the authoritative therapist, but rather at facilitating change. The client, not the therapist, defines change for her.

The feminist therapist listens to and believes in the strength of her client as well as all women. There is no room for rigid doctrine into which human experiences must be fit and packaged. How many incest victims are never heard because the therapist imagines that the client's revelation is imagined rather than real? How many women are never asked about the violence in their lives or are blamed for the violence they do experience? Rogers (1968) speaks of unconditional positive regard, the ability to see and appreciate the value in all people. Feminist therapy enhances this concept by respecting the expertise of clients as those who know, better than anyone else, what the quality and experience of their life has been.

Further, the gap between client and therapist is lessened by the feminist practice of appropriate self-disclosure. Women therapists share with their women clients the experiences of being second-class citizens. Thus, "by sharing our personal experiences of women's oppression, our struggles to overcome internalized fears, doubts and anger, and our growth to our present consciousness, the client begins to see that there is not the distinction between 'sick' client and 'healthy' therapist" (Smith & Siegel, in press).

Feminist therapy then involves a redefining of therapy. It demands new and innovative approaches. Rigidity is anathema; flexibility is a requirement. Like the figure/ground in a gestalt framework, feminist therapists need to learn to look and see differently, willing to believe that other images exist that have been there all along, but that we have never seen because our attention was focused elsewhere. An example of this type of rethinking, or cognitive restructuring, as it is called in behavioral terms, is: I was called by a local business group and asked to speak with management about leading a group for the depressed wives of about-to-be-transferred executives. Instead, it was my suggestion that I meet with the group to discuss the process of how decisions were made between husband and wife about transfer issues. I redefined the problem from one of what to do with the depressed wives after they had been moved to rather how to help them be clearer about the decision-making process before they moved.

Using cognitive restructuring techniques in therapy helps women redefine their environment to be more validating and supportive.

WHAT IS "MENTAL ILLNESS"?

Feminist therapists believe the whole arena of what has been traditionally defined as "mental illness" needs to be reconsidered. Kaplan (1983), in a provocative critique of the diagnostic procedures of the DSM-III, raises a critical issue: "masculine-biased assumptions about what behaviors are healthy and what behaviors are crazy were codified in DSM-II and are now codified in DSM-III, and thus influence and will continue to influence treatment rates" (p. 788). Using as an example the disproportionate amount of depression experienced by women, Kaplan says that such unhappiness for a woman "and her label of 'depressed' may be manifestations that she is scapegoated for society's illness, its unjust sex-role imperatives" (p. 789). Further, Kaplan raises the profound dilemma, also confronted by feminist therapy, that "it is difficult to say when society should be labeled as 'unjust' and when an individual should be labeled as 'crazy' (p. 789). Kaplan's argument is not whether there is a general tendency for all major categories in DSM-III to be given more frequently to women, as Williams and Spitzer (1983) argue in their rebuttal to Kaplan's article. Her issue is the assumption of sickness and the unwillingness, thus far, to equate the behavior described in DSM-III, for both women and men, with a reaction to living in a sexist society. My argument, added to those listed above, is that the value of feminist therapy and the implications of its use is its insistence on not concentrating on diagnosis per se, but rather on the *implications* of the diagnosis: that we treat the *source* of the problem, not merely the *symptoms*. Thus, as Porter (in press) argues, we need to see symptoms as "adaptive solutions to societal oppression rather than as individual expressions of pathology."

To treat the source of the problem, a policy change in the concept of our treatment modality is needed; it should look beyond the label given to a mental health problem to its consequence. If a woman is diagnosed as depressed, what assumptions underlie that label? Is it assumed that women are generally unhappy individuals? Is it assumed that depressed individuals are hopeless? Is the appropriate remedy psychotherapy or chemotherapy or shock treatments? What policy decisions follow the theories held about the causation of depression? A feminist analysis of depression sees it as originating from women's role in society. Radloff and Cox (1981) theorize that depression for women is a sequential model of learned susceptibility and precipitating factors. Therefore it is interesting to note that marriage has a positive effect for men, but a detrimental effect for women. Married women are at greater risk for depression, at the rate of two times that for men (Radloff & Cox, 1981). Thus, assuming her rightful role of mother and wife may be hazardous to a woman's health! A feminist treatment of depression, therefore, centers on an examination of the environmental impact on the woman in treatment, historically and currently. Depression may be viewed as a coping skill (Kaplan, 1983) or as a healthy reaction to an unjust situation. But that doesn't make the depression go away! The role expectations for women in our society and whether a given role is right for any particular woman needs to be critically examined. Feminist therapy aids in the reevaluating and renegotiating of specific roles and the rules governing those roles.

In the endeavor to redefine rules and roles, there are several important topics with which feminist therapy concerns itself. One of the foremost is anger and how women can be encouraged to feel it, recognize it, express it, and deal with it when directed toward them from other people. Sexuality and self-nurturance are other important issues. Feminist therapy respects a woman's self-determination of her own sexual preference and her right to this choice without harassment. Feminist therapy respects that a woman's body is her own and that any attempt to violate it is an unacceptable act of violence. The right of choice around reproduction is an integral part of feminist therapy, extending from a woman's decision whether or not to have children to the need for support for those women who choose to have children and are unable to conceive. Along with sexism, agism and racism are unacceptable. Feminist therapy respects the aging process, the bias against the aged, especially women, and is sensitive to life transition periods and the trauma of loss and separation. Feminist therapy is sensitive to the double burden for women of color. In addition, feminist therapy addresses economic issues such as fee structures that relate to the relative value of the services rendered, as well as the woman's ability to pay.

Feminist therapy changes the concept of treatment by the assumption that behavior that is typically viewed as negative may be valuable. The starting point is a recognition that the client is trying to cope as best she can. This point is well stated by Smith and Siegel (in press) in their analysis of power used by women. Rather than devaluing covert power (i.e., because it is typically feminine and passive), they view it as a viable and effective way of dealing. They help give positive reinforcement to a woman client that she is indeed powerful. They then move on to help that woman be aware that there are other ways of being powerful that she may want to learn, so she can have greater choice in how to create change in her life. Thus, redefining previously labeled negative behaviors as acceptable behavior may produce a society of women who behave differently and will have other policy implications; for example, more women will be seen as unacceptable wives and mothers or may not want to adopt these roles at all, changing the family structure in very profound ways. Science fiction written by feminists such as Ursula LaGuin and Marge Piercy give glimpses of what it could be like.

Too often the focus of treatment has been on what the woman has not done. The battered woman who has not left the batterer is one such example. However, what that woman has done is stay alive, a formidable task for most battered women. The starting point of feminist therapy with such a woman is acknowledgement of those coping skills she has developed. Rape victims are relabeled as survivors, both as a method of avoiding the notion of the woman as perpetual victim and as a way of acknowledging her strength. Not willing to further victimize the survivors of domestic violence and rape, feminist therapy demands a new viewpoint of mothers of incest victims; they are often blamed for not protecting their children, even when they cannot stop the abuse without causing further harm. Current research on domestic violence is illustrating that many mothers of children abused by their fathers were themselves victims of that man's abuse (Walker, 1981, in press). In addition, as Finkelhor (1981) points out, the mother becomes relevant only because the offender has already set off an antisocial train of events.

When women's behavior is reassessed, the notion of passive, "feminine" behavior as second class changes. Choice, a key concept for the feminist movement, is also a key concept in feminist therapy. In my experience, most clients seeking psychological assistance have a restricted repertoire of behaviors from which to choose. It is not that the behavior they possess is necessarily "bad," but, rather it is limited. Women who use therapy to expand their personal growth must expand their behavioral repertoire so they can make more informed choices. Yet, there are consequences to which clinicians must be sensitive. Hence, while women may learn to become more assertive, they may also lose their job or their significant relationship in that process. Fodor (in press), in her critique of assertiveness training, points out that one of the problems with assertiveness training has been insensitivity to the problems greater assertiveness may cause women in the world at large. Thus, without an accompanying policy change to respect assertive women (if such were indeed possible), women who incorporate feminist values and behaviors need to be prepared to deal with the consequences.

Feminist therapy encourages the learning of new behaviors, as well as the acceptance of old behaviors. Since this learning takes place in an egalitarian atmosphere, the views of both client and therapist are equally respected. The ultimate decisions are the client's alone to make. The therapist takes on a new role, though, not found in traditional therapy—that of advocate. Since feminist therapy is based on the commitment to equal opportunity for personal, political, and socio-economic power, the therapist becomes an advocate of social change. This position has raised ethical issues such as asking how the therapist can remain objective and scientific while being an advocate. Dual and multiple role relationships need to be more precisely defined.

FEMINIST ADVOCACY

The meaning of an egalitarian relationship is not that the therapist and client are equal in privilege and power, but rather that the therapist will use her privilege and power for, rather than against, her client (Brown, in press). This interpretation is consistent with the American Psychologicial Association code of ethics, which mandates that psychologists use their skills to be of benefit to their clients. The concept of therapist as advocate is found increasingly in feminist literature. Walker (1981, 1983), has pioneered the field of feminist forensic psychology. Using her own research as a basis for testimony (1979, 1981), Walker, in cooperation with attorneys, developed the self-defense plea used by many battered women who have killed their batterer. Paramount to this defense effort is the necessity of having an expert witness testify to explain the battered woman's syndrome to a judge and jury (Walker, in press). Similar expert witness testimony can also be used to identify and explain Rape Trauma Syndrome and the psychological injury cause by assaults. In a similar vein, I have used feminist test interpretations in court in both criminal and domestic cases to assist the court in its fact finding, whatever issue brought the woman there (Rosewater, in press, a). There is a need to reinterpret traditional personality tests in light of increasing data on the psychology of women (Brodsky & Hare-Mustin, 1980; Franks & Rothblum, 1983; Gilligan, 1982; Miller, 1976). My research developed an MMPI profile for battered women (Rosewater, 1982), which found the battered woman's profile similar to a profile for chronic schizophrenic (Lanyon, 1968), leading me to question whether women previously diagnosed as chronic schizophrenics may, instead, have been battered women. Test interpretation integrating the knowledge base from psychology of women studies will be used to refute a mis-diagnosis (Rosewater, in press, b). Criticism that the mental health system has harmed women (Chesler, 1973; Wycoff, 1977) can be overcome through the use of such advocacy.

Feminist therapists can advocate for clients by helping them decide when to take legal action on their behalf. In Seattle, a lawsuit has been filed at the instigation of a feminist therapist to challenge a state law that gives individuals a limit of one year past majority (age 21) to file lawsuits for injuries that occurred when they were minors (Taylor v. Taylor, 1982). The contention of the lawsuit is that for cases of incest, this law is discriminatory, as many incest victims are not aware or able to realize how they have been harmed until long past age 21. Other groups of women psychologists and women lawyers are considering a variety of policy changes to facilitate healing, compensate women for damages, and, perhaps, deter men from committing such acts.

Sex discrimination and sexual harassment cases provide another avenue for feminist legal action. Feminist therapists whose clients have been sexually exploited by previous therapists can encourage them to explore the options and consequences of filing lawsuits against those men (usually) for punitive damages. Feminist therapists are often willing to testify against their colleagues who sexually exploit clients (see Chapter 11). Physically, sexually, and psychologically abused women may also seek legal redress for physical and psychological injuries by filing civil lawsuits, as well as criminal charges. The emotional strain of a lawsuit is such that many women require supportive therapy while going through it, but, if successful, allows a major resolution difficult to gain in therapy alone.

Feminist therapy includes education for women on issues of rape, incest, body image, self-defense, sexual preference, domestic violence, legal rights, abortion, birth control, pregnancy, childbirth, and divorce. Advocacy programs, such as rape crisis centers, battered women's shelters, self-help divorce groups, and women's centers, initiated and managed by feminists, have successfully created public policy changes in how women are treated: for example, improving police sensitivity and hospital emergency room treatment following a rape; in sensitizing courts to the amount of child support needed by single parents, in identifying physically abused women and children when they seek public or private medical treatment; in instituting state domestic violence laws that allow the battered women with probable cause to have the batterer removed from the home and held in jail for 24 hours. Feminist therapists are both aware of these services and often instrumental in setting them up and directing clients to use them. As a result women do get better services from many institutions designed to help them.

CONCLUSIONS

Feminist therapy has grown and matured. Dogmatic at its inception, like any new philosophic endeavor, the need for a politically correct feminist stance has relaxed to permit a wide variety of acceptable positions. In this maturing process feminist therapy has been rethought and redefined to include some of the concepts discussed in this chapter: feminist advocacy and feminist test interpretation; greater flexibility in the use of sliding fee scales; a reassessment of the methodology of assertiveness training; and a clarification of what is an egalitarian client/therapist relationship. The constant focus of this change has been the advancement toward good quality care for women.

In assessing the implications of feminist therapy for the treatment of women, what is most apparent is the need to understand the developmental processes of women. In the field of psychology, where the research has predominantly normed on male development and male thinking, there is an urgent need to research female development and female thinking. In that same vein, we need to value female process as much as we do male process. Thus all therapists need to consider what their biases are in assessing behavior as positive or negative and how we have arrived at those conclusions.

The value feminist therapy offers to the mental health profession is a new way of looking at individuals—male as well as female—that is more positive and constructive, that equates problems with inequity rather than pathology, that treats the source of the problem rather than just the symptoms, and that values change rather than adjustment. Out of an egalitarian and social activist position, feminist therapy, with its insistence that the personal is political, sees that the sickness lies with the society, not the individual, and hence makes advocacy a vital part of the therapy process.

REFERENCES

Bosma, B. J. (1975). Attitudes of women therapists toward women clients, or a comparative study of feminist therapy. *Smith College Studies in Social Work, 46*,53-54.

Brodsky, A. M., & Hare-Mustin, R. (Eds.). (1980). *Women and psychotherapy*. New York: Guilford Press.

Broverman, I. K., Broverman, D. M., Clarkson, F. E., Rosenkrantz, P. & Vogel, S. R. (1970). Sex-role stereotypes and clinical judgements of mental health. *Journal of Consulting Psychology, 34,* 1-7.

Brown, L. S. (in press). Ethics and business practice in feminist therapy (in press). In L. B. Rosewater & L. E. Walker (Eds.), *A handbook of feminist theraphy.* New York: Springer.

Chesler, P. (1973). *Woman and madness.* New York: Avon Books.

Finkelhor, D. (1981). *Risk factors in the sexual victimization of children.* A paper presented at the National Conference for Family Violence Researchers, Durham, NH, July.

Fodor, I. E. (in press). Assertiveness training for the 80's: Moving beyond the personal. In L. B. Rosewater & Walker, L. E. (Eds.), *A handbook of feminist therapy.* New York: Springer.

Franks, V., & Rothblum, E. D. (Eds.). (1983). *The stereotyping of women: Its effects on mental health.* New York: Springer.

Gilbert, L. A. (1980). Feminist therapy. In A. Brodsky, & R. Hare-Mustin (Eds.), *Woman and psychotherapy* (pp. 245-265). New York: Guilford Press.

Gilligan, C. (1982). *In a different voice: Psychological theory and women's development.* Cambridge: Harvard Univ. Press.

Horner, K. (1967) *Feminine psychology.* New York: W. W. Norton.

Horner, M. (1981). Femininity and successful achievement: A basic inconsistency. In J. M. Bardwick, E. Douvan, M. S. Horner, & D. Gutman, (Eds.), *Feminine personality and conflict.* Westport: Greenwood Press.

Kahn, S. E., & Theurer, G. (in press). Graduate education and evaluation in counseling women: A case study. In L. B. Rosewater & L. E. Walker (Eds.), *A handbook of feminist therapy.* New York: Springer.

Kaplan, M. (1983). A woman's view of DSM-III. *Amercian Psychologist, 38* (7), 786-792.

Lanyon, R. I. (1968). *A handbook of MMPI group profiles.* Minneapolis: Univ. of Minnesota Press.

Lerman, H. (1983). *Criteria for a feminist personality theory: Some rudimentary concepts.* A proposition paper presented at the second annual Advance Feminist Therapy Institute, Washington, DC: May.

Lerman, H. (in press). Some barriers to the development of a feminist theory of personality. In L. B. Rosewater & L. E. Walker (Eds.), *A handbook of feminist therapy*. New York: Springer.

Mander, A. V., & Rush, A. K. (1977). *Feminism as therapy*. New York: Random House.

Miller, J. B. (1976). *Toward a new psychology of women*. Boston: Beacon Press.

Porter, N. (in press). Supervision from a feminist perspective. In L. B. Rosewater & L. E. Walker (Eds.), *A handbook of feminist therapy*. New York: Springer.

Radloff, L. S., & Cox, S. (1981). Sex differences in depression in relation to learned susceptibility. In Cox, S. (Ed.), *Female psychology: The emerging self*, 2nd ed. (pp. 334-363). New York: St. Martin's Press.

Rawlings, E. I., & Carter, D. K. (Eds.). (1977). *Psychotherapy for women*. Springfield IL: Charles C Thomas.

Rogers, C. R. (1968). *Client-centered therapy*. Boston: Houghton Mifflin.

Rosewater, L. B. (1982). The development of an MMPI profile for battered women. Doctoral dissertation for the Union Graduate School.

Rosewater, L. B. (in press, a). Feminist interpretations of traditional testing. In L. B. Rosewater & L. E. Walker (Eds.), *A handbook of feminist therapy*. New York: Springer.

Rosewater, L. B. (in press, b). Schizophrenic, borderline or battered? In L. B. Rosewater & L. E. Walker (Eds.) *A handbook of feminist therapy*. New York: Springer.

Sherman, J. A. (1980). Therapist attitudes and sex-role stereotyping. In A. M. Brodsky & Hare-Mustin, R. (Eds.), *Women and psychotherapy* (pp. 35-66). New York: The Guilford Press.

Smith, A., & Siegel, R. (in press). Feminist therapy: Redefining power for the powerless. in L. B. Rosewater & L. E. Walker (Eds.), *A handbook of feminist therapy*.

Thompson, C. (1973). Cultural pressures in the psychology of women. In J. B. Miller (Ed.), *Psychoanalysis and women* (pp. 69-84). New York: Penguin Books.

Walker, L. E. (1979). *The battered woman*. New York: Harper & Row.

Walker, L. E. (1981). Battered woman syndrome study. Report to N.I.M.H. Grant #R01MH30147.

Walker, L. E. (in press). Feminist forensic psychology. In L. B. Rosewater & L. E. Walker (Eds.), *A handbook of feminist therapy*. New York: Springer.

Wells, T. (1977). Up the management ladder. In E. I. Rawlings & D. K. Carter, (Eds.), *Psychotherapy for women* (pp. 221-249). Springfield IL: Charles C Thomas.

Williams, J. B., & Spitzer, R. L. (1983). The issue of sex bias in DSM-III: A critique of "A woman's view of DSM-III" by Marcie Kaplan. *American Psychologist, 38*(7), 793-797.

Wycoff, H. (1977). Radical psychiatry for women. In E. I. Rawlings & D. K. Carter (Eds.), *Psychotherapy for women* (pp. 370-391). Springfield, IL: Charles C Thomas.

15

MEDIA PSYCHOLOGY AND PUBLIC POLICY

Laura S. Brown

North Americans today take for granted that the media, both print and electronic, have a strong influence and impact on the affairs of daily life. We have become fond, as a culture, of quoting MacLuhan's now hackneyed line that "the medium is the message" as if we were certain that this were the truth. Our legislative bodies have created laws that enshrine popular beliefs about the power of the media to affect the hearts and minds of their audience. Electronic media, for example, are bound by the Fairness Doctrine of the Federal Communications Commission, which requires all radio and television stations to make air time available to all sides of a public debate, be it the presidential elections or a local school levy. The metamessage communicated by the presence of this law is that the electronic media are so powerful that they must be carefully controlled, in order to permit at least the appearance of equal access and impact to all shades of opinion. To judge from what is written about the American media, either by its detractors or its proponents (see any issue of the *Columbia Journalism Review*), it is seen as an extremely powerful shaper of American attitudes and behaviors. The general public has become accustomed to blaming, or hearing others place blame, on the media for the various ills plaguing our country. The enormous stir generated in the federal government by ABC's broadcast of "The Day After," a fictional piece about the potential aftermath of nuclear war, is a case in point. The reactions of the administration and its supporters indicated their judgement that this fictional piece, portrayed on television, could be a powerful shaper of public attitudes and policies regarding nuclear arms and related issues.

In the past, the majority of those practicing the manipulation of public attitudes and behavior via the media were either actors or journalists, primarily the latter. Journalism is a profession that has chronically scored poorly on opinion surveys regarding the respect that a particular profession gets from the general public. Until the Watergate-related heroics of Woodward and Bernstein, most journalists were publically perceived as "hacks." The ability of journalists to influence opinion on matters of public policy was related to their skill as a writer, and to the editorial policies of the medium in which they published. But journalists were not regarded as experts on human behavior. Whenever such expertise was needed, journalists sought a cogent quote from a member of the designated experts, the helping professions and behavioral sciences.

It is in the realm of human behavior that much public policy is made. Governmental programs for the prevention of child abuse and domestic violence, laws prohibiting discrimination on grounds of race or gender, curricula on sexuality in public schools, these and many other things have been legislated to reflect public beliefs on matters that have long been considered the purview of the social and behavioral sciences and/or the mental health professions.

It is thus signifcant that, since the middle of the 1970s, members of the various mental health professions have begun to function as media personalities. Media mental health professionals (MMHPs) perform a variety of tasks. The majority of them work as the hosts of radio call-in talk shows, where the audience can call for direct advice, solutions to personal problems, and referrals to agencies and therapists. Several MMHPs work in television, either doing simulated therapy, or making three minute behavioral science commentaries in the context of news or magazine shows. Others write, replicating Dear Abby, or popularizing the work of the behavioral sciences, as is the case with *Psychology Today* magazine, now owned by the American Psychological Association. Whatever the setting, the MMHP is in a position to directly influence the general public, by being able to share, as an expert, information regarding human behavior. Because MMHPs need not filter their work through other journalists, they are in greater control of what information gets to the public, and thus are a powerful force for influencing the attitudes of the general public in ways that may have implications for the formation of public policy regarding mental health.

The impact that the experts of the social and behavioral sciences do have on public policy can be inferred in a variety of ways. Court rulings on school desegregation, programs such as Head Start, the phenomenon of the community mental health center are all reflections of the body politic responding to the expertise of mental health and behavioral science professionals. Impact can also be inferred from backlash. When Senator Orrin Hatch is moved to write, in the September, 1982 issue of the *American Psychologist* that psychology research and practice must cease to find support for "humanistic" values, and then subtly threatens funding cuts if we cannot lend the weight of our discipline to a more traditionalist value system, he is sending psychology the message that we do make public impact, although not in the direction he would wish. In the past, however, the findings have been perceived, however correctly, as not representing "common sense" or the will of the public, but rather the opinions of only a specially informed discipline. Imagine how much more powerful a stance taken by the mental health professions might be if it were perceived by legislators as representing the general consensus of a large number of voters. The MMHP, by having direct contact with the public, is in a position to catalyse a public groundswell on behalf of a particular issue of mental health policy, and to create support for the policy that would be more difficult for the average vote-eager politician to ignore than it would be if the support came only from a professional association or a group of university professors.

A number of factors enhance the MMHP's capacity for impact on mental health policy. Many MMHPs are at the top of their particular media markets. The proliferation of radio call-in shows reflects the enormous success of the first MMHP, Toni Grant, a Los Angeles psychologist who has been a top ratings getter for almost a decade in the highly competitive LA radio market. MMHPs can find themselves elevated to the status of a local popular culture idol. Listeners and readers may quote the local "radio shrink" or psychology columnist to friends, spouses, and their own therapists, seeing that particular MMHP as the ultimate authority on human behavior because of the power of that person's position in the media. Radio call-in hosts, because of their very immediate and personal contact with their large listening and calling audience, have a particularly great potential for becoming powerful public figures and, consequently, powerful shapers of mental health policy.

The composition of the audience of an MMHP is another factor in the MMHP's potential to shape mental health policy. The bulk of the listeners to radio call-in shows are younger women, mostly well educated, and with good incomes—the cream of the radio advertising demographics markets. Advertisers find such programs to be prime time for their products. Political announcements seem to do well in this setting, simply because the juxtaposition of "Hi, I'm Dr. Radio

Shrink" with "Vote for Jane Doe" has a way of creating a perception in the audience that Dr. Radio Shrink is endorsing Jane Doe (a perception shared by several of my colleagues, who expressed to me their surprise at my "endorsement" of a particular candidate whose ads ran during my program). The audience is intimately involved and affectively stimulated by the events heard on the air during a call-in show; Bruce Marr, the radio programmer who developed the Toni Grant show, and several others, calls it a soap opera with your own life as the main story (1980). The combination of immediacy and emotional arousal creates a sort of electronically enhanced transference relationship between an MMHP and her or his audience, and increases the probability that an already civic-minded group of listeners will develop opinions on matters related to mental health policy. An MMHP's attitudes and on-air or in-print statements regarding current social issues can have a large, although not currently measureable impact, on the mental health policies supported or opposed by an MMHP's audience. The Association for Media Psychology (AMP) has recognized this potential for influence in its code of ethics and standards when it states that "it is incumbent upon the media professional to be knowledgeable in those areas which will inevitably arise, i.e., basic questions about marriage, child care and discipline, sexual relations, contraception, homosexuality, etc. Media Mental Health Professionals are, in addition, sensitive to the needs of minority and special interest groups" (Association for Media Psychology, 1982). The direct and indirect connections between these issues that are commonly raised in the work of an MMHP and legislation that creates mental health policy are observable in eveything from laws defining and mandating the report of child abuse to policies such as the so-called "squeal rule", proposed by the Reagan administration to require family planning programs to report prescriptions of contraceptives to minors to the parents of those individuals. The MMHP, having a combination of implied expertise and media access, is in a position to influence this and similar legislation by having an impact on members of the public and on legislators who are writing public policy.

Some factors may act to limit the usefulness of an MMHP as a catalyst for mental health policy. A station manager or newspaper editor may declare a particular topic off-limits, too "threatening" or "depressing", or not in keeping with the image of the setting in which the MMHP works. An inaccurate picture of who has emotional problems may emerge from a radio call-in show if station policy is to screen out older or obviously depressed callers, as is the case in many settings (Rubinstein, 1981). Or, the MMHP may have complete freedom of speech, and may use that freedom to promulgate attitudes that are neither in line with current research in the behavioral-sciences nor helpful to the "minority and special interest groups" identified by AMP. Lesbian and gay activists have reported the case of one widely syndicated radio call-in host who persisted in telling all gay and lesbian callers that they could be "cured," have their sexual orientation changed, even though the callers had not sought advice on being "cured" and although such a perspective flies in the face of current research on homosexuality. Although it is not possible to measure directly the impact of such MMHP behavior on public policy, it seems possible to infer that listeners who are undecided on the issue of gay rights may turn against it, and even vote against gay rights legislation on the grounds that "Dr. Radio Shrink says that gays can be cured if they want to be."

There is some evidence to suggest that a well-informed MMHP can have a positive influence on public policy related to mental health. A Seattle MMHP, Jennifer James, became active in creating an organization for the prevention of child sexual abuse, an area that had been a research interest prior to her entry into the media field. Her endorsement of the work of this group, the information she gave on air regarding the effects of child sexual abuse and techniques for prevention, and her participation in fundraising activities for work toward the prevention of child sexual abuse created a large amount of public support. Policy changes have included the creation of legislation in Washington state admitting hearsay evidence from social workers and parents when an abused child is too young to be a credible witness in a trial and the inception of a citywide public school curriculum that raises the consciousness of children from kindergarten through high school regarding child sexual abuse. James utilized the electronic transference, encouraged her audience to identify with her concerns on this issue, and made herself physically available as a reinforcer for volunteer workers, with clear and lasting impact on mental health policy.

Having established that media psychology and MMHPs can exercise profound and important impact on issues of mental health policy in general, how then can this potential be extrapolated to understand how MMHPs can affect policies specifically as they affect women? How can feminist psychologists and other mental health professionals concerned with women's issues interact with MMHPs in such a way as to influence their work?

First, it may be helpful to target several subgroups of women who might be more directly affected by public mental health policies. It is such a group of women whose lives are most likely to be influenced by what an MMHP says (or does not say). A group generally benefitted by the work of MMHPs, and one composed largely of women, is the group of present and future psychotherapy consumers. MMHPs generate an interest in therapy, and a demand for high-quality, low-cost mental health services. The admonition to "see a therapist" is probably the most common piece of advice given by MMHPs working in any medium. As a consequence, individuals who might never have considered therapy begin to seek it out.

In addition, MMHPs publicize the existence and content of standards of ethical practice in the psychotherapy professions. They have made the public aware of existing laws regulating therapists, and of the gaps in consumer protection created by the lack of licensure provisions in many locations for nondoctoral-level providers. The MMHP can, and often does, talk about the rights that an individual has as a consumer of psychotherapy. On occasion, callers or writers to MMHPs have inquired as to the ethical nature of the therapy they are currently receiving, only to discover that sexual relationships with a client, for example, are not techniques normally taught in therapy training programs nor considered approved practice by the professions. In such cases, MMHPs have acted as a bridge between an aggrieved therapy client and lawyers or state boards of licensure. All of this can have, and on occasion, has had, a variety of effects on mental health policy, both in general and as it affects women. Audiences of MMHPs are likely to become active in pushing for more funding or low-cost mental health services, or may see therapy as less of a luxury item, and thus more a service that should be easily available. Audiences are also likely to see the need for licensure and other consumer protection legislation as a result of listening to or reading about abuses of psychotherapy via the work of the MMHP. An MMHP can serve as a network resource, announcing meetings and/or encouraging and supporting the formation of consumer groups, and sharing addresses of professional association so that consumers have a target for concerns and/or complaints.

Although it is unclear whether such legislation does indeed protect consumers from abusive therapists, it is clear that consumers become more aware of what constitutes abuses of therapy when, as a result of MMHP educations efforts, the parameters of good and ethical therapy become a part of public consciousness. An example of this process in action can be found in the Seattle-area group called Stop Abuse By Counselors (Stop ABC). Its membership consists primarily of women who had been sexually abused by therapists, and have chosen to turn to activism as a means of preventing further such abuses by other, primarily unlicensed, mental health practitioners. The group's largely female membership reflects the most recent findings on the phenomenon of sexual abuse of therapy clients by therapists (Bouhoutsos, Holroyd, Lerman, Forer, & Greenberg, 1983), where the female therapy client makes up the majority of victims in cases studied. Stop ABC became well-known to potential members and offending counselors both as a result of publicity given to the group by MMHPs. Thus empowered, the group's members have been able to introduce counselor licensing laws at both state and local levels, and have received positive responses to their efforts because there was a groundswell of public support for their work. Rather than being publicly perceived as unusual cases or "crazy ladies" with a vendetta against their therapists (an image insinuated by local non-MMHP media writers covering the group when it first emerged), the group found fertile ground for their legislative efforts and were seen as believable, in part as a result of the educative efforts of local MMHPs regarding the prevalance of abuse in psychotherapy.

Another effect that an MMHP might have on the creation of mental health policy as it affects women, is in regard to funding for specialty training in the area of therapy with women. Graduate programs in the helping professions have begun to tailor the dimensions of training given students to meet with needs for services as defined by funding agencies such as NIMH. For example, current training grants for clinical psychology programs reflect a current federal policy emphasis on working with health psychology, the aged, and young children. If the audiences of MMHPs became aware of the need for eliminating sexism in the training of help professionals, there would be the potential for eventual impact on funding sources. Legislators and potential legislators are among those who read or listen to MMHPs. An MMHP well-informed about developments in the psychology of women could educate those who make policy in ways that could directly affect the allocation of funding. The reader noting the subjunctive case of this paragraph will recognize that, in order to have such influence over the long term, MMHPs must be well educated in the psychology of women. Consequently, it becomes important for specialists in this field to work as MMHPs, or to interact frequently with MMHPs in their geographical areas.

Aside from the large group of current and potential female therapy clients who might be affected by the work of an MMHP, there are several subgroups of women whose concerns surface frequently as topics for media psychology. These groups of women can derive direct benefit or harm from public mental health policies, and are more likely to gain benefit when the public and lawmakers are well informed, rather than working from popular mythologies and misconceptions. These groups of women include: battered women, single parents, displaced homemakers, women working in nontraditional careers, lesbians, and survivors of sexual assault, and their families.

Women in battering relationships constitute a population that is still under identified and underserved. Although there now exists a body of sound psychological research demonstrating the ways in which a woman becomes vulnerable to and then dependent upon a battering man (Walker, 1979), the development of fully funded services for battered women has often been hampered by public attitudes that such women "are asking for it" or "could leave if they only wanted to, if they weren't masochists, and so forth." Spokespersons for the New Right, with Phyllis Schlafly in the lead, have attacked funding for battered women's shelters, calling these refuges, "R and R facilities for lazy or disgruntled housewives" (Schlafly, 1980). Funding for battered women's services is often perceived by legislators as a frill or an extra, serving a small, specialty population.

Well-informed MMHPs can have a positive effect on this phenomenon by using their access to the public ear to make available good and current information regarding battered women. They can cite books by experts, such as Walker (1979) or NiCarthy (1982), can encourage battered women and formerly battered women to call a radio show or be interviewed for a written piece, can publicize the statistics regarding battering rates to make the commonality of the phenomenon more apparent. They can work counter to the trend observed and commented upon by Steinem (1981, 1983), a trend in the media that finds a battered *man* a newsworthy item, but a trend that discards the battering of large numbers of women as the "ho-hum" status quo. MMHPs can clarify for the policymaking public who the batterers and their victims truly are. They can also discuss, in a sympathetic manner, the issue of battered women who kill in self-defense, thus having an influence on potential jurors in self-defense cases. They can use their forum in print or on the airwaves to publicize problems in current public policies as they pertain to battered women. In one such situation, an MMHP called public attention to the murders of two battered women by their battering husbands, and to the fact that both victims had been dropped through the cracks of the local legal system. The publicity resulted in a response from the chief of police in the jurisdiction where the murders had occurred, from a state legislator who had influence on the question of funding for therapy for women on public assistance, and from judges who handed out and enforced no-contact orders on batterers. Policies and procedures for police handling battering complaints were changed to increase the degree of outreach made to a battered woman and enforcement of no-contact orders became a priority. Public policy changed because of the publicity generated by an MMHP.

MMHPs can also have a more subtle effect on public policy related to battered women by bringing the audience into closer contact with the phenomenon. Listeners to a radio call-in show can hear a woman's real pain and dilemmas, and may develop a degree of understanding and empathy that may not have previously existed when the topic of battering was one that they could avoid because it did not enter their own lives. Such heightened empathy has the potential for heightening interest in the issue, and consequently, public policy decisions.

Survivors of sexual assault and their families are a group of women who can be similarly affected by the policies legislated by the public. As battered women, these survivors of rape or child sexual assault have become more publicly visible. This visibility, often in the form of television "docudramas" has raised public awareness, but at the same time, the media have served to implant myths about sexually assaulted women and girls even more firmly in the public mind. A poorly informed or myth-ridden MMHP is particularly in a position to do damage. In one instance, a radio MMHP responded to an incestuous father who had been removed from his home, and who felt misunderstood and victimized by the court system. The MMHP in this case was psychoanalytically trained and proceeded to sympathize on-air with her caller, stating that many reports by sexually assaulted children were false and fantasies, and that the local sexual assault center was, indeed, "unfair" to suspected sexual assailants. Because of the power of the electronic transference, and because of the large number of people in the MMHP's audience, the potential for harm and the destruction of positive public policies was great in this instance. In this case, angered audience members contacted the agency that had been vilified as too victim-oriented on air. Staff members embarked upon an intensive educational campaign, aimed at the MMHP, who recanted her on-air stand several weeks later. Because the agency in this case was publicly funded, its money and services to sexually assaulted women and children could have been jeopardized had sufficient members of the public responded to this MMHP's miseducation.

As with battered women, survivors of sexual assault are often hidden from public view, and thus, can have their existance and numbers ignored. MMHPs who effectively utilize their medium to give the audience direct contact with these women can bring the issue and the consequences of sexual assault into the homes of their audience. As the public learns that women can be raped by their husbands, that rape happens to women of all ages and races, that one-quarter of all girls are sexually assaulted, often by adult relatives, public policy changes may occur to reflect that new awareness. A general public aware of the reality and frequency of marital rape is more likely to press its legislators to enact marital rape laws than would be a general public unaware of the reality and informed by myths.

Women whose lives do not run within the boundaries of traditional role norms may find themselves impeded, not only by the struggles they must engage in within themselves, but also by the lack of social and cultural support systems and the presence of social and cultural barriers. Single parents, women in nontraditional careers, and displaced homemakers have in common that they must continually confront a culture that is critical of their position and/or choices in life. Popular mythology holds that women without men are losers, that they have failed at their task as "nice women," or that they are lazy and incapable of coping with the multiple demands of their roles. Women working in nontraditional jobs are mythologized as wanting to take jobs away from men who need them, or as disturbed in some way because they do not "adjust" to traditional women's interests. Such mythologies can have a detrimental effect on such publicly supported or policy-created phenomena as displaced homemaker programs, day care centers, apprenticeship training programs for women, job sharing and flex-time. Yet all of these are necessary for the mental health of women who, either out of choice or necessity, do not conform to traditional images of women.

MMHPs can shape public perceptions of nontraditional women. They can share information about the success of programs for displaced homemakers, thus encouraging listeners and readers to support new or continued public funding for such programming, which is still regarded in many locales as an unnecessary extra. They can cite data showing the impact of raising children in a home with a mother who works outside of the household, or in a home where the mother is the only parent. MMHPs can respond to the concerns of callers, listeners, and readers about the myths that abound in our society regarding the bad effects of mothers who work for pay. By using their authority as mental health professionals, they can comment on the recent rash of popular parenting books of a neo-Freudian persuasion that insist on a mother's presence at home with her children for the first one, or three, or five years of life. They can speak to the importance of nontraditional career role models in children's career choice, and dispel myths about the relationship of a nontraditional career to an individual's sexual orientation. It cannot be overstressed that the media in general regard women's success in nontraditional careers, women's positive feelings about day care for their children or women's need for job retraining after the loss of a homemaker position, as unnewsworthy items. As with women who are against equality, women who suffer pains of guilt over working outside their homes and women electricians who give it all up for modeling are the targets of popular media. MMHPs, merely by being up-to-date on basic survey research in any of these areas, can serve to reverse the trend. Their status as mental health professionals lends added authority to their words, and to their choice of topics. Those MMHPs who make judicious use of the electronic transference can have an impact on public attitudes regarding nontraditional women. As always, changed public attitudes can result in changed public policy where women's needs and mental health are concerned.

A final group of women who stand to be directly affected by the work of MMHPs are lesbians. Lesbians are as invisible in media psychology as elsewhere in American culture. Several factors acccount for this. There are no openly lesbian or gay MMHPs. This reflects the conservatism of the media business. Although most media outlets are bound by some sort of nondiscrimination clause, either local or union imposed, openly lesbian and gay male media workers are kept out of the public eye with amazing consistency. What is perceived to go down poorly with "middle America" is not admitted to media visibility. Thus, the lack of lesbian MMHPs mirrors a lack of lesbian journalists anywhere outside the pages of *Ms. magazine*. Calls and letters from self-identified lesbians are often screened off the air and out of print, reflecting media management fears of "guilt by association." This invisibility is one of the most potent barriers faced by lesbians when attempting to change public attitudes. If the audiences of an MMHP never hear or read of a lesbian who, like a heterosexual woman, is trying to communicate better with her partner or parent her children more effectively, then they are not likely to see that lesbians and gay men are anything other than creatures of myth. And if an MMHP deals with a parent of a lesbian by sympathizing with this "terrible" thing that has happened, rather than by gently confronting homophobia and offering a referral to a Parents of Gays group, then that MMHP will have contributed to negative public attitudes about lesbians.

MMHPs can educate their audience very effectively about the realities of being lesbian. They can encourage lesbian callers and writers, can speak about research on lesbian mothers, can comment on custody battles that have made local news in a lesbian-affirmative manner. They can dispel mythologies about the etiology of homosexuality, can interview lesbian therapists or activists, and can talk about the positive mental health benefits that accrue from anti discrimination laws and positive lesbian role models for lesbian children and adolescents. The MMHP who encourages lesbian callers or writers who are uncomfortable with their lesbianism to seek lesbian-affirmative therapy and help in dealing with internalized homophobia can confront popular mythology that there are no happy lesbians, or that lesbians can and should attempt to change their sexual orientation if they are oppressed by their oppression.

In reviewing a theme that runs through this chapter, the importance of well-informed MMHPs and the dangers of poorly informed or biased MMHPs become more apparent. The MMHP occupies a territory that is often ignored by colleagues. Few nonmedia mental health workers participate in the audience of MMHPs and many have voiced criticism of the very existence of such a phenomenon (Goleman, 1981; Rubinstein, 1981). This professional isolation, and an understandable tendency on the part of MMHPs to guard their territories (in the media business one is, after all, ultimately replaceable), makes it possible for an MMHP to work with little or no collegial supervision or feedback. An MMHP who is ignorant or misinformed about issues of importance to women has potential to do damage unchecked. And the likelihood is good that any MMHP will at least be uninformed, since most mental health professionals have little training or expertise in the psychology of women.

It becomes apparent that in order to influence public mental health policies via MMHPs in ways that will benefit women, feminists within the mental health professions must actively seek alliances with their colleagues working the media, and/or must seek to function themselves within that genre. It is necessary for interested feminists to initiate contact and dialogue with our media colleagues, and to adopt an educative, nonadversarial stance when we find their sexism, unconscious or otherwise, entering into their work. The MMHP is giving psychology away on a daily basis to people who may never have taken an introductory psychology class, much less a course in the psychology of women. The potential for popularizing and making accessible the work of feminist psychologists is enormous, since the MMHP often acts to fill a vacuum where the audience's data base on this topic is concerned. MMHPs have suffered, and continue to experience, a variety of professional scorn and an outcast status that will be familiar in feeling and process to many feminist psychologists. Thus, the potential for genuine professional empathy, contact, and collegiality exists, if only because media psychology lacks other groups seeking it out.

Feminist mental health professionals wishing to work within the media must recognize that they are entering a context that is more blatantly and comfortably sexist than any other in which they may have previously worked, as well as one that is openly hostile to declared feminists. *A Small But Helpful Manual on Public Information,* prepared by the Division of Psychology of Women of the American Psychological Association, is a prerequisite text for any feminist considering taking her mental health expertise or her research findings to the media (Tavris, Tiefer, Parlee, & Rubinstein, 1983). Strategies that have worked well for feminists within their own professions when attempting to raise consciousness and levels of information can be usefully adapted for a strategic assault on the bastions of the media world.

The field of media psychology, and the role of the media mental health professional, have moved past fad and into an institutional status that does not appear likely to be shaken in the near future. The expansion of cable television, with a concomitant demand for increasing the amount of programming, suggests that there will be more interest in new variations of media psychology over time. The likelihood thus grows that MMHPs will influence an ever-widening audience, and that MMHPs potential as social change agents will expand and solidify. As MMHPs grow in their credibility, both to their home disciplines and to the public, they may also grow in their capacity to influence public policy decisions that will affect women's mental health. As such, media psychology gives feminists both rich growth potentials and complex new problems with which to wrestle. By forging early and meaningful alliances with the field of media psychology, feminists in the helping professions and behavioral sciences will enhance their ability to directly affect public opinions and thus policies that affect women's lives.

REFERENCES

Association for Media Psychology (1982). *Guidelines for media mental health professionals.* Published by the Association for Media Psychology.
Bouhoutsos, J., Holroyd, J., Lerman, H., Forer, B. R., & Greenberg, M. (1983). Sexual intimacy between psychotherapist and patients. *Professional Psychology: Research and Practice, 14,*(2).
Goleman, D. (1981). Will the next problem sign in, please! *Psychology Today, 15* (12).
Hatch, O. (1982). Psychology, society, and politics. *American Psychologist, 37* (9).
Marr, B. (1980). Personal communication.
NiCarthy, G. (1982). *Getting free: A handbook for women in abusive relationships.* Seattle: Seal Press.
Rubinstein, C. (1981). Who calls in? It's not the lonely crowd. *Psychology Today, 15* (12).
Schlafly, P. (1980). Domestic violence bill to increase bureaucracy. *New Orleans Times-Picayune,* February 11.
Steinem, G. (1981). Night thoughts of a media watcher. *Ms. magazine, 10* (5).
Steinem, G. (1983). *Outrageous acts and everyday rebellions.* New York: Holt, Rinehart & Winston.
Tavris, C., Tiefer, L., Parlee, M. B., & Rubinstein, C. (1983). *A small but helpful manual on public information.* Task Force on Public Information, Division of the Psychology of Women of the American Psychological Association.
Walker, L. (1979). *The battered woman.* New York: Harper & Row.

16

PROFESSIONAL PSYCHOLOGY'S RESPONSE TO WOMEN'S MENTAL HEALTH NEEDS

Nicholas A. Cummings

The profession's response to the mental health needs of women cannot be separated from psychology's response to women's issues within the American Psychological Association (APA). Before consciousness could be raised, there had to be a dramatically increased acceptance and participation of women in the governance of the APA. This increase occurred rapidly during the decade of the 1970s, and although for many feminists the progress seemed torturously slow at times, the APA has set a standard for the participation of women in governance that might well be emulated by other national professional societies.

That sometimes clinical understanding is preceded by political awareness in advance of research is embarrassing to the concept of an impartial science and profession. It must be recalled that the decade began with the profession freely invoking the notion of moral maosochism to account for the willing acceptance by women of a role inferior to men (Freud, 1943), while at the same time branding as penis envy any rebellion against that role (Brill, 1938). Sex roles were so thoroughly stereotyped that no one seriously challenged the fact that the most widely administered psychometric test, the Minnesota Multiphasic Personality Inventory (MMPI), standardized its masculinity-femininity scale in part on army sergeants and women flight attendants, called airline "stewardesses" during that era (Sobel & Cummings, 1981). It required that activism of the feminists in APA governance, braving such prevalent appellations as "castrating female" to raise the consciousness of the APA.

I am writing this paper from the perspective of one who lived the decade of change immersed in both clinical practice and APA governance, with the latter culminating in the APA presidency where I was first vilified and then vindicated by the membership for my strong stand in favor of the Equal Rights Amendment (ERA). I, as well as many other professional psychologists, would date my awareness of feminist issues within psychology to the 1972 APA convention in Honolulu. The occasion was the Open Forum, a newly created mechanism that accorded dissident factions within the APA the opportunity to address the Board of Directors. I was speaking on behalf of the Council for the Advancement of the Psychological Professions and Sciences (CAPPS) when two women seized the floor microphone and demanded to know what CAPPS was doing in support of the ERA. I stumbled through a response, but the real answer was that nothing was being done. The CAPPS predominantly male leadership was stunned. Seeing themselves as a group of clinical mavericks who were assaulting the entrenched academic-research controlled APA governance, the accusation that they were an "old boys' club" was a painful one. Before CAPPS could make good its promise to address feminist issues, it was dissolved to make way for the APA-sponsored creation of the Association for the Advancement of Psychology (AAP). But the incident made a lasting impression on the CAPPS leadership, many of whom were subsequently elected to the APA Board of Directors (N. Cummings, 1979) and three of whom (Blau, Cummings, & Siegel) were elected to the APA presidency.

Staff support within the APA Central Office was integral to the profession's ability to influence national policy. Such staff support began modestly in 1969 with the creation of the Task Force on the Status of Women in Psychology, and this support grew as the Task Force evolved into the ad hoc Committee on Women in 1972 and finally the continuing Committee on Women in Pscyhology (CWP) in 1974 (Russo, 1980). but it was not until 1977 when CWP's call for increased staff support was buttressed by the Division of the Psychology of Women that a full-time senior level staff person was assigned to women's issues. It was then that the APA was able to make a significant commitment to women's issues not only within APA, but also to other organizations that looked to the APA to provide leadership, such as the Association for the Advancement of Science (AAAS), the Federation of Organizations for Professional Women, the Association for Women in Science, and the National Coalition for Women and Girls in Education (Russo, 1980). Further, this staff person became a knowledgeable resource on women's issues and acted as a facilitator in identifying and securing expert testimony for the Congress and its subcommittees. In that year the direct influence of the national policy became a significant activity of the APA.

It was also in 1977 that I, as president-elect designate, addressed the Council of Representatives of the APA as it seemed hopelessly deadlocked on whether to cancel its next three conventions in Atlanta, New Orleans, and Las Vegas, all cities in states that had not ratified the ERA. I reminded the Council that I was scheduled to preside over the Atlanta annual meeting, something that my conscience would not permit. I further reminded the council that it had cancelled two convention cities in prior years when a significant portion of the APA membership indicated they could not attend conventions in those cities: Chicago in 1970 when the APA's younger members were dismayed by Mayor Daly's treatment of the Vietnam war protesters; and previously Miami when black psychologists pointed out they would be segregated there. I believed the council should not do less for the APA's women members who would boycott these cities, and I stated flatly that if the APA insisted on holding the 1979 convention in Atlanta I would resign and lead a counterconvention. The Council did cancel those three cities, and the APA became the first national organization to cancel already contracted conventions in non-ERA ratified states. Lawsuits were anticipated, but none materialized, and this gave a precedent followed by more than 150 national organizations as they cancelled existing conventions in states that had not ratified the ERA. I was vilified in the APA *Monitor* for the next year and a half, but eventually in a referendum the membership upheld the council's action. This was in contrast to the American Psychiatric Association (APA) whose cancellation of convention contracts was overturned by a membership referendum. In this strong stand on the ERA, and with its willingness to risk lawsuits by hotels in scheduled convention cities, the APA demonstrated leadership and influenced the policies of many other ogranizations. Gloria Steinem was the invited convention speaker in 1978, and she delivered a major policy address that was widely covered by the media.

Once CWP expanded its original mission which was to represent women members in APA governance (T. Cummings, 1975), it clearly entered the public policy arena. Since the *Publication Manual of the APA* is used by a variety of professional and scientific organizations, an early thrust was the adoption of nonsexist language. To this day the use of nonsexist language remains voluntary, but the incorporation of guidelines for nonsexist language had an immediate and profound impact not only on APA publications, but also on the publications of those other organizations that have adopted the *Publication Manual of the APA* as their own standard.

In 1976 the APA Task Force on Sex Bias and Sex Role Stereotyping in Psychotherapeutic Practice submitted its final report to the Board of Professional Affairs (T. Cummings, 1976), and immediately a storm of protest was unleashed. Psychologists and psychiatrists who were practicing psychotherapy were predominately males treating a majority of patients who were females. They protested that they were not biased, and that they were not dealing with stereotypes but rather clinical truths. Even the profession of social work, which has a better balance between men and women therapists, essentially reflected the decades of psychoanalytic theory that equated passive with feminine and active with masculine (Sobel & Cummings, 1981). The notable exception was the analytic psychology of Carl Jung where women were accorded a more equal status and consequently attracted a larger number of women psychotherapists than did orthodox Freudian theory (Harding, 1974). Interestingly, the changes in the behavior and theoretical beliefs of practicing psychotherapists, and especially of male therapists, came less from the direct assault on sex bias and sex role stereotyping, and more from the steady development of feminist therapy and the extensive reeducation of the female consumer of psychotherapeutic services. As more and more women patients demanded either feminist therapy or bias free treatment from male psychotherapists, what reason could not accomplish economics did.

The APA's role in the development of feminist therapy has been that of a facilitator. CWP published a bibliography of research on issues relating to feminist therapy (APA, 1979), as well as a set of Guidelines for Therapy with Women (APA, 1975). But perhaps the most important single document was the Consumer Handbook: Women and Psychotherapy (Federation of Organizations for Professional Women, 1980), a widely circulated guide prepared by the Task Force on Consumer Issues in Psychotherapy of the Association for Women in Psychology and APA Division 35. This thoughtful handbook nicely separates indications of sexism on the part of the therapist from possible authority and sex problems on the part of the patient, indicating that the differences may not always be clear to the client or the therapist. Although the APA does not maintain a roster of therapists, the Association for Women in Psychology does maintain such a roster that was compiled with the help of the APA.

Recent court decisions have attested to the profession's impact on attitudes toward victims of rape and spousal abuse. For years the judicial system, abetted by expert witnesses from psychology and psychiatry, treated the victims of rape as well as the occasional battered wife who finally struck back as if they were criminals rather than victims. The profession invoked psychological theories of neurotic guilt that ostensibly drove these women to risk rape or enjoy beatings. The fact that abused spouses have difficulty leaving their husbands was regarded as clinical evidence that these women want to stay in the situation. Walker (1979) found that battered women have very low self-esteem and feel powerless to alter the situation. They may be financially dependent on the batterer, or may feel partly responsible for his violence. Or they may fear reprisal on their children or themselves if they leave. These clinical findings are far more appropriate than a metapsychological notion of moral masochism, and provide a valid defense in court for striking back at the batterer. Walker has shown that the battered woman syndrome develops through a series of stages, the final stage being one in which the woman concludes she cannot escape and that her only choices are suicide, endure the abuse, or strike back.

Admissibility of expert witnesses testifying on the battered woman syndrome has been recognized in Alaska, California, Colorado, Georgia, Indiana, Iowa, Kansas, Maine, Michigan, Minnesota, Montana, Nevada, New Hampshire, New Jersey, Oregon, Pennsylvania, South Carolina, Texas, Virginia, Washington, Wisconsin, and Wyoming. In 1983 the APA filed amicus briefs in two jurisdictions, one in New Jersey and another in Florida, where cases are being heard on appeal following conviction in a lower court that did not permit introduction of expert testimony on the battered woman syndrome (APA, 1983). As to whether the battered woman syndrome exists, the APA brief stated that the research in the area employed methodology generally accepted by the relevant scientific community, and that our scientific knowledge is sufficient to permit qualified experts to form a reliable opinion on whether a defendant is suffering from such a syndrome.

Consistently the APA has taken a strong stand on a women's right to an abortion. Recently it published a brochure, "When Children are Unwanted," which cites the research findings of the consequences of unwanted children. Among the consequences cited are unstable marriages and higher illness and death rates of both mothers and children (Russo & David, 1983). the brochure goes on to state the unwanted childbearing restricts a woman's educational and occupational opportunities, resulting in higher rates of poverty. These adverse effects fall more heavily on the poor, black, and young.

Psychologists discovered there is a difference in the manner health care is administered to women than in the way it is applied to men. A woman's physical complaints are less likely to be taken seriously as compared to those of a man, and she is more likely to be given a tranquilizer or referred to a mental health professional (ADAMHA, 1981). This finding has received broad coverage by the news media, and it has commanded the attention of health consumer groups, yet there is no clear evidence that the situation has improved toward women. It would be in keeping with the recent history within health care delivery that if physician's attitudes toward women do change, it will probably be the result of the woman's refusal to be treated as a second class patient.

The APA, through its policymaking body the Council of Representatives, followed by one year the declaration by the American Psychiatric Association (ApA) that a homosexual orientation in an individual does not imply mental or emotional disorder or impairment. And one year after that the Council added that qualification to perform an occupation should not be limited or denied because of one's sexual preference. I recall with amusement an incident in the council. When that body seemed bogged down in debate over the resolution, I stated to the council that I could not think of a single occupation in which one's sexual orientation should be a factor, and I challenged the assembly to name even one such occupation. After a brief silence a council member jumped to his feet and shouted he could think of one—that of locker room attendant. The council members laughed uproariously and passed the resolution by a wide margin. To this day there are members of council who insist I arranged to have that particular member make his outrageous statement toward the view of fostering passage of the resolution.

These declarations regarding homosexuality by both the APA and the ApA have had far-reaching impact on hiring practices, federal guidelines on hiring, and the manner in which the courts respond to and interpret the rights of homosexual employees. Although the issue of homosexuality is not of itself a feminist issue, these resolutions and the consequent changes in societies' attitudes do influence such important concepts as sex role stereotyping, definitions of masculinity and femininity, and parenting. Admittedly, in its report to the APA, CWP has not addressed the plight of the lesbian with the same vigor it has pursued other feminist issues, with the possible exception of its stand in favor of lesbian mothers' rights to custody of their children (Kaschak, 1982). CWP is determined in the future to address lesbian issues more directly.

It is imperative that the APA address the problems raised by patients who have become sexual victims of therapists (Kaschak, 1982). In a survey conducted by the California State Psychological Association it was found that the problem is essentially that of the male therapist with the female patient (Bouhoutsos, 1982). The APA Insurance Trust's decision that the malpractice insurance would not cover judgments resulting from a therapist's having engaged in sex relations with his or her client brought a storm of protest from many male psychologists. Their complaint that this left them vulnerable to false accusation is not valid, since the APA-sponsored malpractice insurance does pay for the defense of a therapist who is accused of sexual impropriety with a patient, and coverage stops only upon having been found guilty by the court.

In another insurance matter, in 1983 the APA Insurance Trust prevailed upon the insurance carrier to define a "spousal equivalent" so that the dependent in a nonmarital living arrangement, whether it be heterosexual or homosexual, is covered by the subscriber's health insurance in the same manner a wife or husband would be covered. The APA has demonstrated bold leadership in this regard, and this action is being followed closely by the insurance industry toward the possible adoption of this definition in policies outside the APA. I sit on the APA Insurance Trust, and as far as I can determine, this action by the APA is the first in the nation. A similar attempt by the City of San Francisco to introduce a spousal equivalent definition in the health insurance for city employees failed by veto of the mayor after the Board of Supervisors had adopted the measure. Again, this matter is important to the concept of sex role stereotyping and whether women have options in life-styles other than the traditional role of the wife who is covered by her husband's health insurance.

A pitched battle has raged for a number of years between those who regard abortion as any fertile woman's right, and those who might be seen as favoring the Right to Life Movement in its opposition to abortion. The APA has clearly sided with those elements of our society that would leave the matter of an abortion to the choice of the individual woman. In keeping with this stance, the APA filed an amicus brief before the United States Supreme Court in the case of the City of Akron v. Akron Center for Reproductive Health (Kaschak, 1982). In 1983 the Court rendered its decision, overturning a city ordinance that required informed written consent of any minor under 15 who seeks an abortion, and further required either the written informed consent of one parent or guardian, or a court order. The ordinance had also required a 24-hour notice to the parent or guardian of an unmarried minor under age 18 before an abortion could be performed. The procedure was found unconstitutional because it did not specify a procedure for judicial review or a "provision for a mature or emancipated minor completely to avoid hostile parental involvement by demonstrating to the satisfaction of the court that she is capable of exercising her constitutional right to choose an abortion" (APA, 1983). This decision would suggest that the high Court might take a different view of its 1981 decision in H. L. v. Matheson, which upheld the parental notification requirement inclusive of mature minors seeking an abortion. The APA had entered an amicus brief in that case also.

Sexism in training, and increasing the opportunities for the training of more women psychologists, has been the joint focus of the CWP and the APA's Minority Fellowship Program (MFP). The APA had revised its accreditation procedures to require that APA-approved programs in clinical, counseling, and school psychology provide relevant information regarding sexism, opportunities for women and minorities, and related matters (Kaschak, 1982). The APA is devising strategy as to how it may effect programs that are not APA-approved training in clinical, counseling, and school psychology, and to further address the issue of enforcement in those programs that clearly fall within the accreditation criteria.

It is clear that the profession of psychology has impacted in a number of significant areas, both internal and external to the APA. Inspite of these influences on national policy and societal attitudes, Hare-Mustin (1979), writing as the chair of CWP and assessing the progress of the ten-year period, was pessimistic:

There continue to be a number of areas that do not reflect sensitivity to women psychologists. These include the lack of substantial changes in the status of women psychologists in research, academia, professional practice, industry, management, and public and community service. For example, the percentage of women in these areas has not changed substantially over the past ten years. Salaries also have not achieved equality with those of men. CWP also noted the lack of responsiveness in publications and in the field of psychology to incorporate knowledge of the psychology of women into the discipline and teaching of psychology. Very few women are editors of major journals. Women are not entering psychology in proportion to their numbers in society.

Interestingly, this same assessment might be applied to the whole of our society, cutting across disciplines and occupations.

How one reconciles our increase in awareness and understanding, and a seemingly significant impact on various sectors of national policy, with the lack of societal change has always been a problem. There is a torturous time lag between discovery and change. For example, the finding almost a decade ago that women offenders tend to be those women who were abused as children by their fathers (Brodsky, 1975) is just now beginning to be addressed by our courts and our archaic correctional system.

The progress and changes in the profession of psychology have proceeded in advance of conclusive research. In her excellent assessment of the issues of sex, race, and class in psychotherapy research, Brodsky (1982) states that methodological problems inherent in all psychotherapy research preclude definitive conclusions as regards these three factors. She, nonetheless, concludes that many studies and much anecdotal evidence exist to demonstrate that personal attributes of race, sex, and social class have an impact on who gets therapy, for which practitioners and for how long, and of which type. Further, the differential impact of these variables appears in interaction with other variables of importance to psychotherapy rather than in isolation as a main effect. And finally, the nature of the impact is not stable, but is prone to change with the shift in sensitivity and awareness of the population of therapists and the acculturation of the population of patients. She goes on to say, "I personally conclude from the literature of both empirical and intuitive accounts that there is sufficient racism, sexism, and classism among therapists to warrant the continued exploration of positive approaches to train therapists to deal with their biases. We do not need more documentation of therapists shortcomings; we need more evaluation of specific approaches with specific patients by specifically trained therapists to improve the therapeutic outcome for minorities and women."

It would seem that on the larger number of issues effecting women, both within and without society, the profession of psychology has taken a position similar to the stance taken by Brodsky (1982) in her assessment of psychotherpy research. The profession has moved to impact on national policy on the basis of awareness, understanding, sensitivity, and some empirical evidence in advance of definitive research findings.

REFERENCES

Alcohol, Drug Abuse and Mental Health Administration. (1981). *Report of a conference on the impact of alcohol, drug abuse, and mental health treatment on medical care utilization.* Washington, DC, DHHS Publication No. (ADM) 81-1180.

American Psychological Association. (1983). *Division of child, youth, and family services newsletter, 6*(3/4), 1-8.

American Psychological Association. (1975). Guidelines for psychotherapy with women. *American Psychologist, 30,* 1169-1175.

American Psychological Association. (1979). *Some information on feminist therapy and counseling women.* Washington, DC: American Psychological Association.

Bouhoutsos, J. (1982). *CSPA president's report.* Los Angeles: California State Psychological Association.

Brill, A. M. (1938). *The basic writings of Sigmund Freud.* New York: Random House.

Brodsky, A. M. (1975). *The female offender.* New York: Guilford Press.

Brodsky, A. M. (1982). *Sex, race and class issues in psychotherapy research.* Master Lecture Series. Washington, DC: American Psychological Association.

Cummings, N. A. (1979). Mental health and national health insurance: A case history of the struggle for professional autonomy. In C. A. Kiesler, N. A. Cummings, & G. R. VandenBos (Eds.), *Psychology and national health insurance: A sourcebook.* Washington, DC: American Psychological Association.

Cummings, T. (1975). *Annual report of the committee on women in psychology.* Washington, DC: American Psychological Association.

Cummings, T. (1976). *Annual report of the committee on women in psychology.* Washington, DC: American Psychological Association.

Federation of Organizations for Professional Women. (1980). Women and psychotherapy: A consumer handbook. Washington, DC: FOPW.

Freud, S. (1943). *A general introduction to psychoanalysis.* Garden City, NJ: Doubleday.

Harding, M. E. (1947). *Psychic energy: Its source and goal.* Washington, DC: Pantheon.

Hare-Mustin, R. T. (1979). *Annual report of the committee on women in psychology.* Washington, DC: American Psychological Association.

Kaschak, E. (1982). *Annual report of the committee on women in psychology.* Washington, DC: American Psychological Association.

Russo, N. F. (1980). *History and current activities of the women's program office.* Washington, DC: American Psychological Association.

Russo, N. F., & David, H. P. (1983). *When children are unwanted.* Washington, DC: American Psychological Association.

Sobel, S. B. & Cummings, N. A. (1981). The role of professional psychologists in promoting equality. *Professional Psychology, 12,* 171-179.

Walker, L. (1979). *The battered woman.* New York: Harper & Row.

ABOUT THE CONTRIBUTORS

ARTHUR H. AUERBACH, M.D. is assistant professor of psychiatry at the University of Pennsylvania, and is currently president of the Society for Psychotherapy Research.

DEBORAH BELLE, Ed.D. is an assistant professor of psychology at Boston University. She is editor of *Lives In Stress: Women and Depression* and coeditor of *The Mental Health of Women.* As director of the Stress and Families Project at Harvard University from 1977 to 1982, she directed studies of low income families, focusing on stress, depression, and social support among low income mothers and on children's responses to stress and to maternal depression.

JACQUELINE C. BOUHOUTSOS is in private practice in Santa Monica and is clinical professor of psychology at University of California, Los Angeles. She received her Ph.D. from the University of Innsbruck, Austria. Chair of the California State Psychological Association (CSPA) Task Force on Sexual Intimacy Between Psychotherapists and Patients (1978-1981), she was president of CSPA in 1981. In 1982 she established a Distressed Psychologist program for CSPA and founded the Post Therapy Support Group at UCLA for patients who sustained damage from sexual relations with a psychotherapist.

JESSIE BERNARD received her doctorate at Washington University, St. Louis, in 1935. She was a social science analyst at the Bureau of Labor Statistics in the 1930s, collaborating in studies of consumer expenditures. She taught at Lindenwood College, St. Charles, Missouri, 1940-1947, and then at the Pennsylvania State University until 1964 when she became Research Scholar Honoris Causa. Since that time she has been engaged in writing and research. She has written extensively in the area of women's concerns, including *Academic Women* (1964), *Women and the Public Interest* (1971), *The Future of Marriage* (1972), *The Future of Motherhood* (1974), *Women, Wives, Mothers* (1975), and *The Female World* (1981).

LAURA S. BROWN received her Ph.D. in clinical psychology from Southern Illinois University at Carbondale in 1977. She is currently a feminist therapist in private practice in Seattle, Washington, where she also is clinical assistant professor in the Department of Psychology at the University of Washington. She hosted a radio call-in psychology show in Seattle for two and a half years.

LORNA P. CAMMAERT currently holds a cross-appointment as a counsellor at the University Counselling Services and as a professor in the Department of Educational Psychology, University of Calgary. She received her Ph.D. in counselling and developmental psychology from the University of Oregon. Her interests encompass female sexuality, sexual harassment, assertiveness, decision-making, and self-esteem groups for women. Dr. Cammaert has served as the national coordinator of the Canadian Psychological Association Interest Group on Women and Psychology and is a coauthor with Dr. Carolyn Larsen of *A Woman's Choice: A Guide to Decision-Making.*

NICHOLAS A. CUMMINGS, Ph.D. is the eighty-seventh president of the American Psychological Association (1979-1980) and only the second independent practitioner to be elected to that office. He is the clinical director of the Biodyne Institute (San Francisco and Honolulu) and the president of the Institute for Psychosocial Interaction (Palo Alto). He served as the chief psychologist of Kaiser-Permanente, San Francisco, the director of the Mental Research Institute, the codirector of the Golden Gate Mental Health Center, and the founding president of the four campuses of the California School of Professional Psychology.

IRENE HANSON FRIEZE is an associate professor of psychology, business and women's studies at the University of Pittsburgh. She received her Ph.D. in personality psychology from UCLA in 1973. Since that time she has worked mainly in the areas of beliefs about the causes of success and failure, achievement motivation, and cognitive reactions of victims. She has also had a continuing interest in career patterns and career decision-making of college educated women.

MAUREEN C. HENDRICKS, Ed.D. is a licensed clinical psychologist in private practice in Denver, Colorado. She is a graduate of the School of Educational Change and Development at the University of Northern Colorado. She is the author of "The Marriages and Adjustment of Resigned Roman Catholic Priests and Their Wives" (Dissertation Abstracts International 40B). Dr. Hendricks is also the Support Group Leader for Resolve of Colorado and a member of Women Church Speaks and the Women's Ordination Conference of the Roman Catholic Church.

MARILYN JOHNSON, Ph.D. is director of the Student Counseling Center and assistant professor of psychology and social sciences at Rush University/Rush-Presbyterian St. Luke's Medical Center in Chicago. She is coauthor, with Mary Sue Richardson, of "Counseling Women," in the forthcoming *Handbook of Counseling Psychology,* edited by Steven Brown and Robert Lent.

ALEXANDRA G. KAPLAN, Ph.D. is co-clinical director and research associate at the Stone Center, Wellesley College, and lecturer in psychiatry at Harvard

Medical School. Her recent presentations and publications center on aspects of women's relational development, including women and anger, depression in women, and gender influences on the client-therapist relationship.

PHYLLIS LYON, Ed.D. is coauthor of *Lesbian/Woman*. She is on the faculty and chair of gay and women's studies at The Institute for Advanced Study of Human Sexuality, a San Francisco graduate school. Dr. Lyon is past chair of San Francisco's Human Rights Commission and is active in civil and human rights issues.

DEL MARTIN is coauthor of *Lesbian/Woman* and author of *Battered Wives*. An activist in women's and other civil rights issues, she served as chair of San Francisco's Commission on the Status of Women and on the California Commission on Crime Control and Violence Prevention, which studied the root causes of violence. Currently she is writing and lecturing.

CAROL C. NADELSON, M.D. is professor of psychiatry, director of training and education, and vice chairperson of the Department of Psychiatry at Tufts-New England Medical Center in Boston. She is a graduate of the Boston Psychoanalytic Society and Institute and was recently the first woman elected president of the American Psychiatric Association. Dr. Nadelson is a fellow of the American College of Psychiatry, a member of the Group for the Advancement of Psychiatry and has been president of the Association for Academic Psychiatry. Dr. Nadelson is the author of numerous books and articles and she has coedited several books including *Marriage and Divorce: A Contemporary Perspective*; *The Challenge of Change*; *The Woman Patient*, Vol. I, II, III; *Major Psychiatric Disorders: Overviews and Selected Readings*; and *Treatment Interventions in Human Sexuality*.

MALKAH T. NOTMAN, M.D. is clinical professor of psychiatry at Tufts University School of Medicine, lecturer at Harvard University School of Medicine, and psychiatrist at New England Medical Center and Beth Israel Hospital in Boston, and formerly liaison psychiatrist to obstetrics and gynecology there. She is currently director of the Women's Resource Center at New England Medical Center and Tufts University Department of Psychiatry. Dr. Notman is a faculty member and a training and supervising analyst at Boston Psychoanalytic Institute. She is a fellow of the American Psychiatric Association and the American College of Psychiatrists and a member of the Group for the Advancement of Psychiatry. Dr. Notman is the author of numerous professional books and articles. Her most recent work includes contributions to *Modern Forensic Psychiatry and Psychology*; *The Challenge of Change*; *The Woman Patient*; and several articles on menopause.

LYNNE BRAVO ROSEWATER, Ph.D. is a licensed psychologist in private practice in Cleveland, Ohio. Dr. Rosewater is one of the founding members and the chairperson of the National Feminist Therapy Institute and is coeditor of *A Handbook of Feminist Therapy* (Springer, in press). In addition, Dr. Rosewater is an expert on domestic violence and feminist interpretations of personality assessment.

NANCY FELIPE RUSSO, Ph.D. is the first administrative officer for women's programs of the American Psychological Association. A former member of the Subpanel on the Mental Health of Women of the President's Commission on Mental Health, she also serves on the Long-Term Research Committee of the Women's Research and Education Institute of the Congresswomen's Caucus and chairs the Mental Health Committee of the Women and Health Roundtable. Author of numerous scientific, professional, and public policy articles, Dr. Russo is a Fellow of the American Psychological Association.

ESTHER SALES is an associate professor at the University of Pittsburgh. She received her Ph.D. in social psychology and social work from the University of Michigan. Her major research interests and writings focus on the impact of women's role choices and experiences on their life course adjustment.

DONNA M. STRINGER, Ph.D. is director of the Seattle Office for Women's Rights. Ms. Stringer is a social psychologist who has spent the past 15 years administering women's programs in social service, higher education, and public sector settings. She has participated in research, teaching, service provision, and policy development regarding issues affecting women, sexual minorities, and ethnic minorities. Her publications include *Battered Women* (Sage, 1979), and over two dozen journal articles on issues icluding violence against women, sex roles, men and women working together, assertiveness, and dual-career couples.

JANET L. SURREY is Assistant Psychologist, McLean Hospital, Harvard Medical School. She is also Research Associate at the Stone Center for Developmental Services and Studies at Wellesley College where her current theoretical work is focused on self-in-relation theory.

LENORE E. WALKER is a licensed psychologist and president of Walker and Associates, a firm specializing in providing clinical, consulting, and forensic psychological services. She was awarded the Diplomate in Clinical Psychology by the American Board of Professional Psychology and is a Fellow of the American Psychological Association. Formerly, Dr. Walker was chairperson and associate professor of psychology at Colorado Womens College and assistant professor of psychiatry at Rutgers Medical School, CMDNJ. She is internationally known for her research on battered women and its clinical and forensic applications in cases where there is violence against women. Dr. Walker was one of the founders and first chair of the Feminist Therapy Institute, a postgraduate training institute in psychotherapy techniques when working with women. Dr. Walker is the author of *The Battered Woman* (Harper & Row, 1979); *The Battered Woman Syndrome* (Springer, 1984);

and is coeditor of *A Handbook of Feminist Therapy* (Springer, in press). She is also the author of numerous book chapters and articles. She travels throughout the United States lecturing and training advocates, lawyers, and psychotherapists who work with battered women.

NANCY R. WELTON is the public information officer at the Seattle Office for Women's Rights. She has been professionally involved in women's programs in governmental, educational, and social service settings for the past nine years. Additionally, she has worked as a lesbian and gay rights activist for the past six years. She is a board member of the Northwest AIDS Foundation and formerly served on the staff and board of the Lesbian Resource Center.